Pamela Weintraub

CURE UNKNOWN

❖

INSIDE
THE LYME EPIDEMIC

St. Martin's Griffin New York

For Jason, who came back to us
For David, who woke up
For Mark

Author's Note

Some patients' names have been changed at their request.

www.stmartins.com

Book design by Kathryn Parise

The Library of Congress has catalogued the hardcover edition as follows:

Weintraub, Pamela.
    Cure unknown : inside the Lyme epidemic / Pamela Weintraub. — 1st ed.
      p. cm.
    ISBN 978-0-312-37812-7
    1. Lyme disease.   I. Title.
    RC155.5.W44 2008
    616.9'2—dc22

                                                2008007816
        ISBN 978-0-312-37813-4 (trade paperback)

First St. Martin's Griffin Edition: October 2009

10 9 8 7 6 5 4 3 2 1

Contents

Acknowledgments

Over the six years of researching and writing this book, I've been helped by dozens of people, far too many to mention here. The first draft of my book, more than twice the length of the current volume, included every person I interviewed and every thought I ever had about Lyme disease and all its coinfections. It sits, now, in a big black binder on a shelf that sags under its weight. The current manuscript has lost many of those original interviews so my own narrative voice could rise up and my story could ring clear—but whether or not you have remained in this version, you informed my journey and investigative arc and the story I tell now.

Special thanks to my gifted editors, Jennifer Weis and Stefanie Lindskog at St. Martin's Press, whose sea of yellow Post-it notes guided me through to a true narrative, and to my agent, Wendy Lipkind, who stuck with me through the maddening saga of Lyme, the book.

Enormous thanks to those who gave my manuscript a technical read, sharing their thoughts and comments: Kenneth Liegner, M.D., of Armonk, New York; Eugene Davidson, professor of biochemistry and molecular biology at Georgetown University Medical Center and department chair from 1988 to 2003; and Carl Brenner, Columbia University geologist, research board member of the National Research Fund for Tick-Borne Diseases, and science historian of all things Lyme. Carl, thank you for talking to me for six years now, for teaching me so much, and for taking me on the world tour of Lyme disease peer-reviewed literature with all your wisdom, humor, and depth.

Thank you, Dr. Sheila Statlender and the whole Statlender family and Dr. David Martz for sharing your lives in this volume.

To the science journalist, Jill Neimark, I can never repay you for coming to my rescue during my darkest hour, when I considered chucking this project; you read every word of my manuscript and sent copious notes so that I could continue—I used them all.

Deep gratitude to my friend, Barbara Goldklang, for opening her amazing historical archives and more impressive heart, and helping me navigate Lyme's rapids when I was so new and even later, when I was "old."

Many academic scientists helped me to think clearly about Lyme research and the very nature of science, most notably, Benjamin Luft, chairman, Department of Medicine, and chief, Division of Infectious Diseases State University of New York at Stony Brook, and Stephen Barthold, director of the Center for Comparative Medicine at the schools of Medicine and Veterinary Medicine at the University of California at Davis.

Other people who provided important help are Pat Smith, president of the Lyme Disease Association; Dr. Russell Donnelly; Dr. Daniel Cameron, president of the International Lyme and Associated Diseases Society (ILADS); Dr. Joseph Burrascano; Dr. Edwin J. Masters; Ken Fordyce; Kerry Fordyce; Phyllis Mervine; Suzanne Smith; Elizabeth Catalano; Heather Florence; and the late Betty Gross, who spent countless hours with me even as she was dying of cancer.

Thanks to Mona Marcus and Sue Sugar of Chappaqua, New York, two soldiers of the suburbs; to Joel Shmukler, Esq., for helping to hone my powers of skepticism; and to Rita Stanley, Ph.D., for her wry, spot-on observations year in and out.

To my husband, Mark, thank you for your eagle-eyed attention to my manuscript, for supporting me in this effort despite all the hits it meant, and for sharing my journey through Lyme.

Foreword

In 1993, journalist Pamela Weintraub and her husband thought they were doing themselves and their two sons a favor by escaping from Queens to the sylvan New York suburb of Chappaqua, a town so famously bucolic Bill and Hillary Clinton made it their outpost after decamping from the White House. In time, however, the deer-friendly backyard where Weintraub's sons spent lazy afternoons building forts turned into the author's personal Love Canal. Tragedy lurked under every fallen leaf. Both her sons eventually contracted tick-borne Lyme disease, as did she and her husband. Their suffering dragged on for years.

The conventional dogma about Lyme disease, according to Allen Steere, the doctor who described it in 1977, holds that a onetime course of antibiotics is almost always entirely curative. But Weintraub quickly discovered that little about Lyme disease was as straightforward as Steere and his supporters in the public health establishment claimed. The tests used to diagnose a case of Lyme turned out to be primitive, sometimes wildly inaccurate, or, at best, unreliable. In addition, the official diagnostic criteria handed down from on high by the Centers for Disease Control and Prevention failed to apply to many patients who the doctors in heavily endemic regions actually saw in their practices.

Instead, as Weintraub discovered, the disease was both a masquerader and a changeling, not unlike another spirochete-induced disease, syphilis, in which overtly neurological symptoms emerged over time such that they were not always understood to be related to the initiating infection—in the case of Lyme, spirochetes transmitted by a tick bite. In fact, as Weintraub was to learn, neurological Lyme disease was a time bomb that, once established in the body, could lead to a host of devastating results from near-crippling exhaustion and nerve pain to memory loss, confusion, and, at its most extreme, a kind of Lyme dementia.

As the years of Weintraub's illness wore on, the quarrels among doctors, scientists, and public health officials became only more bitter and dogmatic, until the mainstream power brokers in medicine seemed to dump those who didn't respond to a short course of standard treatment—the "chronic" Lyme sufferers—into a Bermuda Triangle of diseases. Nowhere is the view of chronic Lyme more hardened and, as Weintraub argues persuasively, unenlightened than in the highest reaches of the federal science establishment. Indeed, as recently as 2006, the federal government endorsed a document stating categorically that chronic Lyme doesn't exist.

To prepare readers for the bumpy ride, Weintraub creates a rich topographical as well as intellectual framework for her, at times, jaw-dropping tale of doctors and scientists behaving badly: the land of Lyme. We are nowhere near the Congo villages of Ebola fame, but, seemingly as dangerous, the backyard savannahs, as Weintraub describes them, of suburban "soccer moms" and "soccer dads" who dwell in false harmony with flourishing deer populations rife with *Ixodes* ticks carrying *Borrelia burgdorferi,* the Lyme spirochete, as well as pathogens causing babesiosis, anaplasmosis, and other infectious diseases in their tiny mouths and guts. Deer lovers stand forewarned: In this author's hands, Bambi just ain't Bambi anymore, but then, that's one of Weintraub's strengths—she takes no prisoners.

Weintraub's journalistic bona fides are impeccable. She's a reporter with twenty-five years of science journalism and editing under her belt, a credential buttressed by solid academic training in her field and apprenticeships with important scientists. Those credits are on full display in this narrative. I suspect, however, that when the nuances of Lyme disease science bumped up against medical dogma that seemed increasingly inapplicable to her own experience of the disease, she must have felt as though she had fallen through the looking glass.

The very people she once might have sought out for definitive quotes on the subject had become unreliable; the scientific literature was increasingly difficult to trust, as well. The more Weintraub investigated, the more virtually everyone with a shred of authority was losing their credibility, from the nation's "expert" on Lyme disease, Steere, to the psychologist at the Horace Greeley High School, who advised her to get her son a good haircut instead of nurturing his fantasy that he was too ill to attend school. As Weintraub would see it firsthand, the so-called "objective" scientists were sending an entire disease down the river and over a cliff for reasons that seemed frequently to have more to do with mere opinion and crass external forces—cash, prestige, careerism—than with scientific erudition.

Happily, Weintraub did not retire to her Victorian fainting couch for the duration, a choice some of the academicians she writes about in *Cure Unknown* surely will rue (and not merely because she was ignoring their recommended therapy for what ailed her). She appears to have tracked down every lead and reached out to everyone with something intelligent to say about this devastating malady. She rejected the science writer's inbred habit of relying on the government official with the highest pay grade or the scientist with a job at Harvard as the final word on a topic.

Instead, she developed a healthy skepticism for the assertions of those doctors whose cozy relationships with the National Institutes of Health or the *New England Journal of Medicine*—not to mention flourishing sidelines as consultants to insurance companies and big pharma— provided them with unchallenged hegemony in the field. In Weintraub's hands, they emerge less as experts than as representatives of the myriad chronic deficiencies in our national defense system against infectious disease. She gives the power brokers their say but then she goes deeper, searching for open minds, not closed ones. When she found them, she gave them her full attention. I think of her, with enormous respect, as a "recovered" science journalist.

The result of her tenacity is *Cure Unknown,* the first major journalistic examination of the Lyme wars and a book solidly in the tradition of the late journalist Randy Shilts's 1987 book, *And the Band Played On: People, Politics, and the AIDS Epidemic,* as well as my own 1996 book, *Osler's Web: Inside the Labyrinth of the Chronic Fatigue Syndrome Epidemic.* Both of those earlier books opened a wide door onto the dangerous and often outrageous phenomenon of doctors, scientists, and federal officials dismissing as folly major emerging diseases. Weintraub follows suit with her impressive contribution to that so-far unique body of literature, offering the third in what is now a trilogy of aggressive investigations into the willfully unchecked spread of infectious diseases in this country.

I wasn't overly surprised by Weintraub's tale, but I was fascinated—in the mournful way one is fascinated by disasters with shocking casualty numbers—by the fact that it had happened again. Most compelling to me, as someone who wrote a book about another disease that was dispatched to the back of the bus in the 1980s, is the clarity with which Weintraub addresses a system of disease surveillance and investigation in this country that is broken in so many ways. She nails the worst of it when she writes near the conclusion of *Cure Unknown* that experts "have imposed a rigid template on an entity they don't fully understand. Because their studies flow from the disease definition, rather than the other way around, they have generated information about a 'disease model' but not the disease itself."

Indeed, when a handful of academic clinicians and federal officials cobble together by show of hands, or a jocular exchange of snail-mail as occurred with "chronic fatigue syndrome," a Chinese menu–style definition of a disease about which they know little, if anything, it is madness, not science. Instead of fostering serious investigation, such definitions spur myth, speculation, and a kind of Tower of Babel confusion from which only scientific errors and misperceptions may flow, possibly for generations. It's no wonder chronic Lyme, chronic fatigue syndrome, Gulf War syndrome, along with several other diseases, tend to be slopped together as if interchangeable. The consensus definitions contrived by federal officials are paradoxically too vague and overly rigid, frequently emphasizing unimportant aspects and putting little stock, if any, in the most salient, distinctive characteristics of each disease.

If it wasn't apparent before, the publication of *Cure Unknown* makes it abundantly clear that we are living in an era of "contested" diseases. In this troubling, even tragic era, people are sick, disabled, and dying from illnesses that the premier authorities in establishment medicine proclaim do not exist as discrete pathological entities but are, instead, a figment of the patient's overactive imagination. All sorts of contorted linguistic anomalies have arisen from the field of contested diseases in the last two decades. Phrases like "medically unexplained symptoms," shorthanded in medical journal articles to "MUPS," "somatoform disorder," "illness attribution," and "sickness behavior" are tossed around as if they have a real grounding in medical science by doctors and especially by psychiatrists, who are having a field day in this new era. These phrases are code for more familiar words like "hysteria," "hypochondria," and "mental illness," phrases doctors prefer not to write in patients' charts.

When these illnesses occur in children, doctors often train their antennae on the parents, who may then be accused of another equally dubious and damning condition known as Munchausen Syndrome by Proxy, said to afflict parents who induce illness in their own children in order to attract attention to themselves. If the parents escape suspicion, the child inevitably bears the brunt, like the wheelchair-bound boy in England suffering from "chronic fatigue syndrome" (or, as that disease is more accurately known in the UK, myalgic encephalomyelitis) who was tossed into a swimming pool by a psychiatrist on the hypothesis that he would find the strength to swim if his life was at stake. The child was fished out before he drowned.

It sometimes seems as if the remarkable technological and scientific advances of the last half century have served to create a medical dead zone in which these contested diseases must languish because the science is still being worked out. Scientists can reconstruct extinct viruses from microscopic fragments retrieved from long-dead corpses; the human genome has been decoded. Yet, a side effect has been that many scientists and doctors—the latter trained to look for horses, not zebras, after all— can no longer allow uncertainty and ambiguity to coexist with scientific fact. This seems to be true even as the science has increasingly resolved the ambiguities and the zebras have emerged as the dominant quadruped in the herd.

The ancient and formerly revered scientific rule known as Occam's razor, which holds that the simplest explanation is probably the correct explanation, has no credence in the Brave New World of contested diseases. Common logic, anecdotal evidence, and on-the-ground clinical observations—by which I mean the simple process of doctors listening to and thinking about what their patients are telling them—are held in disregard by the most powerful players in the research establishment. These power players include pious academicians who have little or no contact with patients who suffer from these maladies, yet form opinions and theories about them that carry far more weight in the medical community than is scientifically warranted. They reduce science to theology, changing the essential question from "What do the data say?" to "Do you *believe* in this disease or do you not?"

They include, as well, medical journal editors who function as gatekeepers of information. Time and again, these editors open their doors wide to putative experts on a particular contested disease because the authors hold high posts in academia or are working under the aegis of federal health agencies like the Centers for Disease Control and Prevention or the National Institutes of Health. In a manner reminiscent of bigoted, stuffy gentlemen's clubs, however, these journals bar their doors to investigators who have actually performed legitimate scientific research in the field but cannot get the requisite traction with the academics and the government because such findings and even their hypotheses run counter to prevailing theory; that is, they are approaching the disease as if its existence is not contested. As a result, their findings are ushered to obscure journals or go unpublished altogether. Progress toward clarifying the disease process, its cause, or, best of all, resolution of a contested disease is inhibited.

One result is that the dreams of researchers who could be helpful to the process are smashed when, year after year, the government rejects their proposals to study the disease. Another is that doctors who want to help their patients with novel drug regimens become too intimidated to even try for fear of reprisals by state medical boards.

These are hardly cordial disagreements. Bodies are strewn everywhere and, for the moment, I am not referring to the afflicted but to the healthy. As Weintraub describes the carnage, doctors shutter their practices and move to distant states; humiliated researchers forswear their interests and retreat into less controversial fields. After the publication of my book, which revealed that scientists at the Centers for Disease Control had created a secret CFS slush fund to misappropriate millions of taxpayer dollars earmarked by Congress for CFS research, the head of the agency resigned and scientists were reassigned—though none fired—depending on which side of the issue they fell. On the matter of contested diseases, public health employees generally raise their fingers to the wind to see which way it's blowing and act accordingly.

Aiding and abetting these power players, if unwittingly, are reporters whose job it is to relay new developments in science and medicine to readers but in doing so rarely step outside the box to solicit interviews with researchers whose work runs counter to the conventional wisdom of federal scientists. In their desire to be "scientifically accurate" or adhere to the much-vaunted journalistic ethic of objectivity, they become stenographers, mistakenly assuming the summary answer to any scientific dilemma can be resolved with a conversation with some government employee in the cinder-block offices of the Centers for Disease Control in Atlanta or on the manicured campus of the National Institutes of Health in Bethesda.

Much like the influential medical journal articles read by doctors in private practice, the mainstream stories that result from such encounters are equally benighted and misleading. They serve to buttress the authority of the "experts" and bring further infamy upon the heads of patients, who tend to be portrayed as people who believe they are ill and—in our P.C. world—therefore worthy of sympathy, but whose maladies have no apparent basis in reality.

In my experience, the last thing patients are seeking is sympathy. What they want instead, quite desperately, is biomedical research. They're often referred to as "stakeholders" by government agencies, as if simply calling them what they actually are, sick people, threatens the established order. In describing what she calls the "Sartre-esque" world of the Lyme-afflicted, Weintraub notes that, often, only the richest and best connected of patients—a "made person," who, for instance, writes books about the (contested) disease or is a leader of a patient organization with access to the rare doctor who will help—actually receive the truly comprehensive treatments required to restore them to health. Even then, help is dicey, with doctors ditching their practices due to burnout or intimidation.

Insurance companies, not surprisingly, are off the hook. After all, if the *New England Journal of Medicine* publishes an article insisting the antibiotic treatment for Lyme disease need not exceed, say, ten days, why should any of the profit-oriented mega-corporations selling insurance policies act in ways that contradict the conclusions of the most venerable medical journal in the world?

Sir William Osler, a clinician of the early 1900s, revered for his clinical acumen, wrote that studying medicine without patients was like going to sea without charts. And yet, that is the cardinal medical sin scientists at the federal agencies and the upper echelons of academia commit in the realm of contested diseases, hiding behind the mantle of "objectivity." When the patients refuse to go away or renounce their "sickness behavior," these scientists convene at the CDC or the NIH to hammer out successive definitions of contested diseases. When their bylines appear at the top of a journal article, the endless feedback loop that props up the system once again anoints them masters of the field despite their being wholly removed from the lowly office encounter between doctor and patient and pathetically unschooled in the entity that has brought that patient figuratively, and sometimes literally, to his knees. In short, they reduce the practice of science to the level of engineering or, perhaps, accounting.

Certainly, medical history is one of myriad cycles of disbelief followed by the begrudging acceptance of scientific truths. In that history, scientific facts long considered heresy are ultimately embraced, but only when the highest authorities in the land get on board, a process that sometimes takes generations. Throughout the last century, for instance, neurological diseases, which have been short on infectious causes, so far, but long on symptoms, have been targets of disbelief. In the early 1900s, multiple sclerosis was known as the "faker's disease." New technologies, such as the debut in 1985 of magnetic resonance imaging, which visualized lesions in the brains of MS sufferers, also have helped to legitimize diseases like Parkinson's, ALS, and Alzheimer's.

But I suspect this particular era will go down in medical history as one of the most contentious. In part, there is the legacy of the 1950s to blame, when, after the development of penicillin drugs, the medical establishment fell into the relaxed stance that infectious diseases had been or soon would be conquered. A bigger problem is that technology itself has removed the workaday doctor in his or her clinic from extended interaction with patients. Economic issues are paramount. Doctors listen to patients long enough to decide which tests to order and the patient is sent packing. But what if the patient is suffering from something for which a test has not been invented or the tests are notoriously unreliable or outdated? When there is a new or emerging disease on the horizon, or right before the doctor's nose, he or she is virtually guaranteed to miss it.

At the moment, even the bedrock discoveries provided by new technologies have not seemed to move the science of contested diseases forward. Weintraub describes in fascinating detail the leaps in understanding the pathogen that can cause Lyme disease to smolder in the body even after treatment and the increasingly sophisticated, if still experimental, technologies that could be marshaled to test for it, as well as antibiotic and immune therapies that may keep the disease at bay.

But, in chronic Lyme, as in other contested diseases, the naysayers at the top of the food chain continue to win the day by shouting down the individual researcher who has made the discoveries. It's particularly easy for those at the top of the scientific heap—such as administrators at the NIH, the CDC, and elite medical schools, as well as journal editors—to silence entire populations of sick people by suggesting patients are malingerers or too wimpy to handle stress when they broadcast their opinions to the mainstream media from their bully pulpits.

It's not only highly placed scientists who determine which disease gets disappeared and which is deemed important and "real." Patent rights that encourage academic researchers to withhold discoveries from public scrutiny for years at a time and internecine politics inside federal health agencies, by which I mean jockeying for hegemony and job security, play a role, too.

The tragedy of contested diseases stems not from any conspiracy on the ground, as Weintraub, who has had years to contemplate the matter, points out. Instead, these tragedies result from a "perfect storm," as she describes it, of flawed science, medical hubris, and moneyed interests. I agree. Yet if one pulls back in a wide angle and with hindsight, occasionally the word *conspiracy* does seem broadly applicable. While I was working on *Osler's Web,* I became friends with a highly respected cancer epidemiologist who sought NIH funding for research in the CFS field and failed, though he routinely received millions of dollars in NIH funding for other diseases. He commented that the tide would turn in chronic fatigue syndrome only when a pathogenic agent was discovered. He added, "Then we will see what was in essence a conspiracy by very rigid people who didn't have the imagination to *believe* this disease exists. They didn't *decide* to do this. It wasn't a bunch of people sitting around a table. It's been institutional sabotage in the broadest sense."

As one of Weintraub's least hubristic scientists notes near the end of *Cure Unknown,* "Some researchers have thrown down their gloves and retreated to their corners, leaving patients out in the cold. But . . . it's not a question of whether you might have to eat crow. We've got to go in and do the right experiments, and then we can look truth in the eye."

The problem is, too many of the power brokers in the medical establishment who launched these faulty definitions and embraced the mantle of "expert" over the ensuing years don't see it that way. To reverse their positions, to admit they might have been wrong, to open up the grant-making process to investigators who have new approaches and ideas, feels very much like eating crow, and few show signs of changing their stance in the future.

There will be those, including other reporters and editors, who will argue that only scientists in the upper echelons of the most prestigious universities and public health officials of the highest rank are allowed the final word in chronic Lyme. As a longtime journalist and the author of an earlier book about another disease that has been similarly deemed not bona fide, I would argue that it is just such thinking that encourages the kind of disastrous public health policies, with their skewed research agendas, that Weintraub describes.

Further, as one who also suffers from the disease I chronicled with kindred passion in *Osler's Web,* I sometimes wonder if the only investigative writers who will possess the necessary temerity to remove the white gloves and tackle these putative experts to the ground will be those, like Weintraub and the late Randy Shilts, whose personal experience demands that they follow the rocky trail that leads to the truth.

—Hillary Johnson

Hillary Johnson's science and environmental reporting has appeared in Rolling Stone, *where she was a contributing editor for ten years, as well as* Mirabella, Life, Self, *and* Working Woman. *Her original reporting on chronic fatigue syndrome for* Rolling Stone *in 1988 was nominated for a National Magazine Award. She has been a journalist for thirty years, reporting for national newspapers and magazines such as* The Wall Street Journal, Vanity Fair, Vogue, Elle, *and* GQ. *She is the author of two books,* Osler's Web: Inside the Labyrinth of the Chronic Fatigue Syndrome Epidemic *and* My Mother Ruth: A Memoir of Love, Loss and Art. *A tenth-anniversary edition of* Osler's Web, *with an update by the author, was recently released.*

Introduction

Navigating by Lymelight

Starting in the early 1990s, after we moved from a city apartment to a wooded property in Westchester County, New York, our family began to get sick. At first the illness was subtle: The vague headaches, joint pains, and bone-weariness seemed par for the course in our busy suburban lives. But as years passed, the symptoms intensified and multiplied, burgeoning into gross signs of disease.

My knees became so swollen that I descended the steps of my house while sitting. Swallowing my food, I choked. My arms and legs buzzed—gently at first, but then so palpably I felt like I was wired to a power grid. A relentless migraine became so intense I spent hours each day in a darkened room, in bed.

My husband, Mark, an avid tennis player with great coordination, began stumbling and bumping into walls. Formerly affable, he began exploding at offenses as slight as someone spilling water on the floor. He was an award-winning journalist with a love of literature and a vocabulary so vast he was our stand-in for the dictionary. But slowly he began struggling with memory and groping for words. Finally, ground to a halt, he left his job as editor in chief of the newsletter *Bottom Line Health* one day after realizing that he'd spent hours trying to read a single, simple paragraph.

Our youngest son, David, began to sleep—first so long that he could not do his homework or see his friends; eventually, so much (fifteen or more hours a day) that he could not get to class. Violating the strict attendance policy at his prep school, he was asked to leave.

Hardest hit was Jason, our oldest, who suffered fatigue and shooting pains starting at age nine, the summer we took up residence in our fairytale house in the woods. The doctors called these "growing pains" normal, but by age sixteen Jason was essentially disabled. He couldn't think, walk, or tolerate sound and light. His joints ached all day long. On medical leave from high school, he spent his days in the tub in our darkened main-floor bathroom, drifting in and out of consciousness while hot water and steam eased his pain. As his condition worsened, as all sorts of lab tests came back negative, a raft of specialists at New York City's top teaching hospitals suggested diagnoses from migraine aura (the dizzying buzz of a migraine) to fifth disease (a swelling of the joints caused by infection with parvovirus). Each diagnosis elicited a treatment, but none of them worked.

"What about Lyme disease?" I asked.

"There are too many symptoms here and he's way too sick for Lyme disease," responded the pediatrician, who declined to even test for it.

But by 2000, with answers still eluding us, the pediatrician drew fourteen vials of blood, testing for hormone imbalance, mineral deficiency, anemia, and a host of infections, including Lyme. A week later he contacted us, baffled. Just one test, a Western blot for antibodies against Lyme disease, had come back not just positive, but off-the-charts reactive. Jason was quickly reported to the Centers for Disease Control and Prevention (CDC) as an unequivocal case of Lyme disease. When the head of infectious disease at Northern Westchester Hospital put his imprimatur on the diagnosis, we had an explanation for Jason's illness and an inkling as to what might be wrong with the rest of us, at last.

Our nightmare had just begun. As with the quest for diagnosis, almost everything about Lyme disease turned out to be controversial. From the length and type of treatment to the definition of the disease to the kind of practitioner we should seek to the microbe causing the infection (or whether it was an infection at all), Lyme was a hotbed of contention. It was the divisiveness surrounding the disease that had caused our pediatrician and the specialists we'd consulted to hold back diagnosis as Jason and the rest of us became increasingly ill.

For patients with early-stage Lyme disease the illness tended to be mild, and a month of antibiotic treatment usually offered a cure. But for those who slipped through the cracks of early diagnosis, for people like *us,* infection could smolder and progress, causing a disabling, degenerative disease that confounded doctors and thrust patients into the netherworld of unexplained, untreatable ills.

Despite the effectiveness of early treatment, withholding therapy had become increasingly common as a battle royal over Lyme's essence spilled from medical centers and clinics into the communities where people got sick. The same doctors who routinely doused acne and ear infections with years of antibiotic often would not prescribe even ten days of such treatment for Lyme unless proof of infection was absolute. Meanwhile, the few doctors willing to treat the sickest patients with longer-term or higher-dose antibiotics could be called up for trial by medical boards, putting their practices and licenses at risk.

The war over Lyme had raged for twenty-five years when it swept us up in its madness. On one side of the fight were university scientists who first studied Lyme disease, initially writing it up in medical journals as an infection of the joints. The disease they described was caused by the spirochete *Borrelia burgdorferi* and transmitted to people by the bite of a deer tick. It was hard to catch and easy to cure no matter how advanced the case when first diagnosed. Late disease was rare, these academics said, because Lyme was recognized easily through an oval rash—the so-called bull's-eye—and a simple, accurate blood test. Rarely was their version of the disease seen outside the Northeast, parts of California, and a swath of the Midwest.

To the horror of these scientists, the circumscribed disease of their studies had been hijacked by "quack suburban doctors" who saw Lyme everywhere, from Florida to Texas to Missouri, invoking so many signs and symptoms that they included every complaint under the sun. These heretical doctors, the scientists charged, were dispensing antibiotics like water, all the while raking in money from patients too deluded to realize they didn't have Lyme disease at all. The patients had other things, the scientists said: sometimes mental disorders, but also chronic fatigue syndrome and fibromyalgia, illnesses with no known cause or cure.

On the other side of the fight, far from the ivory tower, the rebel doctors and their desperately sick patients insisted that Lyme and a soup of coinfections caused a spectrum of illness dramatically different from the one the scientists described. Knees didn't always swell and the rash (rarely a bull's-eye) often wasn't seen. Instead the patients were mostly exhausted, in chronic pain, and dazed and confused. The mental condition they called "Lyme fog" robbed them of short-term memory, stunted their speech, and crippled their concentration. Brain infection could inflict a host of frank psychiatric problems from bipolar disorder and depression to panic and obsessive-compulsive disorder (OCD), they said, and Lyme could trigger what looked like autism or be confused with amyotrophic lateral sclerosis, known as Lou Gehrig's disease, or ALS. Because their illness differed profoundly from the disease described in textbooks, because it often eluded blood tests, the patients went undiagnosed and untreated for years. As they struggled for answers, once-treatable infections became chronic, inexorably disseminating, and causing disabling conditions that might never be cured. If treatment was to work at all, the heretic Lyme doctors said, it required high-dose antibiotics, often in combination or delivered intravenously, sometimes for months or years.

The patients, for their part, tried to comprehend why the academics dismissed their cases as false. The scientists were promoting an impossibly narrow version of Lyme disease to protect their early work and secure a windfall from Lyme-related patents, some patients believed. A flow chart entitled "The Wall of Power" began circulating around support groups, connecting some of the researchers with U.S. patents and federal or industry grants. Other patients complained that university physicians consulted for managed care, making hundreds of dollars an hour dismissing Lyme diagnoses and advising rejection of their claims. The academics advanced their agendas, the patients charged, by reporting the doctors who treated them to disciplinary boards.

As medical tribunals swept through the Lymelands, primary care physicians became ever more cautious about treating or even diagnosing Lyme disease for fear of becoming targets themselves. Stepping into the breach, a few doctors—Ed Masters of Missouri, Charles Ray Jones of Connecticut, Ken Liegner and Joe Burrascano of New York—went to the mattresses for the patients, but with the Lyme war so brutal, thousands of cases were missed.

Lyme or not Lyme? Diagnoses could get mixed up. Dueling brain tumor stories make the point. A young woman from Australia went hiking in California. From that trip on her health declined. She eventually experienced such pain, disorientation, and inflammation that doctors thought she might die. She returned to the U.S. for treatment, and neurologists in Manhattan diagnosed a brain tumor. They actually operated, but when they opened her up, there was no tumor. It turned out the young woman had Lyme disease. She was treated with antibiotics and cured. A young man from New Jersey was diagnosed with Lyme disease and treated with antibiotics for months without impact. Finally he was sent to a local medical center, and further testing was done. Doctors discovered a brain tumor and operated to remove it. The boy from Jersey, like the girl from Australia, got well.

The more I investigated, the fuzzier the whole thing seemed. Various strains of the spirochete caused different flavors of Lyme disease, so diagnosis could miss the mark. Doctors and labs reported more than 27,000 cases falling within the CDC's circumscribed definition for Lyme disease in 2007 alone—a number the CDC estimated could be 10 percent of the total such cases in the United States. With more than an estimated 270,000 new cases meeting the CDC's narrow definition each year, Lyme had become one of the fastest-spreading infectious diseases in the United States. But how many bona fide Lyme disease patients fell outside that umbrella? Thousands? Hundreds of thousands? More? With so many patients failing to see a rash and the blood tests so equivocal, and with new strains reported every year, it was impossible to say.

The line blurred still more because other ticks and infections contributed to the epidemic called "Lyme." *Babesia,* a malarialike disease of fevers, headaches, sweats, and profound exhaustion, was almost as prevalent as Lyme disease itself in many areas. Patients sick for years despite aggressive treatment for Lyme disease "miraculously" recovered once *Babesia* was treated. Intracellular bacterial infections like anaplasmosis and ehrlichiosis, found in a quarter of Lyme ticks in Connecticut, New York, and many other places, including the South, could cause a draining, painful illness marked by fevers, headaches, confusion, and occasionally a rash. Many an "incurable" Lyme patient had been found to have such second, lurking infections; these patients were treated with doxycycline and generally got well. Added to the triad of Lyme-babesiosis-anaplasmosis/ehrlichiosis are other suspect pathogens also inhabiting the same ticks: among them, forms of the rod-shaped bacterium *Bartonella* and *Mycoplasma fermentans,* both sometimes invoked as causes of neuropsychiatric symptoms and chronic fatigue.

Finally, a series of newly discovered spirochetes inhabiting a diversity of ticks have been implicated in a "Lyme-like" disease, including the classic Lyme rash, in regions overlapping with and extending way beyond traditional Lyme zones. The upshot: an illness that was a ringer for Lyme disease—except that sufferers didn't test positive because they weren't infected by the same spirochete as the one causing Lyme disease. With so many cases of true Lyme disease falling short of the CDC definition, and with emerging infections, real and potential, at the periphery of the hostile debate, chaos reigned.

In all the Sturm und Drang, anyone who fell ill could get caught in the mania. Sure, there were those diagnosed with Lyme disease who did not have it. But the more contentious the fight became, the more doctors were targeted for diagnosing outside the CDC definition or treating beyond official guidelines, the more the balance shifted the other way. All you had to do was live in our neighborhoods and meet our families, our children, to grasp how many had waited months and years for diagnoses that should have been rendered swiftly, missing the window of opportunity for early treatment and cure. Adding insult to injury, so many of those who were missed, like our son Jason, had textbook-perfect cases of classic Lyme disease in proven Lyme zones. They, too, were denied. First thousands, then hundreds of thousands, perhaps a million or more fell victim to the war over Lyme disease as the fight raged on.

I was a patient and a mother, but also a science journalist when my family was swept up in the Lyme war. The winds of that war carried us far from normal reality to a twilight zone of double-talk, an inside-out world with layers of obfuscation, where disease was dismissed as delusion and nothing was as it seemed. How had an affliction so cruel and insidious gripped the underbelly of the suburbs? How had so many patients of relative sophistication wound up victimized by a fight between doctors, ridiculed and marginalized as illness destroyed their lives? What was the truth about Lyme disease? Would I discover the answers in Lyme's past or from present-day scientists toiling at the workbench, far from the maelstrom of the fight?

Because I was sick myself, my job as a journalist was complex. Some of the experts I interviewed would have deemed me suspect had they known my status, so I strived to draw the line between my life and my job. I attempted to do that which was almost impossible in Lyme: to lead a double life and inhabit two worlds. In the first I was one of the chronic patients, in the midst of a suspect illness. In the second I was a science journalist, discussing, with equanimity, the notion that patients like me were false.

"You cannot argue on the basis of anecdote and individual case history and speculation," insisted Leonard Sigal, the New Jersey rheumatologist and Robert Wood Johnson Medical Center professor, insisted when I asked him about our ilk. "This way lies madness. Where is the evidence?"

On the beat I looked for evidence, but within myself I felt what Sigal doubted taking hold. Without antibiotics I was sick but with them I was getting well.

As I fought Lyme in my life and struggled to restore my family's health, the questions and contradictions haunted me. For the mother and patient, Lyme was an albatross, but for the science journalist, it was the story of a lifetime. I couldn't walk away from it, not when it devastated my family, not when it inhabited my woods.

Prologue

Second Journey Out

In my first encounter with Lyme I was swept from a healthy, exuberant life to the distant, lonely shore of a controversial disease. As the exhausted, symptomatic wife and mother of Lyme patients, one of them desperately sick, my struggle to beat back illness was initially consuming. Trapped in a new reality, I learned the complex idiom of illness, but all I really wanted was to find my way home.

My second journey through Lyme, ventured as a journalist, was far more strategic than the first. Instead of an unwitting mother negotiating a disputed diagnosis, I was a professional investigator, a science journalist— the job for which I had been trained and paid by the top science magazines in the country for twenty-five years. My personal experience had been frightening, but as a longtime science journalist, I knew it was subjective. Subjective experience is powerful, but ultimately anecdotal. Those trained in the scientific method, and those who report on it, understand that subjective experience falls far short of proof. Proof in science means validation by experiment. Yet to be valid, the experiments themselves must be free of bias and must be of adequate scientific design. I would have to look into all of this—carefully, and with expert input—to understand the research framing Lyme.

A journalist doesn't report only on studies, of course, but also on people—what they experience, say, and feel. Laboratory science is rarely adequate to distill the fear and betrayal felt by patients when misunderstood. Even when blessed with empathetic natures, biomedical scientists may not readily grasp a patient's journey through the desolate outback of a disease. So my job was not just understanding the science, but also reporting back from the front, from the cul-de-sacs, split levels, and toy-strewn yards of the suburbs, where patients got sick and endured the illness itself.

The more people I interviewed, the more I realized that the distance between the scientific studies and the patients' lives was vast. Peer-reviewed articles dismissing the Lyme patients' mental impairment as "mild," for instance, did not remotely capture the experience of having a brain infection—the angst of falling behind in school or feeling perpetually foggy and confused. A young woman forgot how to dial home on her cell phone and found herself stranded. A boy did his math homework each night, but by morning his knowledge was a blur. The clinical language of many studies made Lyme fatigue seem minimal, while patients crashed with an exhaustion so profound they could not sustain employment or care for their children and homes. Memory loss calibrated in percentage points was presented as mere annoyance in the studies, but it translated, in patients' lives, to hours spent navigating local highways, lost in their own neighborhoods, or forgetting a frying pan on the stove and setting the house ablaze. A programmer could no longer hold codes in his head—an office manager could not keep files straight.

As I interviewed patients, I found they were often most disabled by the very problems mainstream studies had tossed out as too subjective or vague to count as Lyme disease. Headache, fatigue, and mental confusion were just too broad, too general, to be of relevance in actually diagnosing Lyme disease, the Infectious Diseases Society of America (IDSA) said in its 2006 guidelines. These symptoms were the same as those found in chronic fatigue and the pain syndrome, fibromyalgia, the Centers for Disease Control and Prevention added—how could you tell the diseases apart? Unless a patient had measurable *signs* of Lyme disease—the very ones used to define it in mainstream studies, like swollen knees, heart inflammation, and quantifiably damaged nerves—the mainstream experts wouldn't concede that the patient had the infection at all.

A contentious tug-of-war over what a Lyme patient looked like had spurred the battle from the start. Because those doctors first describing the illness were trained in rheumatology and dermatology, the objective signs they recognized included swollen joints and the classic Lyme rash. Later, neurologists joined the team, adding such specialty-specific signs as encephalitis or meningitis (swelling of the brain or its lining) and nerve damage. As these signs of disease intensified, according to such experts, so did antibodies in the spinal fluid and blood.

The view was at loggerheads with the experience of the sickest of the patients, who lacked the sanctioned signs and failed the designated tests. Falling outside the mainstream construct they defaulted to Lyme doctors, mostly ensconced in the suburbs. In this alternate Lyme universe, *symptoms* like confusion and fatigue, along with partially positive tests, were factored into the equation, serving as justification for treatment with antibiotics, often for months on end. Rejected as false by mainstream medicine, said to have fibromyalgia, chronic fatigue syndrome, or simply depression by the Centers for Disease Control and the National Institutes of Health, the patients nonetheless sought treatment for the only thing they felt they'd been exposed to—Lyme disease. After treatment with antibiotics, many eventually got well.

Did these people really have Lyme disease? Were they actually sick? Did they *count*? Those were the questions swirling around the Lyme debate.

On one side of the equation are people like C. Ben Beard, Ph.D., chief of the Bacterial Diseases Branch of the Division of Vector-Borne Infectious Diseases of the CDC. "These people are very sick, and we feel great compassion for them. Their lives have been destroyed," Beard says, "but based on their symptoms, we're just not convinced that they have Lyme disease."

Seeing things differently are physicians like Brian Fallon, a psychiatrist and director of the Lyme and Tick Borne Diseases Research Center at Columbia University. "Patients without objective signs can still have symptoms of Lyme disease—cognitive problems, fatigue, joint pain, mood swings," he states. "Because those symptoms weren't objectified early in the history of the disease by the specific specialties first involved, many doctors still think they don't count," he says, but they do. "There are other ways of defining illness and objectifying signs and symptoms of disease."

"If a doctor asks the patient whether he's tired and the patient responds, simply, 'yes,' without any detail, there is nothing objective to report," explains Harold Smith, a Pennsylvania physician who treats Lyme disease. "But if the practitioner asks for objective information, he can elicit it: Does sleep restore you? Is your sleep associated with drenching night sweats that soak your hair and pajamas? Does it take days to recover from raking a twenty-foot patch of your yard? There are corresponding physical exam findings to go with such answers, including loss of muscle bulk, lowered body temperatures, slow heart rates, and abnormal hormone levels, among many others. These impairments can be objectively measured and, with the right treatment, reversed."

Yet even patients with *accepted signs* of Lyme disease, with the exception of the rash, don't qualify for treatment unless they have positive blood tests to back them up. And the fuzziness of the testing opens another can of worms.

One part of the problem stems from the lack of a direct test for Lyme disease. There's simply no way to learn whether a patient is currently infected because as Lyme progresses, spirochetes leave the bloodstream and gravitate into solid tissue. This obviously makes it exceedingly hard to culture living organisms through an ordinary blood test. Instead of detecting infection in blood directly, therefore, doctors test for Lyme's fingerprints—the antibodies formed in the spirochetes' wake. Manufactured by our immune systems to try to fight the infection, Lyme antibodies are detected as literal bands on a test known as the Western blot. Because these antibodies can linger even when infection is gone, they indicate exposure at some point in the past, but do not confirm that infection is active at the time.

Another part of the problem stems from the imperfect antibody pattern chosen by the CDC and other experts to indicate a so-called positive. The pattern of Western blot bands endorsed by the CDC was determined by analyzing blood from a group of classic Lyme disease patients, those with swollen knees and measurably damaged brains and nerves. The test, therefore, reinforced the mainstream presentation of a disease with blatantly measurable signs while excluding patients who had only subtle symptoms like memory loss or subjective complaints like exhaustion and pain.

Yet the Western blot pattern endorsed by the CDC has been subject to furious debate ever since it was voted in amidst a firestorm of protest at a conference in Dearborn, Michigan, in 1994. The pattern was determined by matching antibodies in human blood with a single strain of *Borrelia* from Europe, ignoring the full range of proteins expressed by the hundreds of strains reported in the United States and worldwide. Of the many antibodies expressed, just ten were deemed diagnostic. Chosen statistically, these included some so common they were found widely in the healthy population while excluding others specific only to Lyme disease.

Indeed, it's beyond dispute that patients with confirmed Lyme infection can fail the test for a host of reasons: Antibodies can stick to proteins in human blood, preventing them from floating free to interact with the test. Some strains literally lack all the proteins being tested for. And when patients with undiagnosed early Lyme have been treated with antibiotic for something else, like an ear infection, that treatment may be insufficient to cure the Lyme yet may suppress the antibody response to it forevermore. Even Immunetics, the company that manufactures the blot, selling it to Quest and LabCorp, has found that alternate Western blot banding patterns turn up more real Lyme disease patients, and are more precise.

The bottom line is this: Patients with the Lyme disease *signs* that mainstream experts say count—the swollen knees and frank meningitis—often pass the test with flying colors. Patients suffering mostly from the so-called *symptoms* of Lyme disease, the fatigue and confusion, often fail. Like a castle on a hill surrounded by a moat, the mainstream definition of Lyme disease is a monument to itself: It houses within its impervious walls patients who fit its paradigm, leaving the rest clamoring for recognition at the gate.

The more I looked into it, the more I concluded that the very scaffolding of Lyme science was flimsy as a house of cards. Take the simple issue of how many Lyme disease patients get the famous rash. As I read through years of literature in medical journals, including the early work, I found the estimate ranged from 40 to 90 percent. The different statistics resulted, largely, from entrance requirements for the studies themselves. Where the rash was required for diagnosing Lyme in a given study, authors invariably concluded that most patients had the rash. Where patients were diagnosed based on other factors, for instance, positive blood work, the percent with the rash dramatically fell.

The more I investigated, the more I started to feel that Lyme was not so much a disease as the definition of a disease—a complex calculus that compensated, clumsily, for all that was still unknown. One could be infected with the Lyme spirochete, *Borrelia burgdorferi*, one could even be sick from the infection, but if one did not fit into this or that statistical group or have this or that presentation, one would not have "Lyme disease." I thought the mainstream scientists would be offended when I broached my interpretation based on my read of the medical journals. But instead, to my utter shock, most of them agreed I had pegged it right.

What was Lyme disease? That was a question I asked a lot. There was the official disease definition used to train our pediatricians, our family physicians and internists. But as I conducted my interviews, the scientists themselves told me the definition was limited and flawed.

Lyme or not Lyme? With so many possible infections, known and unknown, tick-borne and not tick-borne; with so many strains of Lyme itself; with tests so equivocal; with each patient's genes and immune system so variable; with the possibility of side effects from treatment; and with diagnostic guidelines statistically determined and then artificially narrowed to eliminate all the vagaries, it seemed impossible to know.

It was the dispute over the disease definition—between those who sought to narrow it and those who sought to broaden it—that formed the first part of the Lyme war. The conflict was distilled for me in a *Philadelphia Inquirer* story about a patient named Amy, who had experienced chest pains, heart palpitations, dizziness, and vision problems. First, she was diagnosed with Lyme disease and treated, and got well. But a few years hence she fell ill once more, this time reporting extreme weakness and intermittent jabbing muscular pain that waxed and waned. Amy sought the help of five neurologists, four internists, and several infectious disease doctors, cardiologists, and neuroophthalmologists, to no avail. Finally, a rheumatologist sent her to Drexel University's Center for Behavioral Medicine and Mind/Body Studies, which focuses on symptoms that are "medically unexplained." After treatment there, the *Inquirer* reported, Amy felt much better, "not because her symptoms are gone, but because she has learned to cope."

The article sparked the ire of Massachusetts Lyme disease patient Alan Stone: "We in the Lyme patient community are only too familiar with having our symptoms explained away as stress, or hysteria, or otherwise 'in our head,'" he wrote. "Until today's physicians can put their egos and arrogance aside and become comfortable with the idea that current medical technological capability is picayune compared to the virtually infinite variety of problems that nature can produce, long-suffering individuals like Amy will be the worse off for it."

The counterpunch to Stone came from Professor George E. Ehrlich, M.D., of the University of Pennsylvania and chairman of the Expert Advisory Panel on Chronic Degenerative Diseases for the World Health Organization (WHO). "What is described may be many things," Ehrlich wrote of Amy, "but it's not Lyme disease." Alan Stone's letter, in particular, he added, "echoes the scientifically erroneous claims" of women who say they were poisoned by silicone breast implants: *I am the evidence*. We would all be better off without the patient advocacy agencies that have sprung up for chronic Lyme disease, fibromyalgia, chronic fatigue syndrome, and other fictitious illnesses. . . . As Leonard Sigal, a real Lyme disease expert, states, 'The romanticism of practice by anecdote, speculation, and "my experience" is not a viable alternative to the rational practice of evidence-based medicine.'"

Skeptical of chronic Lyme disease as an explanation of ongoing symptoms, Sigal often diagnosed such patients as having fibromyalgia, a pain syndrome, instead. But wasn't fibromyalgia the very diagnosis that Ehrlich now threw in the wastebasket as bogus, along with chronic Lyme? While rheumatologists put stock in the fibromyalgia diagnosis—and say it can be treated—many experts, for instance, Ehrlich, contend it is a sham. A survey by the New York State Legislature found fibromyalgia to be the most commonly reported misdiagnosis experienced by patients before being successfully treated for Lyme disease.

The exchange in the Philadelphia press caused such a ruckus that it reached the desk of Lyme disease patient Miguel Perez-Lizano across the country, in Battle Ground, Washington. Perez-Lizano decided to alert Geneva-based Lee Jong-wook, director-general of WHO. "A doctor claiming to be chairman of the Expert Advisory Panel on Chronic Degenerative Diseases for the World Health Organization has made biased and serious misrepresentations to the American public in a major newspaper," Perez-Lizano complained in his letter. Specifically, he pointed out, Ehrlich had asserted a WHO affiliation while disparaging as "fictitious" three diseases—chronic Lyme disease, chronic fatigue syndrome, and fibromyalgia—all recognized by the National Institutes of Health. The affiliation, wrote Perez-Lizano, "gives the impression that WHO endorses these views."

About a month later, Perez-Lizano received a response in the mail. "We perfectly understand your concern," wrote Dr. Tikki Pang, WHO's Director of Research Policy and Cooperation. Pang assured Perez-Lizano that WHO would be contacting Ehrlich "to ensure that in the future no reference is made to his relationship to WHO."

The debate over Amy and other persistently ill patients diagnosed with Lyme disease rages on: Are these patients sick because they are hypochondriacs, because their Lyme disease has triggered an immune reaction (or unexplained syndromes like fibromyalgia), or because the spirochete, *B. burgdorferi,* lingers on?

This question gets to the heart of the second part of the fight over Lyme. Can infection persist after standard antibiotic treatment of a month or two? Do some patients need longer courses of antibiotic treatment at higher doses to beat the illness and get well?

As I made the round of interviews, I found few mainstream researchers who felt that a month or two of antibiotic treatment always eradicated infection in late-stage, long-untreated Lyme disease. The question to most of the mainstream researchers, rather, was this: Following standard treatment for late-stage Lyme disease, was persisting infection the rare exception or the frequent rule? If infection lingered, was it now so dormant or

sequestered that antibiotics, which target reachable, actively dividing organisms, couldn't help—or were the wrong antibiotics being used?

Beleaguered by the battle, the National Institutes of Health had, in
1998, launched three Lyme studies to resolve the debate over treatment: In
2007, all the results were in, but most experts cited the studies selectively,
depending on their points of view. The first study, conducted by Lyme's
hard-liners at Tufts, a group with an autoimmune theory of the disease,
showed extra treatment did no good, none whatsoever. A second study
from the middle-of-the-roaders at Stony Brook showed an advantage to
the extra treatment, but hedged their finding by citing side effects. A third
treatment study, out of Columbia, showed improvement in memory and
fatigue—but after the treatment stopped, improvement in memory was
not sustained. Why the mixed response? Was ten weeks' treatment sufficient for the body but not the brain—or was the antibiotic, in the mode of
some psychiatric drugs, altering neurotransmitters only as long as it was
actively in use? Each expert had an opinion, based on preconceived no-
tions, but since the question hadn't been asked *experimentally,* no one
had *evidence* for his or her stance—no one really *knew*.

Swept into this vacuum of knowledge were the patients. I had personally met hundreds of individuals saddled with diagnoses of chronic fatigue
syndrome, fibromyalgia, coronary artery disease, and multiple sclerosis
who, when treated with antibiotics for Lyme disease for months on end,
finally got well. Some patients shared my personal experience: On the medicine they were fine, but off it they felt sick. Scientists said such anecdotes
were the problem with Lyme—that testimonials weren't proof. But for me,
the journalist on the beat, the anecdotes assumed more relevance once the
disputed nature of the research was revealed.

Given all those shades of gray in Lyme disease, why was diagnosis
(yea or nay) in our doctor's offices usually so absolute? The devastating
consequence of untreated Lyme was undeniable and uncontroversial—
mainstream studies themselves documented, again and yet again, that
some 20 percent of those infected for more than a year never got well.
Given the dismal outcome, the whole-body pain, the confusion, and the
fatigue, why weren't we giving our children, our soccer moms and soccer dads, a few weeks of early treatment when cure was almost certain,
in other words, the benefit of the doubt?

One day, sitting with Peter Krause, a pediatrician at the University of
Connecticut, I mentioned my concern. Like many academic experts,
Krause was cautious—but like most of them, when chatting off-the-cuff,
acknowledged the cracks in Lyme: "I will say, having spent a fair

amount of time in this, that the truth is very complicated and we certainly do not have all the answers." For instance, while the classic diagnosis of Lyme disease (in the absence of a rash) calls for specific, objectified signs confirmed by two consecutive blood tests, Krause himself would treat a child from an endemic area that presented subjective symptoms (like headache and fatigue), even if evidence on the blood test was just equivocal—even if the child had just two specific bands on a Western blot instead of the requisite five. "It can be a bad illness, if untreated, and the treatment in early cases is usually benign," he says.

Why, then, didn't academicians train our family doctors to do the same? Why didn't they broadcast to the rafters that late-diagnosed patients—a shocking 20 percent of them—might stay sick for life?

You can't train doctors to treat a disease without evidence to back them up, Leonard Sigal told me. "That would be unconscionable," he said, adding that in his personal practice he behaves like Krause. "One of the problems that we've had over the course of the years is that honesty in medicine requires equivocation. There are very few absolutes in this world when it comes to medical care. Pneumococcal pneumonia requires antibiotics," he explains, "but is that what it is? If you spit up sputum and it's full of pneumococcus and a whole bunch of white cells and nothing else, it's pneumococcal pneumonia. But usually it is not that clear. There is no sputum to evaluate. The chest X-ray is atypical. It's not the kind of sputum that you would have expected. There is no such thing as an absolutely classic case of anything. For you to tell me, absolutely, this is Lyme disease, usually you can't make that kind of statement. Instead, you can say, 'I think it is likely that this is Lyme disease and the likelihood of response is very high.' Can you guarantee that this will be cured?" No, Sigal says, because "Lyme diagnosis is never 'black and white,' but rather, 'shades of gray.'"

Others disagree. Eugene Shapiro of Yale, who's trained a lion's share of the nation's pediatricians at Lyme seminars and Grand Rounds, is such a stickler for the exact definition that he won't treat a child who's tested positive for Lyme disease on a Western blot if all the child has is, say, a headache, muscle aches, and fatigue. The child must have the rash or wait until he develops one of the verifiable, objective signs, be it grossly swollen knees or meningitis, before Shapiro will call the episode Lyme disease and step in with even ten days of antibiotic to stave off worse illness up the road.

"What of the twenty percent who don't get well if treatment is delayed?" I asked Shapiro during an interview with him.

"We find that children do better than that," Shapiro said.

But even experts who have documented the damage and don't contest the numbers think that sticking to the formula is best. Raymond Dattwyler, an immunologist now of New York Medical College, has done studies showing that 15 to 20 percent of the late-treated patients never recover with his treatment approach. Yet Dattwyler has other studies showing that subjecting hundreds of thousands of possible Lyme cases to millions of tests and hundreds of millions of doses of antibiotics would be more expensive and more dangerous, overall, than letting the 20 percent slip through the cracks to a treatment-refractory form of the disease. During an interview, Dattwyler picked up a marker and wrote his calculations on a whiteboard. "It is a matter of economic medicine," he explained. According to Dattwyler's calculations, the rashes and yeast infections, the stomachaches, the infected intravenous lines resulting as side effects of antibiotic treatment all took a hefty toll.

Others point to superbugs—the fear, ever more heightened in recent years, that by exposing germs to myriad antibiotics for extended periods of time, we'll breed a new generation of bacteria resistant to them all. Phillip J. Baker, the avuncular microbiologist who served as Lyme Disease Program Officer at the National Institutes of Health until his retirement in 2007, explains. While *Borrelia burgdorferi* itself doesn't seem to become resistant to antibiotics, he says, Lyme patients on long-term antibiotics could develop other resistant infections, and those could be spread to the public. "Some of these patients could be carrying antibiotic-resistant staph in their nasal passages. It might not be hurting them, but if it gets into someone else, it could cause a raging infection, unresponsive to most of the antibiotics we have. There is a lot of concern. The drug companies aren't interested in developing new antibiotics, because of the huge investment required for research and passage by FDA." Baker makes a comparison: "The most likely place to pick up an antibiotic-resistant infection is the intensive care unit of a hospital because those patients are on long-term antibiotic therapy." But in the world outside, there are other risks. One is the use of antibiotics in poultry and livestock. But another is the breeding ground within ourselves, embodied in the patient on long-term antibiotics for Lyme. It only makes sense that Baker, who spent years focusing on anthrax and threats of bioterrorism, would have this perspective—especially since he thinks there's little chance that long-term antibiotics will help. So passionate is Baker about this message that after leaving NIH he assumed directorship of the American Lyme Disease Association (ALDF), a nonprofit formed largely to argue against long-term treatment and espouse the mainstream view of the disease.

Indeed, on the issue of the human fallout there was a clear philosophical divide: Thousands of cases of nausea or other, more serious complications might be costlier to society than one ruined life—but to those whose lives were ruined, the triage (even if it carried risk of antibiotic-resistant germs) seemed cruel.

These are the types of differences that have fueled the fight over Lyme disease, whipping it into one of the most vicious medical wars we've ever seen. The boycott of each school of thought by the other is said to be based on scientific dispute. Yet after talking science with dozens of these experts and clinicians for years, I've concluded that I am witnessing not so much a scientific impasse as an ancestral feud—a biomedical reenactment of the Hatfields and McCoys.

It's as if a kind of psychopathology has washed over the Lymelands, paralyzing the experts with disdain for one another, just as brain fog has paralyzed the patients they endeavor to serve. There is no better way to discredit one's adversaries in Lyme country than to suggest that they are emotionally imbalanced, delusional, insane.

It came to a head one Sunday morning some years back when Lyme disease patient Robyn Greco opened the *New York Times* to learn she had been characterized as mentally ill by the rheumatologist who first studied Lyme in Connecticut, Allen Steere. Profiled in an article entitled "Stalking Dr. Steere Over Lyme Disease," the rheumatologist had reflected on his "journey" from his early days as medical hero to his more recent role as a bulwark between clamoring patients and the long-term antibiotic therapy they were fighting to obtain. Whatever patients thought, Steere said in the article, he was actually defending them, and the integrity of science as well, by limiting the treatment they received. Yet in doing so, he feared, he was putting his life at risk.

Patients had started calling his office, Steere told the *New York Times*, telling him he was responsible for their suffering, their pain, fatigue, depression, and anxiety, in some cases their loved ones' deaths. Patients had begun showing up at his public engagements, Steere complained, holding signs that read "How many more will you kill?" and "Steer Clear of Steere!" "They depicted him in the media as a demon, worse than the spirochetes, the tick-borne bacteria that they claimed inhabited their bodies and that, because of his restrictive diagnosis, they could not eliminate," the *New York Times* said.

As Steere sat behind his desk at the hospital chatting with the *Times* reporter, he explained that many of the so-called Lyme patients just didn't have Lyme disease, but rather fibromyalgia or chronic fatigue syndrome—and some were mentally ill. To illustrate this last point, Steere pulled out a letter he said was typical of many patients receiving the Lyme diagnosis when something else was clearly wrong.

"I am twenty-nine years old. I live in northern New Jersey and have been suffering with Lyme disease for seven years," the letter began. The letter writer said she had been treated with antibiotics and tranquilizers for more than a year, but remained "unable to work, to socialize, and unable to perform most daily tasks. I still have the majority of symptoms." On the back of the letter she provided a symptom list: worsening dizzy spells, severe fatigue, muscle pain, low-grade fevers, intolerance to heat or cold, hot flashes, weight gain, weight loss, numbness and tingling in skull and limbs, seeing black spots, sinus infections, constant infections, palpitations, severe digestive disorder, high-pitch ringing in both ears, leg jerks, poor sleeping habits, food allergies, severely altered balance, mood swings, deteriorating handwriting, to name just a few. "What do I do to be well again?" the writer asked. "My life has been turned upside down by Lyme."

"What I suspect," Steere told the *Times*, "is that she doesn't have Lyme disease but some kind of psychiatric illness."

The letter writer was not some disembodied voice from the void, however, but a flesh-and-blood person, a *sensitive* person. Greco, a former auto-body shop manager, was bitten by a tick in the Jersey woods in 1990, and experienced symptoms of nausea and elbow pain within weeks. After testing positive for Lyme disease, she was treated with oral antibiotics for a few weeks, and seemed to get well. But slowly symptoms returned. Headaches, dizzy spells, and nausea gave way to severe heart palpitations, muscle and joint pain, and overwhelming fatigue.

By 1994, sicker than ever, Greco finally found a doctor who said she still had Lyme disease, in fact, neuroborreliosis, an infection of the brain. Because she hadn't responded to the oral treatment, the doctor put her on IV. Finally Greco started to feel better and, with ongoing treatment, continued to improve until, in 1996, the doctor started getting nervous about a possible investigation of his practice and stopped her treatment, again. In 1999, as her beloved mother lay dying, Greco was increasingly symptomatic. Abandoned by her doctor and with nowhere to turn, she sat down to write the letter to Steere.

Publication of her letter in the *Times* in 2001 cut to the quick, Greco says today. "It created so much stress it made me ill, and put me in bed.

What kind of a doctor diagnoses a total stranger with mental illness in the newspaper, without ever having seen that patient?" she asks. "What kind of a *person* releases a patient's personal medical history, recognizable to family and friends, to the *New York Times*?"

Psychoanalysis at a distance (like clairvoyance and reading palms) may be just a parlor game, but in Lyme country, everyone plays. In line with the idea that "what goes around comes around," patients pay Steere back in kind. Stay on for dinner after any patient conference, and you'll find the psychoanalytic deconstruction of Steere and his colleagues a favorite pastime. Why has he turned against them, patients ask, why has he dismissed their suffering, denied they are even sick?

One night after a conference sponsored by the patient advocacy, I sat around a table having coffee with a group of aggrieved patients—a Ph.D. pharmacologist who had conducted research at a major university, a professor of literature (also a Ph.D.), and a psychiatrist. All three spent the better part of two hours attempting to comprehend the inner life of Allen Steere. He was honestly deluded in the belief he was right, the pharmacologist opined. No, argued the English professor, he knew he was wrong, but could not renege on so many years of work, so he let patients suffer instead. They were both mistaken, countered the psychiatrist: It was Steere's unconscious that made him who he was. "He must have been traumatized, perhaps abused, as a child," the psychiatrist theorized. Then there was the Monday-morning quarterback, an embattled Lyme physician who, overhearing the debate, added his special spin: "Steere suffers characterologic disorder and rigidity of thinking," he said.

Exposing the Lyme scene and the quirky players propelling it may seem like mere gossip, but that would miss the point. Emotional discord between scientists and their subjects compromises the scientific method and thus the conclusions reached. How can science objectify a disease so politicized that the vast majority of patients central to the dispute reject involvement with the scientists? Objective science requires that we remove the experimenter from the experiment. But here, hostility between researchers and their subjects has drawn the scientists into a swirl of subjective emotion, preventing the requirement from being met.

Medical science demands that we find a better answer to the question "What is Lyme disease?" Conversely, Lyme disease demands that we answer the question "What is medical evidence?" As consumers of medical information, we take for granted the idea that if a study has been codified in a medical journal, it is probably correct. But Lyme disease teaches us something else—conclusions may be oversimplified, exaggerated, or widely disputed. Data might be massaged. Results might be embraced, but turn out to be false. When proponents of a viewpoint chair the ad hoc review committees of almost every major medical journal, they become gatekeepers of information and de facto arbiters of "Truth." If we are rejecting patient anecdote for the "higher truth" of evidence-based medicine, shouldn't we make sure that the evidence is solid, objective, sound? Don't we need to know whether experimenters have included all the evidence, or just part of it, or whether the references cited to make an argument say what the authors contend? Don't we need to look at the methodology? After hearing the results of a study, don't we need to ask the next hard question: Is the study subject to circular thinking? Is the evidence any good?

As I made my way through the Lymelands, I was instructed by the skeptics' mantra: Extraordinary claims require extraordinary levels of evidence. Long trained as a science journalist, I started by looking for evidence in the science. Despite my personal experience, I truly believed that the patients, not the researchers, deserved my skepticism most. I started out as a journalist in search of the evidence but found the evidence convoluted, twisted, misleading, vague—subject to continual change and challenge not just by patients and their treating physicians, but by many experts in the academic mainstream. Is evidence of this quality more compelling than tens of thousands of anecdotal reports, especially when those reports are so disturbing and so widespread? Should we dismiss patient experience because it isn't "evidence-based" while embracing as absolute—for purposes of diagnosis, treatment, and insurance coverage—experimentally derived evidence which, when scrutinized, is so disputed, lacking in context, and incomplete?

In the end, I'm left with the patients. Many barely sick a day in their lives until bitten by a tick, they are now caught in the crosshairs of a fight between doctors. The victims of others' hubris, their diagnoses are put off for months and years because they fail to meet a controversial, intentionally narrow disease definition or pass a series of embattled, statistically derived, and flawed diagnostic tests. Long-untreated, infection blurs their vision, swells their joints, inflames their hearts, and sends shooting, stabbing neurological pain boring through their arms and legs. Exhausted and confused, the patients visit doctor after doctor without resolution, remaining undiagnosed as infection settles in the brain, affecting memory, cognition, and the balance of the emotional self. If untreated for more than a year, as so many are in the midst of the roiling controversy, a significant number, an alarming 20 percent of them, fail to respond to the normal course of treatment and stay sick. Saddled with a suspect illness, they're mocked as fabricators—malingerers, hypochondriacs, perpetrators of Munchausen Syndrome by Proxy, or simply insane. Responding to antibiotics but relapsing without, they continue treatment endlessly, ignoring risk of superbugs or deadly yeast infection because, they reckon, Lyme disease is worse. Running afoul of mainstream medicine and, often, insurance coverage, they must pay their doctors in cash. These physicians, the controversial Lyme doctors, themselves are targeted and often brought up on charges for overtreating Lyme disease, their licenses and livelihoods at risk. They, too, are more conservative and withholding when dispensing antibiotic treatment than they've been in the past.

Reporting on Lyme has meant reporting two realities. The first reality is neat and outwardly consistent, but it derives from a disease definition that has a partial relationship, at best, to the experience of that disease in the world. What's more, it fails to account for other factors—particularly, other infections, including other *Borreliae*—which, while artificially removed from studies in the lab, cannot be removed from our lives. The second reality, the alternate one, is messy and chaotic and awash in confusion. Its language is the language of Babel. Yet the flawed Reality Two—an open system that acknowledges the vast unknown—seems the better place to start.

PART ONE

DOORS OF PERCEPTION

*There are things known and there are things unknown, and
in between there are the doors of perception.*
                                            —Aldous Huxley

1

Into the Woods

Chappaqua, New York, 1993–2000

In the year 1993, I spread a map across the sunken living room of our co-op apartment in Forest Hills, Queens, and marked a bull's-eye at Grand Central Terminal, where trains come in from the 'burbs. I drew a circle of fifty miles radius around the spot, and spent the next three months searching, with my husband, Mark, for a house inside the curve. We sought top-rated schools for our two little boys, proximity to a train on direct route to Manhattan, and an ample yard. One weekend we toured the toy-town streets of Millburn, New Jersey, the next, the wide-rolling lawns of the Long Island town Dix Hills. As chance would have it, we ended our hunt at the most devastatingly beautiful of spots, a winding country road abutting a spruce forest in the tony suburban hamlet of Chappaqua, in Westchester County, New York.

It would be the biggest mistake of our lives. If only we'd known how infected we'd get living on that land and how much skepticism we would face from the local schools and doctors, if only we'd understood that we, ourselves, would be the bull's-eye, we never would have left Queens. But hindsight is 20/20. At the time, the move to Chappaqua seemed like the answer to our dreams.

Hailing from the hills of Brentwood in Los Angeles, Mark had come of age in the fifties and sixties, atop a canyon, with miles of wooded nature spread out before him and the twinkling lights of the city beckoning below. My background was less lofty, but not less intense. While Mark was running those hills, I was growing up in the housing projects of East New York, Brooklyn, where I shared a claustrophobic room with my kid brother, Alan, and hung out with friends on dicey city streets. I spent my childhood playing tag in the stairwells and scraping my knees on concrete, all the while dreaming of the lush lawns and deep driveways I'd seen only on television, in *Leave It to Beaver* and *Donna Reed*.

Fast forward to the eighties. After college and then graduate school in journalism, I moved to Manhattan and, after a few years building my portfolio, was hired as staff writer on the new science magazine, *Discover*. Mark was finishing an M.F.A. in fiction writing at Columbia when we met in a workshop at the 92nd Street Y. By 1990, we were married and living in Forest Hills with our two little boys. We made our way as writers, specializing mostly in health and science stories for the national magazines in New York.

Thinking back, those long-ago happy days feel like a dream. Blessed with the flexibility of writers, we had abundant time to spend together with our boys. We read books, spent hours at the park, vacationed at the shore, saw movies and friends. It was a rich, creative, fascinating life—it should have been enough. But I longed for that lawn and driveway, and Mark wanted a return to the wide-open nature of his youth, with room for our boys to run.

Chappaqua fit the bill. Countrified in appearance, it was nonetheless urban in sensibility owing to an influx of professionals from Manhattan. It was an easy commute to the city, with a school system so stellar that 15 percent of graduates went on to Ivy League schools. In Chappaqua you could find a taxi company run exclusively for children and a health food store whose work-for-hire clerk knew as much about supplements as a nutritionist with a Ph.D. The hamlet's compact main drag was a potpourri of gourmet food, real estate agencies, and antiques, all of it anchored by a Starbucks—a nod to the fact that, underneath all the *haute*, it was really a brand-name town.

Chappaqua had a way of attracting attention and getting into the news. Whether it was the high school football team partying with a stripper (at an event hosted by one of the fathers) or a Little League coach breaking an umpire's arm, if it happened in Chappaqua it was reported nationwide. When the Clintons vacated the White House, they followed our lead and moved to Chappaqua, a mere two blocks away from us. The day they arrived, reporters chased me down my driveway for quotes.

Chappaqua was one of those *ubersuburbs* where homes segue into forests, rock faces, and fish-filled ponds: The modest raised ranch we bought was no exception. Our front yard, a tangle of lofty pines, led down to a towering spruce woods out back. A fairy-tale forest that stretched beyond our view, those woods provided haven for an abundance of wildlife, including squirrels, skunks, raccoons, white-footed mice, and deer. Residing in one of about two dozen houses that ringed this wonderland, we felt privileged to own a piece of it.

For years, from the time we moved there in late summer of 1993, our children, Jason and David, spent carefree days in the woods. Along with their friends, they constructed a fort, an arboreal Rube Goldberg made of moist, leafy branches and decaying logs. The contraption was well stocked with plastic action figures and draped, haphazardly, by a tarpaulin cloth. At the edge of the forest, just where the woods gave way to our backyard lawn, we hung a swing from the branch of a tree.

Watching my children play in the shadow of the woods, I passed the time plunging my fingers into the dark brown soil of the rolling backyard lawn, easing out crabgrass by the roots. Mark tended the autumn leaves, gathering them with a rake, piling them onto a drop cloth, and dragging them out to a pile of mulch deep in the backyard woods. My home office overlooked the forest, and often, as I wrote, I glimpsed deer, usually in groups, traipsing past my window and traversing from one part of our property to the next. For a city girl from Brooklyn, it was an otherworldy scene.

Sure, we sometimes thought of Lyme disease. Everyone knew you could get it in Westchester County, especially the forested sections home to deer. But for us, it wasn't of great concern. As health and medical journalists, we had investigated the risk before purchasing our house. What we read in the popular press and, especially, in the major scientific journals, put our minds at ease.

One study, published in the *Journal of the American Medical Association* in April 1993, called Lyme mild and curable, except in the rarest of cases. Those who didn't respond to treatment for Lyme disease usually didn't have it, said Dr. Allen Steere, who'd studied the very first patients in Lyme, Connecticut, while working at Yale.

How, then, to explain a tinge of worry expressed by some of our friends when they came to our home? That, too, was clarified by experts, this time in a June 1993 issue of *Science,* a journal I read every week. The article, titled "The biological and social phenomenon of Lyme disease," invoked the specter of a strange new phobia gripping the suburbs, reminding me of the irrational fear of witches in generations past. Otherwise normal, intelligent people were paralyzed by fear of infection, an edginess only heightened because the young nymphal ticks spreading Lyme were so tiny they couldn't easily be seen. The real disease was fear, the *Science* authors said. What a pity, they lamented, that irrational fear of a disease, especially one so mild and treatable, had sparked "a negativity toward deer" and "a new sense of conflict between humans and nature" in "some of the most desirable residential areas of the Northeast."

Reading the *Science* article, I got the impression I was surrounded by a secret cult of Bambi-haters—folks I had yet to meet—who could ruin the value of my hard-earned Chappaqua house with their paranoid, hysterical talk. The *Science* authors placed the blame squarely on the backs of patient support groups and their leaders—misinformed advocates with missionary zeal, who spread nightmare stories of a progressive, *incurable* infection driving overwhelming fatigue, disabling pain, and devastating psychiatric disease. These claimants suffered not from chronic Lyme disease, the scientists wrote, but rather, from "premorbid personality" and the "tendency to somatization," which meant they experienced even the mildest or most ordinary of symptoms with the heightened perception of pain.

What more did I need to know? A new resident in the forested suburb of Chappaqua, I could add Lyme disease to my list of nonworries—it was hard to catch but easy to recognize and treat, so that if you actually became infected, you could be swiftly and completely cured. And all the noise about Lyme disease? It came from a small group of malcontents, I decided, a club of the disordered or exceptionally neurotic, those attracted to the idea of sickness or looking for some excuse.

Though I didn't know it at the time, scientists had long since chronicled the devastating neuropsychiatric fallout sometimes seen when Lyme disease went untreated for months and years. I would have had to dig deeper for those reports—but why would I? Not one to dwell on disease unless forced to, I put worry aside.

It's easy to see why we had such a cavalier, even reckless, attitude toward the environment, and why, at first, we chalked our older son Jason's flu, cough, and joint aches up to ordinary childhood ills. Our pediatricians at the Mount Kisco Medical Group, northern Westchester's largest medical practice, said all of it was routine. We were concerned, in 1995, with the onset of shooting pains through Jason's arms and legs, but the doctors said these "growing pains" were normal. By 1996, in the sixth grade, Jason's knees had become so swollen and achy he could not climb steps, and the middle school, responding to a note from our pediatrician, gave him a coveted key for the elevator earmarked for handicapped students. With his knees in so much pain, Jason had to give up the vaunted position he'd earned on the Chappaqua traveling basketball team because he could barely run. Perhaps such swollen knees should have been a tip-off to Lyme disease—but the doctor who wrote the note seemed blithely unaware. As time passed, pain manifested as well in Jason's elbow. We went to a doctor billed as the top elbow expert in Manhattan, who performed an MRI and could find nothing wrong. Along with these joint problems our boy experienced increasing fatigue, so that sometimes he could barely get up in the morning and out of the house unless we physically dragged him and even dressed him. The head of pediatric rheumatology at the Hospital for Special Surgery reviewed the case and told us it was probably parvovirus, an illness that is usually benign. Tylenol was the therapy he thought to recommend.

By 1997, Jason had suffered a heart irregularity his pediatrician and a consulting cardiologist could not explain and advised us to ignore. He underwent a seizurelike incident that caused his eyes to roll back in his head as he stumbled around his classroom and ultimately passed out. A pediatric neurologist at New York University, herself a resident of Westchester who knew just where we lived, told us this incident was probably a "migraine aura," experienced by boys who had migraines without the pain. Unless it happened again, we needn't be concerned, she said. By early 1998, Jason's knee and elbow pains had intensified, and traveled from joint to joint. Though traveling joint pain is a classic sign of Lyme disease, neither our pediatricians nor the Manhattan specialists we consulted viewed Lyme as a probable cause.

The reason they dismissed the Lyme diagnosis had to do with the tests. In the course of these events Jason was, naturally, tested for Lyme disease a number of times. But each time his test came back "negative." A negative test, our doctors told us, meant Lyme disease had been excluded as a diagnosis—even though our house bordered a forest that was home to ticks, field mice, and deer. It was only later I realized that the tests contained mounting evidence for Lyme in the form of specific Western blot bands that had increased in number and intensity over time. The CDC required five of ten bands, each representing an antibody against the spirochete, for an absolute positive—but the experts I later interviewed told me that changing band patterns offered evidence of active, morphing infection as well. Jason had 3 bands in 1995, 4 in 1997, and then, finally, in the year 2000, on a test done at LabCorp, the unequivocal 8. If only our doctors had tracked our boy's *pattern* of antibody bands, they might have seen the evidence. If only they'd viewed the test results in the context of our backyard woods and Jason's swollen joints and other signs and symptoms, they might have seen the light.

But missing out on the chance to treat Lyme disease in these early years paled beside what happened next. I will never forget that October day in 1998 when Lyme disease announced itself loudly, indisputably, across Jason's torso with what any physician should have recognized as its hallmark—a large red rash with spaces of white clearing, called an erythema migrans and published widely in medical texts. Unnerved at the look of the huge, mottled rash—something I now realize must have come from a recent tick bite—I called the Mount Kisco Medical Group, described it in detail, and suggested I bring Jason in.

"Don't bother coming," I was told by a senior member of the nursing staff, on phone duty in the pediatric department that day. Since I couldn't see a literal bull's-eye, she assured me, it couldn't be Lyme disease.

That's when Jason came down with what I call his "great flu": a fever, cold, hacking cough, and deep exhaustion that caused him to miss two full weeks of school. Slowly the "flu" went away, but Jason never got well. He now had pain that traveled around his body from joint to joint, constant headache and stomachache, a hacking cough, and inexplicable insomnia and fatigue. His neck hurt so much that sometimes he could not lift his head from his pillow for days. He dropped from all his sports activities—they were simply too exhausting for him. He stopped doing his homework. He refused to see friends, even his two best friends. On more and more days he could not get up for school.

Despite the swollen joints and the rash, our pediatrician at the Mount Kisco Medical Group resisted running any more blood tests for Lyme disease. Jason just had too many symptoms now, he explained to me, while Lyme was limited to just a few. To emphasize his expertise he told me he had trained in seminars at Yale.

As Jason continued his alarming decline over the next year and a half and as we fruitlessly sought an explanation, the diagnosis our pediatrician came to favor was depression. One day, some time after Jason had stopped going to school regularly, the pediatrician took him into a private room and encouraged him to talk about his life at home. After ten minutes of chat, the doctor emerged from the room and said, "It seems he argues with his father. This could be the reason he feels so ill. You had better do something about it," he warned me, "because if he doesn't start going to school he's going to be held back."

No, he would *not* do a blood test for Lyme disease, he said again. Instead, he urged us to find psychiatric help and sent us on our way.

We were fortunate because the psychiatrist we found, a renowned expert in his own right though with little knowledge of Lyme disease, did not buy into the "psychiatric" diagnosis. In fact, our psychiatrist had never seen a psychiatric illness like this in thirty years—and why was a pediatrician diagnosing psychiatric disease without any training, and without having completed a full battery of medical tests?

Outraged, the psychiatrist phoned the pediatrician to demand that he be more thorough. And so the pediatrician, finally, reluctantly, drew fourteen vials of blood. "We are testing for every disorder possible, just to make you feel better," he assured us at the time. Just to placate us, he even tested for Lyme disease. (Despite the fourteen vials, he would not, I later learned, test for the tick-borne coinfections anaplasmosis and babesiosis, one prevalent in Westchester County and the other found commonly on Cape Cod and Eastern Long Island, where we'd spent summers and vacationed many times over the years.)

Even so, at last we hit bingo. In February 2000, Jason finally tipped the scales for Lyme disease on a Western blot, a test for detecting targeted antibodies in blood. To validate a case as late Lyme disease, the CDC required the blot detect five of ten specific antibodies formed to fight the spirochete. And, in what I will always consider a gift from the gods, Jason had eight. The laboratory, LabCorp, duly reported his case to the CDC, but even then, the pediatrician would not concede that Jason definitely had Lyme disease.

Instead, he sent him on to the head of infectious disease at Northern Westchester Hospital, Peter Welch, known for his view that Lyme disease was vastly overdiagnosed. Welch nonetheless told us that Jason had slipped through the cracks and was a bona fide case of late-stage, disseminated Lyme disease, meriting a month of intravenous Rocephin, the big-gun antibiotic for Lyme in the brain. Welch's Lyme disease diagnosis was something for which we would always be grateful. With so many Lyme patients relegated to the gray zone, we found the Welch imprimatur a valuable commodity when dealing with our insurance company and other M.D.s. Getting the diagnosis from such a skeptic was convincing to us, as well.

When Jason was sicker than ever at the end of the treatment, Welch said that it might take a while for the treatment to work. But if Jason didn't get better, if the treatment didn't work, he warned us, then whatever was ailing him wasn't actually Lyme disease, after all. As weeks passed, as Jason's illness only worsened, Welch's ominous words came home to roost. In due course, the diagnosis of "Lyme" was revoked and Welch sent us packing. Back at the Mount Kisco Medical Group, the pediatrician (along with a neurologist he'd brought onboard) returned to psychiatric theories for Jason's ills.

Too sick to go to school and too confused to do his schoolwork, Jason was immobilized by his brain fog and pain. But what psychic switch had been flipped to prevent our former basketball star and straight-A student from standing or even sitting up in bed; from focusing enough to read a paragraph, let alone a page? What caused him to writhe in pain whenever anyone jostled him, to demand near-darkness before opening his eyes, or to appear so twisted and bent? This "psychiatric disorder" had no name, and could not be found in DSM-IV, psychiatry's diagnostic bible. Nor could it be validated by our psychiatrist, a university scientist who remained skeptical of these doctors to the end.

We managed to obtain a prescription for an additional four weeks of Rocephin from another, more open-minded physician—Daniel Cameron, a good-humored, kind-hearted Mount Kisco epidemiologist-turned-family-practitioner who saw merit in longer treatment. But in April 2000, after the extra treatment had run its course, Jason was so disabled he could no longer walk. I pondered what to do next. Now wracked by so much pain he could barely sit up, he spent most of each day lying in the bathtub, generally half-asleep, running hot water from the faucet so that it filled the room with a thick gray fog. The soothing water and steam offered the only relief from agony he could find. I kept constant watch over him for fear he could lose consciousness, slip underwater, and drown. The bathroom reflected the state of our lives: The mirror, the countertops, the floor were coated with mist. The hot steam made the drywall crack so plumbing was visible, and caused tiles to blister off the floor. The streaming bathwater created a backdrop of sound, like a white noise machine with the dial set somewhere between "waterfall" and "rain."

As the water ran and Jason lolled back in the bath, I phoned the Mount Kisco neurologist in one last-ditch plea for help. Had he ever seen this kind of thing? What could it be? "I can't tell you what it is," he said tersely, "but one thing I can tell you is that if he's still sick after two months of Rocephin, it's not Lyme disease."

"Should I put him in the hospital?" I asked. "That's entirely up to you," he said, before quickly excusing himself, and hanging up the phone.

2

A Place in the Whirlwind

Various places in Massachusetts, especially Framingham,
during the 1980s and 1990s

Sheila Statlender was completing her doctorate in clinical psychology when she met an athletic young medical resident at the wedding of a friend. It was 1980. Sheila was the maid of honor and Russ, the best man. They shared a lot: Academic stars from working-class backgrounds getting through on scholarships, they were both, by nature, practical yet caring, a combination that led to the selection of careers in health. Russ had already been to Israel twice and Sheila, by then the wayward Jew, found his interest compelling; a path to adventure and a sign that he might be someone who could share the kind of responsible yet open life she'd dreamed of since she was young.

Married in 1983 at age thirty, the Statlenders moved to the suburbs of Boston, where Russ was pursuing a residency in orthopedic surgery while Sheila worked at the outpatient psychiatry department of a suburban hospital and built a practice of her own. Their firstborn, Seth, a sparkly, gregarious baby, was born in 1985. Then, in 1987, came Amy. Healthy and adorable, Amy's predilection for dresses and dolls during her early years amused her feminist mom.

Sheila was soon juggling a job counseling law students at Harvard with a private practice and motherhood. "I specialized in dual-career families like mine, lots of women's issues," she recalls. Russ signed on as orthopedic surgeon with a nearby health maintenance organization.

By 1990, they'd purchased a spacious contemporary Cape Cod house with a luminous great room whose rear glass wall faced a personal savannah and woods. That gorgeous manicured lawn, all three acres of it, was bordered by fourteen acres of undeveloped woodland, a virtual deer preserve that served up nature's panorama with each morning meal. "We were thrilled in those early days to see not only deer but also wild turkeys, a few pheasant, a beautiful red fox, and an irksome woodchuck, along with the more mundane squirrels and scores of chipmunks," Sheila recalls. Their street was just blocks away from caves where the Salem witches once hid, lending a touch of the subterranean and unknown.

"We split our work commute and did the nanny thing," says Sheila. "I loved having young children. It was like redoing my own childhood and making it fun." As if all this bounty weren't enough, they had another child, a blond-haired, blue-eyed boy, in 1992. Like his siblings before him, he walked early and eagerly took in the world. They named him Eric.

To outsiders it looked like Sheila Statlender had it all—until the day her best-laid hopes and dreams went up in flames. It was a morning in August 1996 when, listening to the radio, she learned that while she'd slept a fire had ravaged a summer camp at the New Hampshire border, along the coast. Seth, then age eleven, was a camper there. Rushing to her car and making the trip up, Sheila arrived to find Seth standing on a hillside overlooking his bunk. He'd awakened to enormous flames leaping from a nearby building, and had alerted others. Evacuating their bunks, he and his fellow campers heard the arts and crafts building explode around four A.M.; they stood outside through the night while fire devoured the recreation hall and bunks. Miraculously, no one died.

Back home the next day, Seth was clearly ill. Already having spent much of the month in the camp infirmary, he had a sore throat, swollen glands, and a fever. He was sick for the next few weeks and Sheila couldn't help but wonder whether the explosion had released something toxic. Yet it didn't seem likely because, while other campers had suffered sore throats and colds, he was the only one they knew of who had stayed ill. As the start of the school year approached he seemed to recover, but his health was never the same. Unlike before, he now suffered intermittent nausea and fevers as well as recurrent swollen glands, sore throats, sinus problems, and aches and pains. His most oppressive symptom was an ever-worsening headache. The year before, he'd been a soccer star on the traveling team, but now he had trouble playing. He was often out of school sick.

"We knew something wasn't right with him," says Statlender, "but we didn't know what. This was not our kid."

As a physician family, the Statlenders attacked the problem systematically, visiting the best and brightest the medical community of Boston and its environs had to offer. Only one doctor, a neurologist, had an explanation: Their son was having rebound headaches from the over-the-counter analgesics he had been using, and now he would need to go cold turkey. But even after the analgesics were pulled, the problems remained.

Then, that Christmas, he was hit in the back of his head with a snowboard. At first he appeared fine. But in the weeks that followed, his headaches worsened, progressing to full-blown migraines. He started seeing spots, couldn't tolerate light, and the overwhelming pain kept him up at night. One doctor attributed his headaches to the onset of puberty. Another doctor, harkening back to the snowboard incident, thought he could be suffering postconcussive syndrome.

It would have made sense if he'd been fine before the snowboard accident, says Statlender. "But he wasn't." By now it was 1997 and Seth, twelve, was so sick he couldn't regularly attend school. He bravely tried to play soccer but felt so sick during one game that he threw up in front of the team. Eventually he left the town's top traveling team for a less competitive group, struggling to keep his spot there, too. It was hard to be an all-star when your body just wouldn't cooperate and you were in so much pain.

The Statlenders trudged from their pediatrician at the Fallon Clinic to the University of Massachusetts Medical Center to Tufts–New England Medical Center to Children's Hospital to Massachusetts General, from a series of neurologists to infectious disease specialists, seeking a diagnosis and cure. Diagnostic studies included all manner of blood tests (including Lyme disease tests) and brain scans, even a sleep study. Treatments included every category of migraine medication as well as biofeedback, Benadryl, prednisone (a steroid), and, when his headache lasted for seventy-two hours straight, intravenous Compazine. The Compazine relieved the headache, but as a side effect, caused akathisia—an inability to sit still; it hit him in the middle of a Friendly's restaurant, where they'd stopped on the way home from the treatment itself. To treat the akathisia, the doctor prescribed Ativan—but the dose was so high that Seth staggered as he walked and almost passed out.

It was a nightmare of futile treatments and guesswork, largely to no avail. A year and a half had passed since the campground fire, and Seth, who had ever more trouble focusing, was now often too tired to get out of bed. By this point, placed on homebound instruction, he still tried valiantly to get to school, if only for an hour or two each day. Always a gregarious, popular, and active child, he was lonely and hated the isolation imposed by his illness.

Even so, since no one could find anything wrong, and none of the therapies worked, one physician, a Tufts University neurologist, suggested a battery of psychological tests. Sheila was flabbergasted.

"Why would you do that?" she asked.

"You're a psychologist—you figure it out," the neurologist replied.

While Sheila and Russ had no doubt that their son was seriously ill, the neurologist wanted to rule out the possibility that the problem could be psychiatric. The Statlenders briefly considered the personality testing. "But when we learned that they were to be administered by a student intern," Sheila reports, "we came to our senses. Seth was clearly medically ill. He was a bright, well-liked child who never met a sport he didn't enjoy. He had nothing to gain and so much to lose by being ill like this. It was clear to us that they were clutching at straws, and that, in his condition, it would be cruel to put him through a battery of tests that were unnecessary."

The next specialist was another neurologist from another pediatric teaching hospital across town. Considered an expert in pediatric migraine, he offered the opinion that many such headaches are driven by occult viruses, and suggested a pulsed course of steroids.

Russell, from his perspective as an orthopedist, had seen permanent hip damage result from steroid treatment. But the prescription was "time-limited and pulsed in decreasing doses," the neurologist assured him. "I don't think you need to worry."

They followed his recommendation with a mixture of trepidation and hope. But when Seth only seemed to get sicker, they had trouble reaching the neurologist by phone. Ultimately, in the follow-up appointment, he chastised them for calling his office too often and quickly resorted to the psychiatric explanation as well. "This isn't a migraine, this is depression. He needs Prozac," he barked.

"One of the worst parts," Sheila notes, "was the complete cluelessness on the part of so many professionals and acquaintances, which often shaded into skepticism. Maybe he wasn't motivated enough to get well, or just wasn't trying hard enough—or maybe we were being too soft on him."

One neurologist asked why they took his temperature so often; another wanted to know what kind of thermometers they used. One time Seth, under the care of a cognitive-behavioral therapist, was encouraged to sit through school despite his complaints. By the time Sheila finally arrived for him in her waiting room, his fever had soared to 103 degrees Fahrenheit. Sheila was furious. "I'm pulling the plug on this therapy," she said. To her credit, the cognitive-behavioral psychologist wholeheartedly endorsed the decision; this child, she concurred, was truly ill.

Another time, a doctor suggested that the vomiting was really bulimia. "I'm a trained psychologist," *Dr.* Sheila Statlender responded. "Throwing up in front of his entire soccer team and a crowd of spectators doesn't fit the profile. Bulimics purge in private."

Finally, in a last-ditch effort to find an explanation, they took Seth to an immunologist at the University of Massachusetts Medical Center. After reviewing the chart the doctor said Seth had been so thoroughly worked up he didn't think he would find anything new. Moreover, he added, in light of the record, the treatment had been appropriate. The immunologist did not even bother with a physical exam of his own. Instead, he sat the Statlenders down.

"There is this illness called chronic fatigue syndrome," he told them.

"But he seems so sick," Sheila Statlender replied.

"Indeed he is sick," the immunologist agreed. "Chronic fatigue syndrome is a real medical condition, but we don't know what causes it." Without a known cause, there was naturally no cure, but he could take drugs for insomnia and pain.

"Essentially he told us, don't call us, we'll call you," Sheila says. His office was hooked up by computer to the NIH, alerting him to new treatments, should they emerge. When medical science found a cure for the mystery illness afflicting their son, the doctor assured the Statlenders, he would give them a buzz on the phone to let them know.

And that's when their daughter, the middle child, Amy, then in the fifth grade, started getting sick. Early on, it was just a cough on the soccer field, something the Statlenders' pediatrician thought might be a seasonal allergy that would soon go away. But the cough continued, taking on a chronic, crouplike quality that was not relieved by nebulizers or other treatments aimed at allergies.

Finally she was seen by a pulmonary specialist at the University of Massachusetts, who, finding nothing amiss, suggested cognitive-behavioral therapy for the cough. But Dr. Statlender, the psychologist, pointed out that Amy coughed throughout the night, in her sleep. "If you cough in your sleep," she explained, "it's unlikely to be due to a cough habit," which is what cognitive-behavioral therapy would treat.

Besides, other symptoms had emerged. The croupy cough now was joined by stomach problems so severe that Amy doubled over and began missing school. Soon the Statlenders were trucking from doctor to doctor with their second child just as they had done with the first. Amy had not been at the campground blaze, nor had she been hit in the head with a snowboard. Nonetheless, as her symptoms intensified they became ever more like her brother's—an exhausting, multisystemic illness that never went away.

Looking back, Sheila and Russ now realized that Amy had been declining gradually over the course of a couple of years, but had somehow managed to push through. By the spring of the fifth grade, she'd come down with a flulike illness that kept her home for three weeks, but she struggled to find the energy to return to school. A top student, she was highly motivated: She loved her bilingual English-Spanish program, missed her friends, and was eager to present her fifth-grade project, which she had been preparing for most of the year.

By sixth grade, at age ten, Amy was barely hanging on. That fall, as she embarked upon her first year of middle school, she continued to be wracked with stomach pain and other digestive disturbances. A test for lactose intolerance was negative and then, finally, a pediatric gastroenterologist at the University of Massachusetts Medical Center performed an endoscopy, detecting the helical bacteria *Helicobacter pylori*, often a cause of ulcers.

Sheila started to cry. "Do we finally have an answer?" she asked the doctor hopefully. "I doubt the infection is causing all this, but she has to be treated anyway," he said.

Placed on two antibiotics and a proton pump inhibitor, however, Amy not only got sicker, she also experienced excruciating pain. No one mentioned the possibility that symptoms might temporarily worsen with antibiotic treatment of another bacterial infection—Lyme disease—which, given the dozens of deer living on the Statlender's property, could easily have been at the root.

Amy never seemed to recover from the treatment for *H. pylori*. She remained weakened and fatigued, and her digestive problems continued.

Placed on a homebound academic program for the remainder of that school year, this book-loving, intellectually curious, dedicated student struggled from home to keep up, never losing hope. A soccer player like her older brother, she insisted that her parents purchase the new soccer uniform adopted by her team for the following fall.

3

❖

Son of a Preacher Man

Illinois and Colorado, 1947–2000

Dave Martz, age seven, lived in a small Illinois town in a small house with a highway right out front. It was July 3, 1947, when a speeding gravel truck crushed his scooter, causing a skull fracture, a concussion, and burns across his face. He was unconscious for a day, but when he came to, his father, a Baptist minister, was there to explain what had occurred. If the truck had been going faster, or struck at a different angle, he might have died. "Six more inches and you'd have been history. There must be a plan for your life," his father observed. From that point forward Martz celebrated his personal "glad-to-be-alive" day ahead of the nation's birthday. "I'd been given my life back, and I knew I couldn't waste it," he says.

One day, while walking young Dave to first grade, his father stopped for a talk. "Son, you're a bright kid and you'll need to go to college," he said, "but I don't have the money to send you." Indeed, there was only one way Dave would ever get there—by remembering the *V* word—valedictorian. If he got even *one* B, someone else would claim all the A's along with the title, the scholarship, and the college dream. It was a few years before Dave could even pronounce "valedictorian," but he never forgot the concept, or his responsibility to excel.

And so it was that Dave Martz passed through childhood and adolescence. A good-looking, affable kid who made friends in every town (a new one every three or four years, as the minister transferred from church to church), Martz played the trumpet, shot hoops, and collected those A's. His efforts paid off—graduating high school in the tiny, arid town of Las Animas (the Spirits), Colorado, he was named valedictorian and received a full scholarship to the state flagship university in 1958.

At the University of Colorado at Boulder, Martz decided his summer jobs would be test balloons for his future—whether medicine or the ministry, he'd try it on first. His first year, the summer of 1959, he worked as an orderly at the tiny Las Animas hospital, where he was told he could observe the surgeries in exchange for providing bedside care in the men's ward. It wasn't much of a trade: While there were just three minor operations all summer, he was given the arduous daily task of caring for a man with advanced amyotrophic lateral sclerosis (ALS). The neurodegenerative disease, also called Lou Gehrig's disease after the baseball player who brought it into the spotlight in 1939, attacks both upper and lower motor neurons, ultimately causing paralysis and ravaging the spinal cord and brain. Completely paralyzed except for his eyes, the Las Animas patient needed total-body care. So it fell to his orderly, David Martz, to suction the mucus from his tracheotomy every fifteen to thirty minutes, eight hours a day, five days a week, for three months. Even though the cause of ALS was unknown (and remains so today), even though contagion through bodily fluids was theorized as possible, protective barriers weren't standard for those who did this work in 1959. "The secretions got everywhere," Martz recalls.

The next summer he served as associate minister for youth at a church in Denver, and though he enjoyed the work, by the end of the season he knew that medicine would be his personal path. Still the boy with all the A's, Martz did so well in college that he was able to enter medical school at the University of Colorado at the end of his junior year.

There he spent his weekends and vacations doing medical research, ultimately landing two plum assignments: an internship at Washington University in St. Louis and a residency at Stanford. But in the end he rejected high-profile academic job offers to return to Colorado, where he took a position, in 1970, with a group specializing in internal medicine and hematology-oncology at the base of Pikes Peak.

The summer as orderly by now a distant memory, Martz devoted himself to his work. "An eighteen-hour-a-day man, a guy with no limits," he absorbed the *V* word as part of his essence, and eventually became one of the top oncologists in the state of Colorado, as well as a leader of other doctors: president of the Colorado Medical Society and the force behind a movement to deal with HMOs.

As the years passed, Martz got married, had two children, got divorced. By the early 1980s, he'd met a grief counselor, a woman who handled her own beloved husband's terminal leukemia with such depth of feeling and compassion he couldn't help but be impressed. By 1988, he'd married that grief therapist—a woman friends called Dee—knowing her qualities would complement him well.

Yet slowly, and by degrees, things in Martz's world changed. More and more, he found, he couldn't offer treatment to some cancer patients, even when the chance of success was good, because insurers wouldn't pay for it. By the year 2000, as our son Jason was being diagnosed, at last, with a classic case of Lyme disease, the oncologist from Colorado was deciding he couldn't stand the position insurers were putting him in. Unable to live with it, he up and retired from oncology, taking a job as the director of a hospice.

Instead of trying to save patients, now he softened their passage by treating their physical pain and reframing their sense of hope. "All things work together for the good to them that love God" was his favorite Bible quote. "I told them it was more important to achieve peace, to embrace forgiveness and friendship and love, than enter another useless clinical trial," says Martz.

He never thought, not once, that some internal ticking time bomb would threaten to cut his own life short. He never saw the fragile thread connecting him to a long-dead man he'd tended during a summer of his youth in a dusty Las Animas back ward. The shepherd of others' graceful passings, Dave Martz couldn't have fathomed that when his time came, he would dig in his heels and, rejecting his doctors' diagnoses, not just pray but fight for his life on Earth. *Had* he known all this, he *still* couldn't have imagined that he would come to suspect a link to a new disease out East, a controversial entity his colleagues were fighting over, something called Lyme.

4

❖

Connecticut Genesis

In the spring of 1956, a young artist from Manhattan was commissioned to paint the portrait of a little girl in rural Essex, Connecticut; but over the course of weeks, as the artist completed her painting, she felt a sickness and malaise take hold. A portrait painter with pageboy-style hair the color of corn, the artist, Polly Murray, was pregnant. Could her rashes, headaches, and swollen joints be due to *that*? When the symptoms abated, she thought no more of them, not at first.

Instead, enthralled at the beauty of the community in southeast Connecticut, she moved there. Ensconced in a large white colonial nestled in the woods of a town called Lyme, close to the Long Island Sound, Murray and her young family—three sons, a daughter, and her artist-husband, Gil—reveled in nature's splendor: Polly spent hours tending her garden while Gil led family hikes to "Deer Patch," a grove of soft moss and cedar trees that served as haven for sleeping deer. The Murray children spent countless hours playing in secret forts deep inside the woods. Inspired, Murray painted happy, impressionist flowers and dreamy pastel scenes of the shore.

The idyll was not to last because, by 1965, Murray's health problems had returned with a vengeance. Now she also suffered memory loss, nausea, shooting pains throughout her body, and unremitting fatigue. Realizing she was sick but not knowing why, she consulted the great medical centers of Boston and New Haven.

No one could figure out what was wrong, and eventually Murray was dismissed as psychologically, not physically, impaired. "You know, Mrs. Murray, some people subconsciously want to be sick," a physician from Boston advised. She became still more suspect when the rest of her family came down with the same bizarre set of ills. By the late sixties, her sons and daughter also had rashes, headaches, and gastrointestinal problems. Two of the boys had knees so swollen they required crutches to get around. One doctor, guessing that Murray's children were imitating her, took umbrage when she suggested all of her family members suffered from a single disease. "Why, they might even call it Murray's disease," he said.

While the doctor was being sarcastic, his words were prescient: Not just an artist but also once employed by the World Health Organization, Murray was familiar with epidemiology and knew when medical clues might warrant a careful look. Like the pioneering environmentalist Lois Gibbs, who documented chemical toxins in Love Canal, the unassuming artist would indeed discover a new illness cluster. Lyme disease would be named after the town in which she lived.

At first, Murray pressed on alone, haunting the medical library at Yale and collecting a list of neighbors whose stories were much like her own. She was especially disturbed at the diagnosis of juvenile rheumatoid arthritis, or JRA, in her son, Todd. The disorder was exceedingly rare, yet Murray knew of eight neighboring children with the same set of symptoms. As with Todd, their "arthritis" was often accompanied by severe headaches. Without the presence of an infectious agent, she wondered, what were the odds of such a disease cluster? On October 15, 1975, her notes and documentation in order, Polly Murray finally picked up the phone and called the Connecticut Department of Health. It wasn't until she began dialing that the loneliness of the journey ahead truly hit her. Would her call for help lead nowhere? Would she be misunderstood?

Though Murray didn't know it, she wasn't alone. There was another mother from Lyme, Judith Mensch, whose eight-year-old daughter, Anne, came home from school with a swollen knee. Mensch thought the swelling was due to a fall, but when it did not abate she took Anne to an orthopedic surgeon. The doctor placed Anne in the hospital, drained the knee, and sent the sample off to test for infection. Waiting for results, he placed Anne on antibiotics, just to be safe. But when tests came back negative for infection of any kind, Anne was taken off antibiotics, instructed to take aspirin, and sent home in a wheelchair with the diagnosis of JRA.

Mensch, like Murray, had her doubts. JRA was rare, yet she knew of four other neighborhood children diagnosed with it, too. "I was amazed at personally knowing five people, four living on the same street," who had the disease, she recalled. She, too, finally placed a call to the Connecticut Department of Health.

Then there were the researchers William E. Mast and William M. Burrows, an internist and dermatologist, respectively, from the Naval Submarine Medical Center in Groton, not far from Lyme. In a study of four patients thought to be bitten by ticks, the doctors recorded a mix of symptoms: first, a rash, then severe malaise including fever and headache. To get to the bottom of the mystery, the navy doctors reviewed the medical literature and discovered that physicians in the United States and Europe had described the same type of illness dating all the way back to 1883. Reports mentioned that antibiotics generally resolved the illness, which the European literature referred to as "erythema chronicum migrans." So the naval doctors followed suit, reporting success for the treatment in the *Journal of the American Medical Association* in August 1976.

While Polly Murray and Judith Mensch were busy collecting evidence and the navy doctors in Groton were treating their odd new patients, a doctor in Hamden, to the west, had observed the strange disease, too. Charles Ray Jones, age forty, was a tall, friendly pediatrician with thick glasses and a stream of zany jokes that made his young charges laugh. But he didn't find it humorous when, in 1970, he noticed a disease resembling JRA in Hamden. Unlike the prototypical JRA he'd studied in med school—the one that was rare and progressive and had autoimmune markers like those seen in lupus—the Hamden disease was common, and in any given child could ebb and flow. Unlike classic JRA, it was accompanied, much of the time, by headache and fatigue and lacked the immune markers typical of JRA.

Even without a name or suspected cause for the disease, Jones stumbled upon a treatment. By coincidence, a few of the children with the strange new condition simultaneously contracted strep. He treated the strep with antibiotics. When he did, the odd new arthritis went away as well.

Though the disease remained unexplained, Jones's clinical strategy could not be clearer: He tracked his young patients, recognizing signs and symptoms of the strange new syndrome early in the game, and then treated with a week or two of antibiotics, strep or not. "It seemed to me that on ten to fourteen days of medication, they all got well," Jones recalls. Clearly, he reckoned, he was dealing with a bacterial infection. And based on the timing of most of the cases, which seemed to cluster in the fall, he theorized that infection was transmitted by some sort of insect.

Jones had started out hoping to become a member of the clergy, not a physician. As a first-year student at Boston University's divinity school in 1954, he had been drawn to activism. Along with Martin Luther King Jr., his classmate and friend, he attended weekly meetings with Jewish students from Hillel and worked for civil rights. But a twist of fate would cause Jones to seek his ministry in medicine, not the cloth. "The divinity school was oriented toward social action," Jones explains. "One afternoon a week we went around to see people who had requested a ministerial visit. One day it fell to me to visit a woman of eighty, someone mentally vital but withered by rheumatoid arthritis. She came up to me, grabbed my hand, and said, 'Help me in a *real* way.' But as a divinity student, I couldn't provide the help she truly needed—medical help. That's when I decided to have a different kind of ministry, a medical ministry. I felt that was the way I could contribute best."

Drafted into the army, Jones managed both his passions with aplomb. He secretly left base to march for civil rights with his friend Martin, even at the risk of a court-martial. And he spent his evenings at Georgia State and Emory taking courses in premed. By the time Jones was discharged from the service a couple of years hence, he'd married his college sweetheart, Margery, and had a letter of admittance to New York Medical College in New York City. It was 1958, and he was twenty-nine.

After Jones finished medical school in 1962, he secured a coveted internship at St. Luke's–Roosevelt Hospital. With an interest in pediatrics as well as research, it naturally made sense that he would go on to specialize in the hot field of the day—oncology—at the top institution for such work, Memorial Sloan–Kettering Cancer Center, in New York.

Doing research at that biomedical juggernaut, it didn't take long for Jones to become expert on an obscure but confounding disease most Lyme patients have never heard of: Langerhans cell granulomatosis, characterized by lesions in bone and soft tissue. While physicians of the day were treating the condition with whole-body radiation, it was Jones—today, ironically, accused of *overtreating* disease—who rang the alarm bell that aggressive therapy was far worse than the condition itself.

But the time demands of academia took too much of a toll on Jones's family. He rarely arrived home before 10 P.M. So in 1968, pushing age forty, he decided to buy a pediatric practice from a retiring physician in the bucolic Connecticut town of Hamden, where he hoped for a saner, more manageable life. Little did Jones realize he had purchased not a country paradise, but a residence in the whirlwind, at the epicenter of what would become one of the most bitter medical fights in modern times.

The first salvo was launched quietly in October 1975, when Polly Murray placed her critical call to the Connecticut Department of Health. Both she and Mensch were eventually referred to Allen Steere, a former CDC investigator and by then a medical fellow in rheumatology at Yale.

5

⁘

A New Disease and
a Ring of Fire

A gentle, music-loving, bowtie–wearing rheumatologist, Allen Caruthers Steere was the first doctor to give Lyme disease patients credence, the first to believe them and tell the world they were real. Yet Steere would later become Lyme's antichrist, so hated by the very patients he hoped to help and enlighten that he received death threats and worked under the eye of security, at times fearing for his life.

Steere wanted to be a violinist. A student at Columbia University in New York City, the young man from Indiana was so gifted that he played with Itzhak Perlman and trained with Ivan Galamian, head of the violin department at Juilliard. But it was not to be. After a basketball accident injured his tendon, Steere was forced to forge another path, and chose medicine. He felt the choice would work: In both music and medicine, intuition, creativity, and empathy were needed, and in these things, Steere felt, he excelled.

And so it was that Steere attended medical school at Columbia. Right from the start, he had an interest in infection, spending part of his final year in Liberia, where infectious disease was rife. Like Charles Ray Jones, he completed his residency at the St. Luke's–Roosevelt Medical Center in Manhattan. He rounded out his training with a stint at the Centers for Disease Control, where he joined a team of infection sleuths known as the Epidemic Intelligence Service, or EIS.

Essentially the CIA of the CDC, the EIS was established in 1951 following the start of the Korean War as an early warning system against biological warfare and man-made epidemics. Composed of medical doctors, researchers, and scientists who served in two-year stints, the Service ultimately became a surveillance and response unit for all types of epidemics and disease. But Steere had come to the CDC with an unusual frame of reference, "the heretical idea" that he would go into rheumatology. For Steere, infectious disease was most compelling in the context of the immune system—the body's defense against outside invaders. When such defenses went awry, diseases might result.

By 1975, Steere was a rheumatology fellow at Yale, but his project—basic research on white blood cells—seemed boring after sleuthing for the CDC. So when he received a call from the Connecticut Department of Health alerting him to the arthritis clusters in nearby Lyme, he wanted to get involved.

Allen Steere's formal investigation kicked into high gear on November 20, a month after Polly Murray's call. That's when Murray handed him a list of thirty-seven potential patients laboring under a potpourri of diagnoses, ranging from JRA and ringworm to lupus and multiple sclerosis. Mensch contributed patients to the study group as well.

Steere's first epidemiological decision was coming up with a disease definition. Since arthritis was a common denominator for his patients and since Steere was, after all, a fellow in rheumatology, it's no surprise that, initially, the only factor required for entry into the Yale study was the odd arthritis, characterized by brief, recurrent attacks of swelling and pain in a few large joints. Studying a group of thirty-nine children fitting the description, he was finally able to rule out the diagnosis of JRA, which appears randomly in the population with a frequency of 1 to 10 per 100,000 children. This new disease, whatever it was, struck a hundred times more frequently than that. Conducting formal patient interviews, he also documented what Mensch and Murray had reported: "geographic clustering within the communities, as well as seasonal and familial clustering." Half the patients lived on only four roads, and most had fallen ill in the summer or early fall.

One of the first things Steere pondered was the mode of transmission. He could find no common exposure, like an immunization, a swimming place, or a particular food. The disease did not seem to be airborne or passed from person to person, because residents living close together, even those in the same family, often came down with the illness in different years. Given the clustering in a rural area, the seasonal onset, and the hit-or-miss pattern within families, Allen Steere suspected the disease was transmitted by some sort of arthropod, probably a tick. Aside from the swollen knees, Steere soon recognized another, earlier symptom—one that would "brand" the disease and give it a pop identity: a red rash with central clearing or, as Yale's public relations department declared, a "bull's-eye."

What caused the mysterious illness? The Yale scientists considered, briefly, the notion that whatever it was, it was the same thing that caused erythema chronicum migrans, a chronic spreading rash with a host of other symptoms long documented in Europe and thought to be caused by a spirochete and transmitted by ticks. Sure enough, the Yale scientists found several paragraphs describing the European disease in a textbook, *Fitzpatrick's Dermatology in General Medicine*.

But this didn't convince Allen Steere that the two diseases were the same. His major rationale was the presence, in the Connecticut patients, of arthritis, relatively unusual in the European patients, whose symptoms seemed more neurological. Instead, Steere concluded, the cluster in Connecticut represented the holy grail for any research physician—an entirely new disease.

In the wake of his discovery, Steere's findings emerged rapidly. The disease had an "enlarging clinical spectrum," he said in the *Annals of Internal Medicine* in 1977. Arthritis was just one of several possible outcomes following the rash, and no longer a strict requirement for the disease. Reporting on thirty-two Lyme patients with arthritis, the rash, or both, he recorded a host of broad symptoms: malaise, fatigue, chills and fever, headache, stiff neck, backache, myalgias (muscle aches), nausea, vomiting, and sore throat. He also established what he viewed as more specific signs of disease: migratory joint pains, neurological and cardiac abnormalities, and elevated markers in the blood. The symptoms were so diverse and general that they could not be used, in and of themselves, to diagnose Lyme disease, Steere said. "The diagnostic marker is the skin lesion," he instructed physicians. "Without it, geographic clustering is the most important clue."

But could patients from Connecticut be treated with antibiotics, like the patients from Europe? Here Steere and his navy colleagues parted ways: If Lyme was truly a new disease, after all, there was no reason to presume it would mimic the rash illness from Europe. So while the navy doctors treated their patients with antibiotics, the Yale team held back. In the end, Steere made no bones about the fact that in rejecting antibiotics he was bucking the overwhelming preponderance of worldwide medical literature to date. But he was adamant and held his ground: If Lyme disease and the European disease were different, then why would anyone treat them as if they were the same? He felt more than justified in dismissing the old, European studies in favor of his new clinical observations at Yale. Eight Yale patients had received antibiotics for their rashes before entering his study, Steere pointed out, yet seven of them went on to develop arthritis and sometimes neurological or cardiovascular symptoms nonetheless. Antibiotics didn't seem to work in these patients at all, insisted Steere. Until the drugs proved effective in formal controlled and blinded studies, he held, he couldn't endorse their use. Instead, he meticulously recorded the natural history of the disease, studying the progression of the erythema migrans rash *prospectively* and producing a series of finely wrought papers describing the arthritic and neurologic picture of full-blown Lyme. He rejected for the children and adults participating in some of his early studies the antibiotic treatment recommended by other researchers, addressing their symptoms from the rheumatologist's black bag: aspirin for minor aches and, for the sickest patients, steroids like prednisone to suppress the immune system and the inflammatory response responsible for so much pain.

It was only in 1980, after observing patients for four consecutive summers, that Allen Steere changed his mind about treatment—to a degree. The Yale team had treated rash patients with seven to ten days of antibiotic medication during the summer epidemics of 1977 and 1979, but not during 1976 and 1978. Now, with 139 patients to pool in a single study, comparison was possible and the results were incontrovertible: The Lyme rash resolved more than twice as rapidly in treated patients, who also got arthritis at less than half the rate of untreated ones.

Given the findings and patients' word-of-mouth, people began clamoring for antibiotics. But aside from treating the rash with penicillin, the team at Yale would not sign on. After all, Steere pointed out, many treated patients still developed subsequent arthritis, and ten days of medicine did nothing at all for Lyme in the nervous system or heart.

There were two ways to view these facts. Doctors like Jones had begun to treat longer, eliciting better results. But Steere saw little reason to treat after the earliest stages of disease. It would not be necessary to treat Lyme patients longer or at higher doses, not necessary to treat late Lyme disease at all, he explained, because neurological, cardiac, and arthritic problems were "post-infectious." Any problem remaining after a week or so of treatment was caused not by a microbe, but by an immune reaction triggered by the microbe and now running amok.

It was a rheumatologist's view of the disease, based on the same type of autoimmune theory used to explain lupus, rheumatic fever, and some forms of arthritis—standing in stark contrast to the aggressive treatments prominent in the rest of infectious disease. Of course, if, as Steere suspected, the Connecticut disease was actually different from the European one—if it were viral, say, and not bacterial—then the case could be made that antibiotics wouldn't work, and that Steere's approach was right.

Many people encountering the Lyme scene find it difficult to understand the depth of the rancor between the sides. But students of Lyme disease history, who have observed the unfolding of events, trace the origin of the conflict here, to the early work, which defined the disease. Before Allen Steere came along, virtually no one in the medical establishment had listened to the cluster of patients with the bizarre set of symptoms by the Long Island Sound. It was Allen Steere who explained that they were not disturbed, not crazy, but truly sick.

Yet Steere's specific point of view and set of circumstances had set the stage for a blood feud between him and the patients he hoped to help: In opposition to an extensive body of published research, the earliest Lyme disease patients often received no medication save steroids, which reduced inflammatory symptoms by suppressing the immune response, allowing active infection to proliferate out of control. Many of the sickest Lyme disease patients today are those treated with steroids in the early years, before doctors understood the damage that could be done. As more became known, those patients, many of them vocal, charged that they were sacrificed to hubris—the desire to believe a new disease had been found when it had not. Other patients accused the scientists of heartlessness: knowing antibiotics would help, but nonetheless withholding them to study the natural course of the disease.

As differences in perspective mounted in subsequent years, patients and their treating physicians sparred furiously with academicians over the length and intensity of antibiotic treatment. When newer research proved that neurological and cardiac symptoms were infectious and *could* in fact be prevented or reversed with longer treatment at higher dosages, the original conflict was stirred up, again and again.

The problem, says Raymond Dattwyler, today a professor at New York Medical College in Valhalla, New York, is one of perspective. "It's unfortunate that in the U.S., the rheumatologists studied Lyme disease first," he says. "Lyme disease is a multisystemic infectious disease that impacts many organs. But because the early work was done by rheumatologists, the prism through which we viewed the disease was artificially narrow, and impeded research for years."

Robert A. Aronowitz, a professor of the history and sociology of science at the University of Pennsylvania, agrees. Aronowitz saw, in Lyme disease, a pitfall that biomedical scientists must always be on the lookout for if their work is to stand the test of time: The risk that a researcher might unwittingly impose his or her personal worldview or training on a system under study, thus biasing experiments and influencing the outcome without quite realizing it had occurred. Not only did the Yale researchers view a multisystem illness through the prism of rheumatology, they also failed to factor in a hundred years of research from Europe, including descriptions of the rash, the tick vector, the neurological complications, the curative power of penicillin, and even suspicion that a spirochete was at the root.

Lyme hadn't really been discovered and studied, said Aronowitz, but constructed from elements having more to do with the scientists than the disease. "The construction of a categorically new disease was built implicitly and incrementally from a number of interacting factors, not as a self-evident reflection of the biological and epidemiological facts." Because of this odd beginning, beliefs and attitudes—as opposed to fundamental biological reality—"shaped almost every aspect of medical practice and lay response."

Sometimes relationships just start off on the wrong foot. Despite Allen Steere's early best intentions, that is what happened between him and the patients with the disease he described. Like an allegory from the ancient past, the story of the early days in Lyme, Connecticut, passed down from one generation to the next. Academicians celebrated the pinnacle of achievement, the discovery of a new disease. Patients mourned what they saw as jockeying for turf (at their expense) and the history of a mistake. As new generations slipped between the cracks of the negotiated disease definition, the early days of Lyme assumed the stigma of original sin. The ring of fire through which they all had passed, the story became a symbol of betrayal and a rallying cry around which patients could rise up and fight back.

6

Finding Lyme's Counterculture

Farmington, Connecticut, 2000

The opposition to Steere had started quietly in the southeast corner of Connecticut, but over the years, as his theories and guidelines spread worldwide, the patients' protest grew to one of the angriest medicine had ever seen. Like all Lyme patients shown the door by mainstream medicine, it didn't take long for me to find the protesters: They were on the Internet, in my neighborhood, holding a conference at a Marriott up the road. Like most Lyme patients still sick after the standard treatment, like most mothers of such patients, I found hopelessness in the establishment viewpoint but the glimmer of salvation in the counterculture it spawned.

By April of 2000, we had exhausted whatever establishment medicine had to offer our boy. From the infectious disease expert at our local hospital to our personal pediatrician to a range of specialists in the great teaching hospitals of Manhattan, there was no answer for, and no interest in, our desperately sick son.

I was casting about for an answer when Jason's Spanish tutor mentioned another Chappaqua family with children disabled by Lyme disease, who had run afoul of mainstream physicians and the schools. The children were now better, the tutor told me, and the woman had a phone number dedicated to Lyme disease inquiries. Perhaps I should give her a call. That woman, Mona Marcus, responded to my story in a tone so indignant, so strident, that had I not lived through the past few years, I would have dismissed her as nuts. "Lyme is a political disease," she said over the phone wires, her emphatic New York accent rattling my brain. "There are treatments for your son!" Mona was just the sort of support-group person our pediatrician had emphasized it was important to avoid. But after the pediatrician and his minions, including a dozen high-powered Manhattan specialists, suggested Jason's illness was all in his head, it was Mona I believed.

Later that week, while searching the Internet, I discovered an upcoming Lyme disease conference sponsored by the Lyme Disease Foundation, a national patient-advocacy organization. The next weekend I headed north to a Marriott ballroom in Farmington, Connecticut, a suburb of Hartford, another area rife with Lyme.

The conference was unlike any scientific meeting I had ever attended—and as a medical writer, I'd been to many. Instead of the sober, dry, aloof affairs to which I was accustomed, this gathering had a heightened emotional pitch, a palpable heat and light that made it feel more like an antiwar protest from the sixties than a forum for research. It wasn't just that many attendees were patients. The professionals leading the talks—and I noted many from elite academic and government backgrounds—projected something beyond enthusiasm and different than passion, a kind of smoldering anger and contentiousness that had long been brewing, and might at any second explode. A scientist from a drug company, for instance, gave a talk on the attributes of a Lyme disease vaccine he was studying. No sooner had he finished than a senior scientist from the National Institutes of Health stood up to accuse him of twisting the facts. I was too much of a novice, back then, to grasp the nuance of her argument. But while the meaning may have eluded me, the affect was clear. Waving a fistful of papers, she upbraided the researcher at length, firing a volley of angry questions—Was he sure his lab tests were accurate? How did he measure adverse reactions?—to which he could barely respond. In talk after talk, presenting scientists were interrupted by rounds of applause. In all my years of medical reporting, it was something I'd never seen.

Fireworks notwithstanding, I found myself surrounded by academic experts who profoundly disagreed with our pediatrician and neurologist, with the specialists we'd consulted at teaching hospitals around Manhattan, and with the experts writing for *Science* and quoted in the *New York Times*. A scientist from Cornell, Reinhard K. Straubinger, presented an experiment with infected dogs. After what was thought to be thoroughly adequate antibiotic treatment, Straubinger had, upon autopsy, found *B. burgdorferi* DNA and living spirochetes in their organs and even their brains. Other researchers explained that coinfections—a host of microbes sharing the tick with Lyme—were also infecting patients. When present along with Lyme disease, coinfections could cause a form of illness that was especially long-lasting, difficult to treat, and severe.

I was alarmed by a group from Columbia Presbyterian College of Physicians and Surgeons in New York, introduced as world experts on central nervous system Lyme disease. They found that children with Lyme had impaired attention, short-term memory loss, and drops in processing speed. They had scanned the brains of adults with persistent symptoms and histories of Lyme disease, and found blood flow was decreased—a possible explanation for the patients' new psychiatric complaints. Yet most psychiatrists didn't understand the neuropsychiatric fallout of Lyme disease any better than rheumatologists. This was a problem, said Brian Fallon, a Columbia psychiatrist, because those treated late might respond to short-term antibiotics but just in part, with symptoms such as memory loss or confusion persisting after fatigue and pain have resolved.

In contrast to what I'd read, such chronic patients—products of widespread misdiagnosis on insensitive tests—were abundant, at least according to Kenneth Liegner, a Lyme doctor from Armonk, a town east of Chappaqua. A member of the conference treatment panel, Liegner had been described by patients I met as the most rigorous of all the "LLMDs"—the initials stood for "Lyme literate medical doctor," a term used by patients to describe the physicians who viewed their illness as chronic persistent infection, thus treating them with antibiotics for longer periods of time. Meeting up with Liegner during a coffee break, I related my experience with the Mount Kisco Medical Group and Peter Welch at Northern Westchester Hospital, where Liegner was affiliated as well. He listened to my story, and then turned so red I thought steam would rise out of his head. For years he'd been seeing desperately sick Westchester County patients told they didn't have Lyme disease, and had been "scraping them off the sidewalk," he said. By the time these people got to him they were "so disabled they could barely think or walk."

I'd thought we were an anomaly. But if my table at the LDF luncheon was any indication, there were many patients far sicker than Jason. Across from me was a man whose wife, once a clinical psychologist, had become so light- and sound-averse she had to wear an eye mask and earplugs in the house. No one was allowed to watch television, or even speak, in her presence. Not that it much mattered, he said, because, though once brilliant, she had become so cognitively impaired she couldn't understand even the simplest TV shows, or the meaning of the words her family spoke. She appeared to have dementia, he said.

Especially harrowing was the story told by Kay Lyon, a mother from Wenham, Massachusetts. Lyon described the decline of her previously healthy, normal daughter from 1995 through the summer of 1998, when she was locked in a pediatric psychiatric unit for three and a half weeks. She had just turned nine. "She was paranoid, delusional, psychotic, suicidal, homicidal, and having visual hallucinations while partially blind," Lyon told me. "She suffered severe confusion, and pain in large and small joints."

Saddled with numerous diagnoses, including bipolar disorder, schizophrenia, and mitochondrial disease (difficulty in burning food and metabolizing oxygen for energy), the girl was treated with a cocktail of psychoactive drugs that caused massive weight gain and dulled her mind. Lyon had been frantic. The child's IQ had dropped forty-five points in six months, and a scan with magnetic resonance imaging (MRI) revealed multiple lesions throughout the brain, predominately in the frontal lobes. "Our daughter was a patient of sixteen doctors," Lyon told me over a box lunch, "but not one of them knew what was wrong."

That had been a year ago. Now, having been treated with a combination of oral antibiotics by Charles Ray Jones, the girl was getting well. Back in fourth grade in the regular public school, she did her homework, and had friends.

At dinner that night I met two Michigan women dressed in pants suits who asked me why the idea of treating beyond a month had become so controversial. "I'm new here," I told them. "I don't really know."

Also at the table was a beautiful young woman with straight black hair and tight slacks who looked like a model. "I've graduated," she told me. "I'm finally healthy." She had been receiving intravenous and intramuscular antibiotics for eight years, but now she was off the meds at last. Her story made sense to a New Jersey physician who said he'd had his medical license suspended for treating Lyme disease. Karen Forschner, cofounder of the LDF, came by our table at one point and asked him if he would care to speak to reporters about his travails. "Tell them to go away," he said. "They never get it right." I saw no need to mention that I, too, was a journalist. At the moment I was not a reporter, just a mom.

In that role, I could not help but feel horrified by an overweight woman to my left. Hidden by layers of loose clothing, a soft plastic pump, resembling a spaldeen ball, was attached by tube to the inside of her chest. She fingered the pump throughout dinner as she ate. "It's the latest model," she explained to me. "Really state of the art."

A science journalist with the most skeptical of mind-sets, I wanted no part of these extraterrestrial patients and their alien treatment cocktails. I did not care for outlaw physicians the state hoped to put out of business or in jail. Yet now I'd also met scientists from Columbia, Cornell, and even the NIH who supported these rebels and pariahs.

In the aftermath of the conference, my personal choice was clear. With mainstream doctors dismissing Jason's illness, we faced a tunnel of darkness involving psychiatric hospitals, antipsychotic medication, and a notion we found impossible to accept: that our straight-A, basketball-playing son, after contracting Lyme disease, being misdiagnosed for years, and finally receiving antibiotic therapy for two months, now had developed a bizarre, unrelated psychiatric disorder whose symptoms were, coincidentally, exactly the same as the symptoms of Lyme disease. Perhaps it is possible to believe this kind of explanation when served up by experts talking about other people's children; but it is the rare parent who would accept this decree for a child of his or her own, no matter how illustrious or expert the source. In this case the sources were questionable—those who insisted on the psychiatric explanation had many fine credentials from rheumatology to infectious disease, but none whatsoever in psychiatry. Our psychiatrist, on the other hand, had never seen this form of psychiatric disease.

In the end, the path we chose despite our personal skepticism offered hope. After all, if Jason still had Lyme or one of the other diseases transmitted by the ticks on our wooded property, then he might ultimately be treated and cured. So in June of 2000, with the doors of the medical establishment slammed shut, we took the only route still open to us. Following the advice of my new friend, Kay, and with our psychiatrist's medical blessing, we set off for New Haven and a consultation with the maverick pediatrician, Charles Ray Jones.

7

Hide in Plain Sight

Framingham, Massachusetts, 1998–2000

In her relentless quest for answers, Sheila Statlender began to learn all she could about chronic fatigue syndrome—or, to those who recognized the immune component, chronic fatigue and immune dysfunction syndrome (CFIDS). Her research and contacts eventually led her to David Bell, the pioneering physician who had recognized one of the first clusters of the illness in rural Lyndonville, New York.

Flying from Boston to Rochester in the winter of 1998 with Seth and then driving an hour west to Bell's office, the Statlenders felt as if they had entered a time warp. With its rural population and rundown buildings, Lyndonville seemed, at first, more like the backdrop for the Bates Motel than a center of high-tech healing. It felt strange for this medical family, trained by the denizens of modern research, to abandon the great teaching hospitals of Boston for the ramshackle likes of this. Seth was so sick (Sheila feared he might be dying) and the journey so hard on him (he had barely been able to walk from the plane to the rental car) that part of them wondered what they were doing here at all.

Yet they knew that they had to come, and that in seeking alternate solutions, they were doing the right thing. "We never felt like we were going down the back alley for an illegal abortion," Statlender explains of her family's search for answers. "We knew that our kids were sick—very sick—and became grateful for thinkers who would venture outside of the box. Perhaps because of the fact that we had trained in academic medical centers, as much as in spite of that fact, we knew that the emperor often has no clothes."

Indeed, Bell offered something important that the powers in Boston did not: a place of compassion and a refuge from the slings of the skeptical world. Although Seth's erratic low blood pressure had caused frequent, alarming blackouts, once sending him down a flight of stairs, Bell was the first doctor to provide a real explanation: "dysautonomia," a dysfunction of the autonomic nervous system often seen in chronic fatique. It was Bell who sent Seth on to a cardiologist at the Children's Hospital in Boston, where "tilt table testing" yielded results considered classic for the dysfunction, leading to treatment with Florinef, a corticosteroid that helps the body retain fluid and, hence, maintain blood pressure. Bell confirmed for Seth, who was by then in seventh grade, the diagnosis of CFIDS originally suggested by the immunologist at the University of Massachusetts Medical Center some time earlier.

A little more than a year later, Bell would make a provisional CFIDS diagnosis for Amy as well. Though Amy didn't want to believe that she suffered the same illness that brought her older brother down, as time went on she only got sicker. So during the summer of 1999 it was decided that she would go to Lyndonville to see Bell, too. At first, noting Amy's chronic cough, Bell thought she might be suffering from some kind of infection and treated her with antibiotic. But she reacted much as she did when treated for *H. pylori*—she got much sicker. By the fall, having just started seventh grade herself, Amy's health plummeted dramatically. Like Seth, she developed dysautonomia, but also a tremor, balance and gait problems, and what appeared to be Raynaud's syndrome, in which the tiny blood vessels in the fingers and toes constrict in response to cold, and the lips turn blue. "I looked at her as I had looked at Seth before her, and I wondered if my child could be dying," Sheila states.

Hearing about all this during a telephone consult, Bell was concerned. "It's in her nervous system now. Be prepared that she may actually become worse than Seth, at least for a while," Bell said. He immediately referred Amy to the same pediatric cardiologist treating her brother and several other Boston-area CFIDS children for dysautonomia. By this time the cardiologist had put together a loosely organized team of specialists at his hospital, and wanted Amy screened by them first.

That led to a trip to Children's Hospital in Boston, where a rheumatologist, a short, terse man, conducted his exam with a small army of residents in tow. Never making eye contact with either Sheila or Amy, he went straight to work with his instruments, using a magnifying glass to examine Amy's fingers, which cooperated beautifully by turning blue for the residents.

"I'm going to tell you something," he said when he addressed Amy, at last. "You can regain control of your body, but you have to do exactly what I tell you to. No naps in the daytime so that you can get your sleep regulated. You also need to start a program of regular exercise. You can get better, but only if you follow my advice."

Listening with alarm, and noticing that he was ignoring Amy's attempts to speak up, Sheila wondered if he had observed her daughter's tremor and jerking arm movements, or the fact that she couldn't walk straight. "He was prescribing stereotypical cognitive behavioral techniques that didn't fit the symptoms," and hadn't bothered to learn that too little sleep, not too much, was what bothered Amy most.

"Excuse me," Sheila Statlender, Ph.D., said to the doctor, "but as a clinical psychologist as well as Amy's mother, I have some concern about your input here. If you tell patients they can gain control of their bodies when they can't, you may be setting them up to blame themselves if they fail."

"I don't think so," the doctor snapped, arching his back as if to appear taller. He then marched out as abruptly as he had entered, his contingent of residents trailing behind.

Next, as part of the diagnostic screening, they saw a neurologist. Noting the problems with balance and gait, he ordered an MRI to rule out childhood-onset multiple sclerosis, which he said he was seeing more and more of. He also ordered a panel of blood and urine tests to rule out the possibility that Amy's neuropathies were rooted in some kind of nutritional deficit.

Days went by without any word from the neurologist regarding the results of the MRI. The Statlenders called his office to learn the results. When he finally returned the call to report that results were normal, he just left a message with the nanny. Even with Amy so sick, and no explanation in sight, the neurologist thought it unnecessary, he told them, to return before three months. Given the dismissive nature of yet another interaction, the Statlenders never pursued that follow-up. They did, however, continue to bring Amy to the referring cardiologist, part of the same hospital system and even the same CFIDS consultation team, who went on to treat her dysautonomia for another two years.

It was only years later when, preparing for a consult with yet *another* physician, that Sheila and Russ requested the neurologist's notes from that day. They were stunned to read the comment at the end, written almost as an afterthought:

> *Finally, I have discussed the advisability of performing a spinal tap on [Amy], to look for evidence of multiple sclerosis or for CNS [central nervous system] Lyme disease. This does not have to be done currently, but after results of the suggested tests have returned, if symptoms persist, such a test may be warranted. I have made an appointment to see [Amy] again in three months time.*

The Statlenders never saw the note, which had been sent on to their pediatrician as well as their cardiologist—but to no avail. None of these practitioners ever discussed it with *them*. On the neurologist's comment about there being "no rush," Sheila is appalled to this day. "He had this child in his office turning blue, with her body swaying and her arms flailing. I have never understood how he could let her leave in that condition, let alone not plan to see her again for twelve more weeks."

By fall 2000, entering the eighth grade, Amy was too sick to read the books she so loved; instead, she sat in a darkened room watching music videos. For Sheila, the CFIDS diagnosis ultimately bequeathed on Amy by David Bell was some kind of comfort, offering, at least, access to his supportive office, the validation that her daughter was medically ill, and negotiating power with the school. Amy, on the other hand, never quite believed the diagnosis was correct.

Now officially ensconced in the CFIDS community, the Statlenders met other local families with children too sick to attend school or lead normal lives. Each such child was marginalized: Too sick to have friends, cast out by mainstream medicine as undiagnosable and untreatable, many kept a low profile and were invisible to all but one another. Others, like the Statlenders, made themselves known to the medical community and schools. Either way, they formed a close-knit, unenviable club.

Eventually Sheila, together with another clinical psychologist whose son had been diagnosed with CFIDS, organized two support groups for families hailing from the Boston suburbs and beyond. "These were high-powered families," Statlender notes: doctors, lawyers, Ph.D.s. "Very educated and bright, but their children were dreadfully sick, and they did not have any answers."

In one family, for instance, both parents were scientists. Their son, always a very bright and academically ambitious young man, now had trouble concentrating and completing his assignments. He was perpetually dizzy and in constant pain, and for the first time since starting school required academic accommodation.

In a second family, both parents were attorneys. They lived in a heavily wooded neighborhood in an affluent suburb outside Boston and had two daughters, one healthy and one quite ill. To bring the sick daughter back to health, the mother became strictly macrobiotic, ladling soup into the girl's mouth when she was too ill to feed herself. Previously a creative, academic star in the public school, a child so precocious she might have skipped a grade, the girl now was so sick and weak that she had to transfer to a smaller, private school with a physical terrain she could more easily navigate, and which would better accommodate her needs. She finished high school, but it took five years.

A third family included a girl who had once been an honor student, but now, after suffering a debilitating flulike illness, appeared so confused she was taken to Boston's Brigham and Women's Hospital for a neuropsychological evaluation. There, the experts found she suffered from inexplicably slowed processing speed and impaired working memory. They had no explanation for the deficits, and no way to help the girl recover her former self.

And so it went. Sheila joined the CFIDS organizations, hobnobbing with other professionals. She attended meetings of the American Association for Chronic Fatigue Syndrome, first in Cambridge and later in Seattle, and made friends with the experts and advocates, many of them professionals who had been diagnosed with the mysterious ailment themselves. Twice she went to Washington to lobby for increased funding and patient rights.

In their past lives Sheila and Russ had drawn society from the soccer field, often splitting up so one parent could go to Seth's tournaments and the other to Amy's. Now they were part of a different social set, a subculture of parents with children who were inexplicably sick and frighteningly untreatable.

8

⁂

The Epidemic Spreads

Some time after Allen Steere's first articles were published, he and Charles Ray Jones met at the hospital, by chance. "I remember the talk as bittersweet," says Jones. "Steere was obviously studying the same disease I'd observed for years. He thought it was spread by ticks, I thought mosquitoes or gnats. I thought the infection was bacterial, based on my treatment success with antibiotics, but he thought a virus might be the cause."

The main difference between the children of Lyme and the children of Hamden, as Jones saw it, was that the children living in Lyme were sicker, by far. Thanks to careful tracking and early antibiotic treatment, Jones's regular patients rarely developed advanced forms of the new illness. The untreated children in Lyme, on the other hand, progressed beyond anything Jones himself had seen.

"I learned about what seemed to be the full spectrum of the illness by reading Allen Steere's papers," Jones said, "but I always treated the children in my practice with antibiotics when they came in with symptoms, so they never got very sick." In the end, many residents of Lyme and other neighboring towns, including those participating in the first classic studies, went untreated for years. It was by studying them that scientists came to document the pathology of Lyme from the earliest, acute stages to the debilitating, disseminated, late stages of the disease.

Throughout the 1970s, the bizarre new illness made an appearance in

Lyme zones across the United States, most notably in Wisconsin and Minnesota, where *Ixodes* ticks like those in the East appeared to transmit Lyme disease, and in California, where a tick cousin named *Ixodes pacificus* would be found to spread the disease. Those who knew Phyllis Mervine in the heyday of the 1960s say she was one of the original California hippies. Today in her sixties, Mervine reflects that spirit. With wire-frame glasses and hair in a pixie cut, she speaks ardently about her many passions, from home-schooling to world peace. But as she raised her family in the mountains of California through the 1970s and 1980s, Mervine's clarity and idealism were shattered by a mysterious, incapacitating disease.

In part her story reflects the era. In 1972, living in San Francisco, Phyllis and her husband, Fred, at the time an engineer for Bechtel, decided they'd enjoy a life "off the grid," far from the power and phone lines rooted to the workaday world. So with other young "back-to-the-landers," they bought property on a 5,300-acre cattle ranch in Mendocino County, northwest of Ukiah, high in the rolling hills of the Coast Range. The sprawling ranch land, with its deep ravines, dense woods, peaceful meadows, and high grass, was home to plentiful wildlife—deer, white-footed mice, squirrels, rabbits, lizards, raccoons, possums, many species of birds, coyotes, foxes, rattlesnakes, mountain lions, bobcats, and bears.

In the earliest years, Phyllis and Fred and their three young children spent weekends in a teepee, cooking their food in a cast-iron pot over an open fire and walking the trails barefoot. By 1975, the Mervine homestead consisted of a large garden and a rustic house, an octagonal structure inspired by Japanese architecture. Off the grid, there was "no running water, no electricity, no telephone." To approximate indoor plumbing, they took a hose from outside and ran it through a hole in the wall, fastening a garden spigot to one end of the rough kitchen counter. "We cooked and heated our house with an antique wood-burning stove and grew most of our own food," says Mervine. "We spent hours each day outdoors while our kids played 'rocket ship' on the logs." The Coast Range community even had its own school, reachable by a deer path that the children traversed on ponies. "The grass along the trail was so high it came up to your eyebrows," Mervine recalls. "We knew we were bitten by ticks. One night our youngest son, Eli, was in bed, between us, and Fred said, 'Look, Eli has a tick between his eyelashes.' It was a tiny larval tick. We pulled ticks out of belly buttons and from between toes."

As the years passed, as Lyme spread through the towns of southeast Connecticut, the Mervines of Mendocino thrived. Her hair tied back in a single, luxuriant braid so long she could literally sit on it, Phyllis put in many hours of work: caring for the children, gardening to grow the family's food, tending the horses, and milking the goats.

Early in the summer of 1977, just as Allen Steere was publishing his very first papers on the strange Connecticut disease he called Lyme, Phyllis Mervine, pregnant with her fourth child, noticed a bite that had swelled up like a sting; a month later, she suffered a severe flulike illness; and then, that fall, her knee swelled. Though the swelling seemed to resolve, after the baby arrived in November, Phyllis was perpetually unwell. Her neck hurt, her body ached, she had joint and muscle pain, and she felt a constant malaise.

By 1978 her neck hurt so much that she could no longer comb and braid her cherished hair, so she cut it off. "I kept it in a drawer, wrapped in a silk scarf," Mervine recalls. As the years passed and the pain and exhaustion increased, she took the braid out occasionally to help her remember her former, healthy life. The new reality was inexplicable, and seemingly without end. Sometimes she had vertigo so profound she couldn't walk forward without holding on to a wall. Her ears rang and she couldn't hear well. She remembers lying on the floor too sick to get up, her children playing around her. Other days she had unexplained attacks of vomiting. Searing pains often radiated down her spine and back.

By the early eighties Mervine had been diagnosed with ankylosing spondylitis, a chronic degenerative arthritis primarily affecting the spine. It explained only part of her worsening malaise. Despite visits to doctors in search of an explanation, only acupuncture relieved her pain. Mervine recalls sitting courtside at a soccer game, watching one of her sons play. She felt so ill that when another parent inquired after her health, she replied, "I don't think I'm going to live much longer like this." She was only forty. And she wasn't alone. Three children in the ranch community had swollen knees and were diagnosed with JRA before doctors realized they had the newly described disease: Lyme disease. Other homesteaders experienced "the encroachment of a kind of mental slowness, a brain fog." But since they owned their land and had no utility bills, since they grew their own food and could survive without much money, many just drifted along.

It would be a decade before Mervine was finally diagnosed, through a positive blood test, with a case of late-stage, disseminated Lyme disease, and many years more before she was successfully treated with long-term doxycycline by Paul Lavoie, a rheumatologist at the San Francisco Pacific Presbyterian Medical Center. Hearing that Mervine had conducted an informal survey of the ailing Coast Range residents,

Lavoie recognized the community as a window into the West Coast version of Lyme. Just as Allen Steere had studied the Lyme, Connecticut, cluster in the East, so, too, would Lavoie and Berkeley entomologist Robert Lane study the Coast Range cluster in the West, ultimately finding different ticks, different host species (including the lizard), and different animal reservoirs of infection.

In 1981—as the Mervines and other Coast Range families succumbed in their infested paradise and Allen Steere searched vigilantly for the origin of Lyme disease, which he thought was probably viral—a young doctor named Joe Burrascano was finishing up his residency at a hospital in Nebraska.

Originally from Montauk, at the very eastern tip of Long Island, Burrascano had grown up loving the ocean. Nebraska didn't have one. So when it was time to open a practice of his own, the athletic young physician with Frankie Valli hair and a degree from New York University Medical School decided to move back East. "I didn't know it at the time, but that part of Long Island, the South Fork, had the highest rate of what we'd eventually call Lyme disease in the world," he says today. Like most of the community doctors who found themselves at the center of the Lyme controversy, Joe Burrascano did not know what he was walking into, at all.

Still, it didn't take long for Burrascano to realize he wasn't in Nebraska anymore. Other local doctors, those practicing in the area for years, quickly filled him in on the medical idiosyncrasies of the locals. One physician, an internist and public health expert named Sidney Robin, had worked at Johns Hopkins but vacationed on Montauk. He so loved the area that he'd given up the high-powered life of a Johns Hopkins professor to become a country doctor, opening a home office in the early 1960s and treating the locals for their everyday ills. It was from Robin that Burrascano learned of the condition called Montauk knee, which we now know as Lyme arthritis. Robin treated the swollen knees (often accompanied by strange, circular rashes thought to be "spider bites") with antibiotics, especially penicillin and tetracycline, and the patients seemed to get well.

Another local doctor, Edgar Grunwaldt of Shelter Island, had noticed the strange erythema migrans rash on many of his patients. Credited by some as the first true discoverer of Lyme disease in the United States, Grunwaldt saw a Lyme rash on a Shelter Island patient in 1975, and another one in 1976. The rashes were so odd that Grunwaldt, like the navy doctors, searched the medical literature, discovering reports from Europe stretching all the way back to the early 1900s. European physicians had connected the rash to the bite of the *Ixodes* tick, and found that treatment with antibiotic was effective. Grunwaldt had been following Steere's papers as well—and realized that he was seeing Lyme disease. Unlike Robin, however, Grunwaldt stopped using antibiotics on his patients in 1978, when a telephone conversation with Allen Steere assured him that the disease was self-limiting. While Shelter Island residents had once been treated for Lyme disease, by the late 1970s, they, like their counterparts in southeast Connecticut, often progressed to endpoint, ultimately adding to the knowledge about the expanding spectrum of disease.

While Robin specialized in knees and Grunwaldt in rashes, Burrascano began to notice an assortment of other strange ailments in the local population—things he'd never seen in Nebraska, and defined by symptoms that went way beyond what Allen Steere described in his papers as Lyme. The bizarre conditions seemed to go back three generations in some families, Burrascano found. "I didn't know what these illnesses were, and neither did my colleagues. These patients were confused and they couldn't think right. They were fatigued and had body pains. Some of these patients I sent to rheumatologists—who either diagnosed them with lupus or said no, that's not lupus, but something very strange, like lupus. No one knew what was going on."

9

Crossing the Line

New Haven, Connecticut, 2000

Diagnosis and treatment should have been easier for Jason, with his classic presentation, than for the bizarre lupuslike patients Joe Burrascano observed in his earliest experience of the disease. We lived at ground zero for the epidemic, at the edge of a deer forest in an area certified as not just endemic, but hyperendemic, by Yale. We vacationed at all the Lyme hot spots, including the eastern tip of Long Island and the Jersey Shore and Cape Cod. From swollen knees to an enormous classic Lyme rash to an off-the-charts positive Western blot at a standard lab, our boy could have been an Allen Steere poster child—until he didn't get well. After failing the treatment, he'd once more become a pariah to the mainstream doctors as surely as if we'd insisted he contracted his infection on Mars. Though Jason had been classic in every way, when his disease didn't respond to the eight weeks of treatment specified as the ceiling in mainstream treatment guidelines, he was cast out of the medical fold again. Unless we wanted to give up on our son, our only choice was to join the hundreds of patients I'd met at the conference in April, crossing the line to seek treatment from Lyme's radical left.

On most June mornings in New Haven, students wander Park Street and Broadway clutching cups of Starbucks coffee, stopping to chat on benches or browse for books and clothes. Walk a few blocks east and you'll find the source of all this charm: Yale itself, one of the most beautiful and august universities in the world.

But there's another, less illustrious route through New Haven, requiring no academic admission save from the school of hard knocks. Just follow Park Street back past the gothic Christ Church, alongside the filling stations and Laundromats, the dilapidated deli storefronts and the children hanging on stoops. There, in the shadows of the Yale–New Haven Medical Center, in a building more notable for its seventies-style blandness than ivy along the wall, is the first-floor office of Charles Ray Jones, the sole U.S. pediatrician specializing in long-term antibiotic treatment of the controversial condition called "chronic Lyme." Keeping his doors open long past the age he would otherwise have retired, Jones was the last-chance depot for kids like Jason who hadn't recovered, the final stop for those en route to the trash heap of unresolved Lyme. His demeanor belied his "finger in the dike" role. The day we arrived, he was there to greet us wearing an acrylic running suit, trifocal lenses that glazed his eyes, and a wide, whimsical grin. Age seventy-one, he had a cane and a limp.

The term chronic Lyme is usually a misnomer, Jones told me that first day, because the disease spectrum includes not just *Borrelia burgdorferi,* the bacterial infection known to cause Lyme disease, but a host of other tick-borne germs. At the top of Jones's list of coinfections were the malarialike blood parasite *Babesia,* and the bacterial infections *Ehrlichia* (today often recognized as *Anaplasma*) and *Bartonella,* the latter an organism he said could gravitate to the central nervous system and brain. "The children who get sickest and who are hardest to treat," said Jones, "may have more than one infection or an immune vulnerability to the disease."

As far as Jones was concerned, moreover, children and teenagers treated appropriately usually kicked the disease altogether, no matter how sick they might be when they walked through his door. "In my practice, at least," Jones told me, "the word chronic usually does not turn out to be correct. We find that children, when diagnosed with the correct infections and treated with the appropriate medication, usually get well."

Jones had long since been maligned by Yale as the Pied Piper of Lyme, a beguiling guru who hypnotized parents and endangered children's lives. "A quack," said Eugene Shapiro, the Yale pediatrician who loudly declared he wanted Jones's head. But Jones would have the answer for us. Sitting in his office for consultation, I realized he had read Jason's medical records so thoroughly he could recite chapter and verse on the sequence of symptoms, diagnoses, treatments, and previous lab results. "What happened here is a crime," he said.

His exam was a four-hour marathon, in which blood was drawn, a detailed history taken, and every inch evaluated. While most physicians considering Lyme look for a rash and sore knees, decades of treating intractable cases and mixed infections had taught Jones to recognize what he saw as more subtle fingerprints of disease, from pain (upon pressure) in the bones of the chest to the telltale sluggishness of a sick child's gait. He also elicited from us a detailed history of where we had vacationed: the weekends at Montauk, the weeks at the Jersey shore and in a cabin in the woods on Cape Cod.

A couple of weeks later Jones called to tell us Jason had tested positive not just for Lyme disease, but also for anaplasmosis/ehrlichiosis and babesiosis. Instead of using more aggressive intravenous treatments, as the mainstream experts had done, Jones now prescribed relatively low doses of three targeted oral medications: To treat both Lyme and anaplasmosis, Jason took a tablet of doxycycline twice a day. For babesiosis, he consumed two teaspoons a day of a thick gold sludge called Mepron, also a treatment for malaria. Because Jones thought spirochetes could be encased in hard-walled cysts, he prescribed a medicine called Flagyl to break them up.

About a week after starting the treatment, Jason's body started to straighten. He pulled himself out of the bathtub, retrieved a basketball from his closet, and threw it across the room. He was, of course, still sick. But at that moment I was so happy and relieved my eyes welled over and I cried. "Please let this be real," I whispered to myself. Jason had spent years in freefall. But now, some six months after finally testing positive for Lyme disease, and after starting treatment for the coinfections *Babesia* and *Anaplasma,* he appeared to be floating back up.

10

❖

The Rocky Road

Chappaqua, New York, 2000

I wish I could report that Dr. Jones's initial treatment was so targeted, so powerful that Jason improved each day in the summer of 2000 until, by September, he was completely well. Not just ready to return to school and rejoin his friends but raring to tip-off in basketball and blaze through the AP classes for which he had been approved—able to pick up where he'd left off in the life of a normal teen.

That was not the case.

Instead, his improvement was partial, his climb back slow. His unending headache was gone—poof! The shooting, jabbing pains had lessened and then vanished entirely, but new, duller aches migrated from joint to joint throughout the night and day. After lolling in the steamy sea of our tub for months, he picked himself up one day and left the bathroom, though still so fatigued his destination was only his bed.

In September 2000, Jason showed up at school to restart the tenth grade, which he'd been too sick to finish the year before. He was still in pain, still fatigued, but he was *there*. The trip back up from the bottom had felt frustrating and slow, there had been setbacks and plateaus, but over the course of three months it was quite clear his improvement, while incomplete, had been vast.

We sustained our optimism through October—he had absences, and required a reduced workload, but appeared to be hanging in and keeping up his grades. Then he got a rash. Could it be an allergy to one of the drugs? Jones took him off all antibiotics. The plan was to let the rash resolve and then reintroduce the three medicines—doxy, Flagyl, and Mepron—one by one and watch to see if the rash reappeared. The process took weeks and although all three medicines eventually passed the test and were exonerated as the cause of the mystery rash, Jason had slipped back down the long Lyme tunnel, until fatigue and pain took him over and school was again just a dream.

It wasn't until December that Jason climbed back up, not just retreading old ground but moving forward: By Christmas he was healthier—stronger, more focused, in far less pain, than he'd been in a couple of years. He returned to school, he saw his friends. His disease was less severe, but even as it receded it morphed: The migrating muscle pains had stopped but the raw grind of bone pain, especially in his chest, back, and shoulders, had by then set in. At least the treatment seemed to be working, at least we saw change. After years of searching we'd found only one road back, and we were on it. It was a rocky road, with untold detours, divots, and blockades. All other paths were paved with hopelessness, so we carried on.

11

Then There Were Three

Framingham, Massachusetts, 2000–2002

When the Statlenders' third child, Eric, began his descent into illness, his slide was so gradual, so subtle, that at first his parents didn't quite see it for what it was—maybe they just didn't want to, and who could blame them? It started not with any physical symptom, but with a cognitive glitch. Always an enormously alert and competent child, Eric all of a sudden stopped grasping the spoken word. "What?" he would ask in response to all manner of comments throughout the day. "What did you say?" He asked people to repeat things constantly, worrying Sheila and Ross and wearing his teachers' patience thin.

Because it was mainly his verbal comprehension that seemed affected, the Statlenders at first thought he might have a hearing problem. The results of a hearing test, however, were normal, so the Statlenders took him to a neurologist at Children's Hospital. That doctor found that Eric required several repetitions before he was able to parrot back a complex sentence. "It takes a while to get in, but once it gets there, he has no trouble repeating it," observed the physician, who diagnosed an auditory processing problem. He could hear the sound, but his brain had trouble making sense of what it meant.

Learning that the Statlender's property bordered a deer preserve, the neurologist wondered if Eric should be tested for Lyme disease. But when Sheila explained that Eric had already tested negative on Lyme tests at the pediatrician's office, the neurologist dismissed ·

the possibility of Lyme disease out of hand. He had no clue as to why Eric, who had understood everything until months ago, now was so impaired.

As time went on and public school became more of a challenge, the Statlenders transferred Eric to a local Montessori school that was smaller and could offer more individualized attention. By then, however, his auditory processing deficit was only part of the problem. Like Seth and Amy before him, Eric had begun to experience an array of physical symptoms. His legs hurt all the time. At the spring soccer tryout, he was unable to muster enough energy to complete a run around the field, holding his sides in pain and dragging himself to the sidelines with a mixture of misery and disappointment. He also was starting to miss a lot of school; he just felt sick, he said, and his stomach often ached.

"He went from sunny to irritable," says Sheila, explaining that his auditory processing problem contributed to this shift in his temperament. "His inability to understand his peers led to misunderstandings." Unable to understand the words spoken to him, he would often misconstrue their meaning or think that his friends were teasing him. Indeed, some of them did begin to make fun of him. As a result, he could get upset or feel hurt.

By the time Eric was in fifth grade the writing was on the wall: He, too, had begun to journey down the path of the sickness without a cause or a treatment or an end. "We didn't want to accept it," Sheila says, "but when we saw it was harder for Eric to walk than it was for Amy and Seth, who were both so sick, we had to admit—we had three."

Was that even *possible?* Sometimes it happened, said David Bell, but for Sheila and Russ, this was the breaking point.

"When we had two, we resigned ourselves to living with it and helping them as best we could. We accepted some sort of status quo, putting whatever supports were possible in place from tutors to assist with academics to palliative treatments that imperfectly addressed their medical symptoms," Sheila explains. "But with three, the drive to get to the bottom of this returned. We couldn't help but think that they must have been exposed to something."

Then one afternoon Eric had two bouts of intense and excruciating chest pain. Clutching his body, he fell onto the bed, writhing and screeching, "Make it stop!"

Sheila was terrified. "Once again, it crossed my mind that my child might be dying—this time, it was my youngest."

First they had the house tested for toxins, but an expensive inspection yielded no findings of any significance.

Then Sheila began calling the CFIDS professionals she'd befriended at the Seattle meeting some years before. "They thought it was suspicious that all three kids were sick," Sheila says. "That made it sound, to them, more like an infection, or some sort of common exposure. Since we lived in the Northeast, they said we should think about Lyme disease."

Going to the Internet, to a mailing list of CFIDS professionals, Sheila posted about the episode. Soon one of the members, a Ph.D. researcher whose wife had been diagnosed with CFIDS, was posting back. "Chest pain like that can be a symptom of Lyme disease," he wrote.

The children have already been tested for Lyme, Sheila posted back.

"Well, those tests are hardly reliable," numerous other posters on the list wrote back.

"I really got a barrage of replies," Sheila recalls, "all urging me to pursue the possibility of Lyme disease."

Following the online exchange, the Statlenders took Eric to a holistically oriented doctor known for treating patients who had slipped through the cracks, someone who had periodically assisted with the care of Seth and Amy after they had been diagnosed with CFIDS, and who knew the family history.

After examining Eric, the doctor turned to the Statlenders and said, "There is something terribly wrong with this child."

"Do you think he could have been exposed to an infection? Because we are ready to go back to square one for all three kids, and we are looking for suggestions," Sheila said.

"It's certainly possible," the doctor said. "One thing I would recommend is to test for tick-borne disease." Sheila had never heard the term before, but now, for the first time, she understood that the ticks that carried Lyme disease could sometimes carry other infections, too.

12

Night Falls Fast

Colorado Springs, Colorado, 2003

Friends joked about the oncologist marrying the grief therapist. Imagine those dinner talks! What kind of life would it be? Folks were more quizzical still when Dave Martz left oncology after thirty years to work at a hospice. But the marriage and the career change felt right. "We understood each other," Martz says. Besides, Dave and Dee Martz, themselves, were in the best of health. "Before we got married, I had a physical to make sure we wouldn't repeat the past." She'd been so devastated when her previous husband, Norm, died of leukemia, and Martz wanted to protect her from another big loss.

So it came as a shock when, in April 2003, Dave, like Norm, started to slide. At first, it was a question of energy. "Just talking for an hour would exhaust me," recalls Martz. Soon his muscles ached and his whole body hurt. Then he got so weak he couldn't lift his heels off the mattress. "I rolled out of bed and crawled to the shower," he recalls.

Long a skilled diagnostician, Martz found himself considering the possible causes of his own disease. His self-diagnoses ranged from polymyalagia rheumatica—easily treated with steroids—to a bizarre form of widespread bone cancer that couldn't be cured. When a couple of weeks went by and he hadn't improved, Martz knew he needed others to chime in.

At Penrose Hospital in Colorado Springs, a team of highly qualified physicians, who were also colleagues and friends, worked him up with what seemed like every blood test, toxicology screen, imaging technology, and form of biopsy known. Ultimately, eight skilled neurologists settled on two possible diagnoses, one fatal and the other offering hope.

The first possibility was devastating: Like the end-stage patient in Las Animas, Dave Martz seemed to have ALS. Keys to the diagnosis included exaggerated reflexes and rippling muscle movements under the skin called fasciculation. Martz had both. This would be early, very early, in the game.

Yet the diagnosis wasn't set in stone because ALS patients usually don't also suffer arthritic pain or severe fatigue—those were more like something rarely diagnosed in Colorado, a disease called Lyme. So a crack team of doctors at Penrose drew Martz's blood and sent it to the Mayo Clinic in Rochester, Minnesota, not once but thrice: And three times running, the blood work came back negative for Lyme disease. Unconvinced, they even sent the blood out to the controversial Lyme lab, IGeneX, in Palo Alto, California, where a different combination of markers were said to find Lyme disease Mayo couldn't—yet IGeneX, too, found the blood equivocal, at best.

That's when the neurologist Steven Smith, a University of Minnesota professor and ALS expert who'd recently moved to Colorado, got involved. Reviewing the history, Smith said the Colorado workup had been so thorough that no one could do better—and it was *time,* not more testing, that would make the call. "ALS is a death sentence," said Smith, "so physicians often wait until even a first-year medical student can call it before we give the label." Two or three more months, he told Martz, and they'd know for sure.

So Martz waited as the fasciculation got so bad his legs waffled like Gumby. To quell the inflammation, his shoulders were injected with cortisone and he took methotrexate. He swallowed OxyContin for the pain. Yet still he got sicker. "I keep wondering if this could be Lyme disease," he said hopefully to Smith.

But Smith had waited long enough: Now, he said, he could tell. "I'm from Minnesota, I see lots of Lyme. This is ALS." What's more, Smith knew the slope of the disease—some folks could drag it out for five or six years, but others declined faster. That was the case for Martz—he had maybe two years to live, and that was the outside max.

So four months after the first of the symptoms, in August 2003, the oncologist and the grief therapist prepared for another death, and planning to die was one of the most oddly fulfilling things Dave had ever done.

He reckoned he had maybe eighteen months more to have adventures, connect with loved ones, and party his way to God.

Since he was losing his mobility, some things had to be done right away: As he'd long dreamed, he flew as a passenger in a glider over the Rockies. And he arranged for a ride in the cabin of a semi, an eighteen-wheeler, to be exact. "I'd tried to get a ride in one of those trucks for years," Martz explains, "but the drivers wouldn't take me, something about insurance." But for the dying man, exceptions were made. A trucker that Dee knew finally relented and took Dave out.

Mostly, his journey was emotional. For one thing, he learned who his friends were: Some of those who had seemed most intimate fell away, while others, those who could empathize with his anguish and struggle, stepped up. Dee kept a list of such friends and told them what they could do to help: One could stop by with a DVD while Dee did the shopping and watch a movie with Dave. As his condition worsened, another could hold a Popsicle so that Dave, his hands too weak and his mouth too parched, could enjoy some cooling licks. He built nurturing friendships with half a dozen men, meeting them for lunch or breakfast, and, for the first time in years, talking, really talking from his heart.

Becoming the great oncologist had consumed his youthful hours and years, but now, working on his relationships, Dave Martz learned how neglected his wife, children, and siblings really felt. He'd been the model of the compassionate physician, extending every sensitivity to his patients, but his family said that 90 percent of his focus went to the job, that he ignored them. "I was stunned and hurt," Martz says. Yet in the little time left, he could make repairs. Had he died suddenly of a heart attack in the middle of some night, he would have walked into his grave having given all his intentional love to strangers. but now he could make things right.

"I was determined not to waste the months of dying," Martz says.

13

◈

Discovering the Spirochete

With the eighties under way, the hunt for the microbe causing Lyme disease was going full tilt. Steere's group at Yale searched high and low for the agent, which they thought might be a virus. From the lofty perch of the 1980s, after all, many scientists believed that virtually all bacterial infections had already been discovered—and that, thanks to the antibiotic revolution, they were all essentially curable. With the advent of AIDS, it was the *virus* that represented the hot new frontier of infectious disease. If a virus was at the root, it would distinguish Lyme disease from the bacterial entity in Europe as something entirely new. It would also validate Steere's insistence that antibiotics, which were biologically incapable of treating viral illness, barely made a dent in Lyme patients' health.

But in the end, the *bacterial* cause of Lyme disease was discovered across the country in Hamilton, Montana, a tiny town in the foothills of the Rockies, in a state without a single reported case. Stationed in Hamilton and responsible for the discovery was the brilliant, exuberant Swiss microbiologist Willy Burgdorfer, an employee of the Rocky Mountain Laboratories of the National Institutes of Health. With his cheerful courtly manner and distinctive wardrobe of vests, the workaholic Burgdorfer was widely considered one of the top tick experts in the world.

For Burgdorfer, whose name was lent to the organism, discovering the spirochete would be a transformative, life-altering event. "When I was a student, I was full of dreams. I would be part of a team," Burgdorfer says. "And I always was, until I found the spirochete. After that, my life was never the same." Dale Burgdorfer, his wife, said that Lyme was a fatal disease, and she wasn't talking about physical death, but the toll it took on her family. She liked to say that Lyme disease had killed her.

Part of the problem, of course, was envy. As with any race to the finish line, the first arrival runs the risk of resentment and a lifetime of jealous barbs. Perhaps that's why, over the years, some dismissive colleagues have chalked Burgdorfer's discovery up to serendipity—to being in the right place at the right time. But Burgdorfer brought far more to the Lyme table than that, including training from the world's preeminent tick and spirochete experts, an in-depth knowledge of the scientific literature going back a century, and extraordinary powers of vision, literally and intellectually. If serendipity means all that, then serendipity it was.

Born in the 1920s in Basel, Switzerland, Willy Burgdorfer had a longstanding fascination with biology. So in 1945, he began graduate studies at the Swiss Tropical Institute, where he specialized in the arcane but up-and-coming field of parasitology. Burgdorfer's mentor was zoologist Rudolf Geigy, director of the institute, whose area of specialization was the role of arthropods—insects, spiders, and ticks—in transmitting and maintaining human disease. As luck would have it, Geigy assigned Burgdorfer the task of investigating the spirochete, *Borrelia duttoni,* the cause of relapsing fever in Africa, transmitted to people by *Ornithodoros moubata,* a tick.

To jump-start the project, Geigy handed Burgdorfer a glass of sand he'd brought back from the Belgian Congo. "This is your material," Geigy said.

Looking into the glass Burgdorfer saw only the light brown granules, and nothing else. "Finally I picked up a pencil and swirled it through the sand," Burgdorfer explains. "There were the ticks—and, it followed, the spirochetes. Sometimes you have to shift perspective. Just because you don't see something at first, doesn't mean it isn't there."

To aid in that perspective, Geigy gave Burgdorfer special tools: a microscope to magnify the organisms and sharpen their contrast and surgical instruments for slicing ticks apart. Burgdorfer used eye scalpels to remove each tick's outer shell, exposing internal organs. He removed the organs with forceps of the sort used to repair Swiss watches.

Over the next three years, dissecting thousands of ticks and examining their organs under the microscope, Burgdorfer learned that spirochetes were ingested during feeding and eventually reached the midgut. There they persisted for a couple of weeks before rapidly multiplying

and disseminating to tissues throughout the tick. The disease was ultimately transmitted to humans by an ordinary bite.

But there was more. Geigy insisted his students immerse themselves in
the literature of whatever field they studied; in Burgdorfer's case, everything about spirochetal infection transmitted by ticks. Thus, Burgdorfer
was steeped in the very studies Steere had dismissed as essentially irrelevant to Lyme disease.

Based on that literature, Burgdorfer felt a disease that appeared to be a
ringer for Lyme had been described in Europe for almost a hundred years.
It was mentioned in the medical journals as early as 1883, when the German physician Alfred Buchwald described it as a red rash that ultimately
became transparent but never disappeared. It was described in 1902, when
physicians Karl Herxheimer and Kuno Hartmann coined the term acrodermatitis chronica atrophicans, or ACA. Chronica stood for chronic and
atrophicans stood for atrophy. Skin with ACA resembled wrinkled ciga-
rette paper, the researchers said. And a disease just like Lyme was reported
in 1909, when the Swedish physician Arvin Afzelius described a ringlike
rash that expanded at its border as its center cleared. Afzelius called the
migrating rash erythema chronicum migrans, later shortened to erythema
migrans, or EM. He suggested it came from the bite of an *Ixodes* tick.

The strange syndrome had already been described in the medical literature many times over when, in 1930, the dermatologist Sven Hellerström of the Karolinska Institute in Stockholm associated the peculiar
rash with central nervous system disease, specifically meningitis
(swelling of the brain's lining) and encephalitis (swelling of the brain itself). He speculated that the culprit was a spiral-shaped bacterium—a
spirochete—transmitted by ticks. Almost twenty years later, at the dawn
of the antibiotic age, Hellerström presented more findings at the forty-
third annual meeting of the Southern Medical Association in Cincinnati.
Not only did he connect the rash, the tick bite, and neurological disease,
he also reported on successful treatment with antibiotics. His findings
were published in the *Southern Medical Journal* in 1949.

Finally, in 1955, a German team provided the first indisputable proof
that the EM rash was caused by an infectious agent susceptible to penicillin. To do their study, the scientists removed pieces of skin from the
periphery of a patient's rash and transplanted it into three volunteers.
Within three weeks all three volunteers developed the typical EM rash.
In each case, treatment with penicillin resulted in the disappearance of
the rash within a few days.

By the time the 1960s rolled around, scientists had recognized ACA and EM as manifestations of the same disease. They had tied the rash syndrome to a spectrum of specific, objective symptoms, including Bell's palsy, meningitis, peripheral neuropathy (dysfunction in nerves located outside the brain and central nervous system, often presenting as buzzing, numbness, or pain), heart abnormalities, and even some cases of arthritis. And they had conducted successful treatment studies using not just penicillin but also tetracycline.

The first American physician to document what would soon be called Lyme disease came not from Connecticut, but Wisconsin. Rudolph Scrimenti, a dermatologist at the Marquette School of Medicine in Milwaukee, was drawn into the arena by a patient, a fifty-seven-year-old physician who had gone grouse hunting in October 1968 in north central Wisconsin. The patient, who recalled a tick bite at the site of what had become an expanding red rash, had been hospitalized for complaints of headache, malaise, and a dull, radiating pain over his right hip. But no one could find the source of the distress.

That's when Scrimenti entered the scene. As a dermatologist with rigorous training, Scrimenti knew that a migrating red rash had been described in Europe for nearly a century. In fact, ever since his student days, Scrimenti had admired the work of Sven Hellerström, who saw the skin as a window to complex disease. And so it was that, years later, when the grouse-hunter entered his office, Rudolph Scrimenti recognized the signs and symptoms of EM. Remembering that the Europeans—Hellerström and others—had successfully treated such patients with antibiotics, Scrimenti decided to do likewise. He treated his patient with intramuscular penicillin, and forty-eight hours later the patient was symptom-free.

Willy Burgdorfer, the brilliant disciple of Rudolf Geigy and an expert in spirochetes and ticks, was well aware of this complex history long before the Connecticut contingent—including Polly Murray, Allen Steere, Charles Ray Jones, and the naval doctors at Groton—had ever considered the concept of Lyme disease. Burgdorfer may have lived across the continent, in Montana, yet it seemed as if he'd been waiting for this moment in the sun.

Fresh from his training with Geigy in 1951, he'd taken an assignment in the United States, at the Rocky Mountain Labs in picturesque Hamilton, planning to stay only a year. But he fell in love with a secretary, Gertrude "Dale" See, and settled in for good. He married, purchased a home two blocks from the lab, had two sons, and became a U.S. citizen.

He even introduced soccer, his favorite childhood sport, to Hamilton, and for decades thereafter was greeted on the streets of the town by many of those he coached when they were boys.

All this offset a grueling work schedule, which often spanned the day from eight in the morning until after midnight. The long days and late nights provided passage through the doors of perception, allowing him to peer at his microbes and tick sections alone. "I made dissections during the day and sat at the scope at night," Burgdorfer says. It was still his job to swirl the sand with a pencil and conjure creatures out of nowhere. It was still his style to shift perspectives when something wasn't clear.

In this way he spent the next couple of decades happily, productively: discovering different disease patterns on either side of the river dividing the Bitterroot Valley in Montana, identifying pathogens in classified projects for the U.S. military, studying Rocky Mountain spotted fever with collaborators nationwide.

In 1981, while Steere and others hunted for the microbe that caused Lyme disease, Burgdorfer was collaborating with the New York State Department of Health on a different task: finding the ticks that spread Rocky Mountain spotted fever, responsible for eight deaths on Long Island in the preceding few years, alone. That October, two New York researchers, Jorge Benach and Edward Bosler, headed out to Shelter Island, in search of the tick that carried the spotted fever pathogen, a rickettsia, in hopes of stamping it out. They collected a batch of *Ixodes* ticks and shipped them off to Burgdorfer, who would slice them, dice them, and search for evidence of the disease.

Burgdorfer did not find evidence of the rickettsia that caused spotted fever in those Shelter Island ticks. But as he examined the ticks' blood under his microscope, he noticed the undulating movements of nematode worms.

For the nematodes to appear so freely in the ticks' blood, they would probably be found throughout the digestive tract, particularly the midgut. But when Burgdorfer dissected the ticks and examined the midgut under the microscope, no other nematodes could be seen. Finally, hoping for a better view, he readjusted his microscope as he had once twirled his pencil through the sand. With the perspective changed, his attention was captured by faintly stained, rather long, and irregularly coiled microorganisms that looked like spirochetes. Other tick tissues, from ovaries to salivary glands, were free of these spirochetal forms. As he watched the sluggish movement of the organisms, he remembered Hellerström's talk in Cincinnati in 1949. He felt sure he'd hit the jackpot—the elusive agent of erythema chronicum migrans in Europe and Lyme disease in the United States. One of the first things he did was call Benach. "Jorge," he said, "we have a hot potato on our hands."

Excitement pervaded Burgdorfer's lab that day. The whole world was searching for the cause of Lyme disease, and he believed that he had it right there. Within hours of the discovery he'd dissected 124 additional ticks and examined their contents. Sixty percent contained the novel spirochetes—only in the midgut, and nowhere else. It took a few more days for Burgdorfer to establish the presence of similar spirochetes in the midgut of the European sheep tick, *Ixodes ricinus*. The related borrelial species found in those ticks—eventually named *Borrelia garinii* and *Borrelia afzelii*—would join the Shelter Island spirochetes as the cause of European Lyme.

In the end, of course, researchers could not merely assume they had found the agent of Lyme disease. Specifically, they had to meet the burden of proof for attributing any given disease to a specific microbe, established at the dawn of the microbial age by the great German bacteriologist Robert Koch. Koch had set four conditions, and the nation's scientists now collaborated to meet them, one by one: The pathogen had to be present in all cases of the disease; it had to be isolated from an infected animal and then sustained in culture; if inoculated back into an uninfected animal, the germ would have to cause the disease; and finally, that microorganism would have to be isolated from newly infected animals and grown in culture again.

Aiming to meet the first condition, Benach contacted Edgar Grunwaldt, the Shelter Island physician who'd been diagnosing Lyme rashes and Montauk knee for twenty years. Grunwaldt had collected hundreds of blood samples from his patients, and quickly donated some to Burgdorfer and Benach. Testing the blood of the Shelter Island patients, they found antibodies made against the new spirochete in every one. That was condition number one.

Then Burgdorfer asked Alan Barbour, a Rocky Mountain microbiologist, to isolate the spirochete from the midgut of ticks and grow it out in culture, right in the lab. Spirochetes are so exquisitely adapted to their living hosts that it's generally difficult to grow them outside, in a petri dish or test tube. Barbour had already cultured another spirochete, *Borrelia hermsii*, in a medium created at the Baptist Memorial Hospital in Memphis by Richard Kelly, a pathologist, and then perfected by Herbert Stoener at Rocky Mountain Lab. Tweaking the solution, Barbour was soon culturing spirochetes in the so-called Barbour-Stoener-Kelly (BSK) medium, allowing Koch's second requirement to be met. (Barbour's medium and the strain he cultured in it were both ultimately distributed worldwide as crucial laboratory tools for studying and diagnosing Lyme disease. Use of that particular strain—called "B31" for Burgdorfer, Benach, and Barbour—as a lab standard has garnered criticism from those who say it is at the root of an especially arthritic form of Lyme disease, including Montauk knee, and can't possibly represent *all* the strains making patients sick, especially with more neurological forms of the disease.)

To meet Koch's third requirement—infecting healthy animals and causing the disease—the scientists placed infected ticks on the abdomens of laboratory rabbits and watched for signs of Lyme. All the rabbits developed circular rashes, and blood tests confirmed that the rabbits had generated antibodies to the spirochete. The results were published in the journal *Science* in 1982.

A final step remained: The spirochete, by now seen by the entire scientific community as the key to the disease, had to be cultured directly from the human host. While culturing spirochetes from ticks was now straightforward, culturing them from patients remained a challenge. Bernard Berger, a dermatologist at New York University, helped by studying his patients' Lyme rashes. Using silver stain, he and his colleagues were able to document spirochetes in the lesions, most often at the periphery. Taking things further, both Benach at Stony Brook and Steere at Yale managed, with great difficulty, to culture spirochetes from human blood and cerebrospinal fluid, satisfying Koch's fourth requirement and proving the spirochetal etiology of Lyme disease. The work was published in the *New England Journal of Medicine* in March 1983.

In a final flourish, one that Koch could not have imagined because he predated the discovery of DNA, microbiologist Russell Johnson of the University of Minnesota Medical School in Minneapolis analyzed the new spirochete's genome and proved it was novel, an entirely new species unlike any previously known.

In 1983, at the First International Symposium on Lyme Disease, held at Yale, a cabal of scientists met in a sequestered room to decide how the spirochete should be named. While a community like Lyme, Connecticut, would rather not lend its name to a disease, for a scientist there is no greater honor. In what was politics as usual in science, Russell Johnson remembers the phone calls asking for his support in the scientific clamor for the name. Some people thought the spirochete should be named after Burgdorfer, and others opted for Steere. Johnson thought it over, and nominated Willy Burgdorfer. Although there were some dis-satisfied customers in the room, the name was approved, and *Borrelia burgdorferi* was placed in the firmament of human disease.

The competition and animosity accompanying the discovery would dis-rupt Burgdorfer's once-copacetic career and peace of mind from that mo-ment on. As the person who discovered the spirochete, and the namesake of the disease, he found himself at the center of a firestorm. Patients at the end of their tether, with no place else to turn, would flip through the phone book and find his telephone number listed. They reasoned that the mi-crobe had his name on it, so he must know a thing or two. He could be reached at the lab, and someone calling the information operator in Hamilton could simply ask for him and get him at home. The calls were frantic and frequent, mostly from patients whose doctors had refused to continue antibiotic treatment beyond a certain point. Some people called at three A.M. because they just couldn't wait.

No, he did not agree that treatment should be stopped when the pa-tient still felt sick, he would tell the caller. He did not agree with what was going on. "I was the one who found the spirochete, and I felt re-sponsible for all of this," Burgdorfer says.

Burgdorfer's stance as a scientist sympathizing with patients when so many scientists were at odds with them emerged from his perspective, his particular point of view. His position was shaped as much by the pa-tients' experience as his fifty-year relationship with spirochetes—first *B. duttoni* and then *B. burgdorferi*—in the lab. His scientific instinct, every ounce of it, had coalesced to help him find the spirochete. Now those same instincts, that same feeling for the organism, told him that a piece of the puzzle remained lost.

It was a vision thing: "What does a spirochete look like?" Burgdorfer asks. "Most physicians say if you don't see helical forms, you don't have spirochetes, but the worldwide medical literature presents powerful evi-dence that spirochetes also assume sporelike forms, especially in re-sponse to stress like antibiotic." When the stress is removed, the spores, also called "cysts," convert back to spirochetes. This could explain why infection treated with antibiotic may survive.

Burgdorfer's work in the lab also helped him view borreliosis as a dis-ease of the brain. As long ago as 1952, his mentor, Geigy, had taught him that the best storage vessels for spirochetes were the brains of mice. "We infected baby mice with spirochetes, and when they were fully grown we removed their brains and fed them to new suckling mice." To keep a given spirochetal strain going, Burgdorfer would just feed the brains of one mouse generation to the next. While spirochetes sustained in a lab dish often mutated or lost their vigor, spirochetes stored in mouse brains remained plentiful and consistently infectious and strong. "Spirochetes have an organic tropism for the brain," Burgdorfer says. "That is consistent with the neuropsychiatric nature of patient complaints."

And there was something else: Like the patients on the phone, Burgdorfer had been buffeted by the same Lyme politics. He'd been working with a Lyme-infected rabbit one day at the Rocky Mountain Laboratories when some urine got into his eye. A few days later he developed a classic erythema migrans rash under his arm. Consulting the academic physicians he was working with, he was told to take penicillin because he clearly had Lyme disease. The rash disappeared but then returned three weeks later, so Burgdorfer was placed on the antibiotic tetracycline. That did the trick. The rash never came back.

But years later, when those same academicians were trying to squelch what they saw as undue anxiety over the illness, Burgdorfer's personal diagnosis was literally revoked. The problem was that someone in the press had gotten hold of the story and wanted to write it up. "What if patients start thinking they can get Lyme disease from urine?" a doctor asked Burgdorfer. Soon enough, old medical records from Burgdorfer's personal file were pulled from the void and his ancient lab results reviewed. It hadn't been Lyme disease after all, he was told. Someone had made a mistake: The antibody levels in his blood had been too low. The same physicians who diagnosed and treated him now claimed he'd been misdiagnosed. Recalling the episode, Burgdorfer sits back and laughs. "What was going on? Did I have Lyme disease or not?"

14

❖

The Chasm Widens

In another time and place, with other protagonists, the discovery of the spirochete might have been a light in the darkness, beckoning the way toward an answer, a cure. But with the discovery of *B. burgdorferi,* the chasm in Lyme only widened. The new spirochete undulated carelessly between two worlds, but few people could inhabit both. The first realm belonged to those on the ground, who experienced the late stages of the disease, that is to say, to the sickest patients and their treating physicians. The second belonged to those in the tower, the scientists, who endeavored to objectify in studies what the patients experienced subjectively, in their lives. The spirochete had burst forth, spawning not just one cosmos but two. The inverse of each other in every aspect, the two realms embodied opposite languages, opposite cultures, opposite histories, and opposite versions of Reality and Truth.

Charles Ray Jones of Hamden was validated in his hunch that Lyme disease was bacterial when Willy Burgdorfer of the NIH identified the spirochete at its root. Evidence in hand, some doctors at Yale began treating more aggressively, recalls Jones. And thus, when his patients became especially ill, Jones sent them on to New Haven. There, Yale doctors used heavy antibiotic artillery, including intravenous treatments administered over the course of months, to beat back the symptoms of Lyme. One child from Jones's practice had Lyme meningitis, and the Yale physicians gave her two months of intravenous antibiotics. When she remained ill, they gave her two months more. For that particular child, four months of treatment seemed to work.

But gradually things changed. As the eighties inched forward, the children coming to Jones's practice were increasingly sick. Often unrecognized and untreated by other physicians, they had progressed beyond the milder illness of his first patients, manifesting the full sweep of signs and symptoms meticulously recorded by Steere and many others as well. The disease could impact almost any organ of the body or the whole body in systemic fashion, Jones found. While many children showed up with the rash and arthritis, cognitive and neurological symptoms were increasingly prevalent. Children found it harder to focus or remember things, and many were too wiped out to get to school or even see their friends. A headache that never left was commonly reported. A few young patients went blind or deaf. Others suffered devastating psychiatric complications: otherwise inexplicable panic or violence, apparent autism, or the sudden onset of OCD.

Jones continued to treat these children with short-term oral antibiotics until, one day, a very ill teenage patient caused him to change his mind. Upon hearing that his two weeks of medication had come to an end, the boy, then fifteen but reportedly sick with Lyme since age ten, posed a question: "I'm getting better, but I'm not well yet, so why not just keep giving me the pills?"

Jones knew from experience that a complete recovery could be elusive for such children. So he agreed to the experiment, and the boy kept improving week in and week out. "It took three full years of treatment for him to become asymptomatic," Jones says, "but he has remained completely well."

After that, it became Jones's policy to treat not for an arbitrary number of days, but rather until all symptoms resolved, sometimes measured in weeks, sometimes years. One child who came to his practice blind had his vision return "one piece at a time" for years. "If I treated until every last symptom was gone, the child was cured."

In this fashion Charles Ray Jones treated from the saddle—a cowboy, other doctors called him—using observation, empirical deduction, and hands-on experience without formal studies to back him up. He still had his regular pediatric practice, of course, but as more physicians and parents sent Lyme children his way, the practice changed. "I was the country doctor on a tangent," he says, "and the tangent was Lyme."

⁘

As time passed, things changed at Yale as well. While Charles Ray Jones pushed the envelope, Steere and other Yale scientists involved in the basic research held the line. They were, after all, academics, and evidence-based medicine—proof generated through studies—was their stock and trade.

Yet in the end, Steere might have been no more objective than the patients. Carl Brenner, a Columbia University geologist who spent five years as patient representative on an NIH advisory committee for Lyme disease treatment studies and currently serves on the research board of the National Research Fund for Tick-Borne Diseases, thinks it's possible that the Yale team suffered from what scientists call "confirmation bias"—the tendency to search for or interpret new information in a way that confirms one's preconceptions. "Sometimes people see what they want to see," Brenner says.

Steere's initial belief that Lyme was viral—and thus invulnerable to antibiotics—jibed with the early results showing that two weeks of treatment barely worked at all. But in 1981, Burgdorfer's discovery of the spirochete, a bacterium, clearly threw a monkey wrench in the works. As with the spirochetal disease syphilis, antibiotics had to be the treatment of choice for Lyme disease. Dismissal of antibiotics no longer made any sense.

So Steere went back to the drawing board, and in the July 1983 issue of the *Annals of Internal Medicine* came out with something else. His new recommendation was based on three more years of data gathered from 1980 to 1982 as he treated patients for early Lyme disease, that is, the rash. The study sought to determine which of three antibiotics—penicillin, tetracycline, or erythromycin—might help the rash resolve most quickly. The researchers treated each patient with ten days of one of the antibiotics, and for those who relapsed, another ten days of the exact same drug. Then, following the patients prospectively, they waited to see which, if any of them, progressed to the arthritic or neurologic signs, or the wide range of other late manifestations of the disease.

Analyzing the new data, Steere now recommended ten or twenty days of one antibiotic—tetracycline. This, he contended, was the best treatment for Lyme disease; this, he suggested, brought a cure.

But many of those who examined the *Annals* study closely were disturbed: According to Steere's own data, almost as many patients reported remaining sick as in the treatment studies published prior to Burgdorfer's find. In light of that, claiming treatment success where once there had been failure appeared especially odd. *What had happened?*

The answer could be found in the study's fine print, under the subhead of *Methodology*: Steere had achieved his new "cure" rate by reorganizing his data and redefining what it meant to be cured.

In the earlier work, before the discovery of the spirochete, Steere had reported that many patients went on to suffer what he called "late manifestations" of Lyme disease—the severe arthritic and neurological signs as well as constitutional symptoms like headache and fatigue. Based on his theory that Lyme was viral and immunological, this had made sense.

But now, with the spirochete in the picture, with the root cause *bacterial,* the outcome didn't wash. If Lyme was caused by bacteria, after all, then one would expect antibiotics to bring a cure. So to cross the chasm between "treatment failure" and "treatment success" from one body of work to the next, Steere made a strategic change. He divided the "late manifestations" into two categories: "major" and "minor." The "major" late manifestations were true signs of Lyme disease, by Steere's reckoning. One such manifestation was "meningoencephalitis," marked by severe headache, stiff neck, and elevated white blood cell count, indicating infection. Another was recurrent arthritis with documented swelling.

The "minor" manifestations included facial palsy, an unusual heart rhythm, also known as tachycardia, and headache or joint pain. Fatigue, even severe fatigue, was labeled minor as was mental confusion and memory loss. In fact, except for a few designated disease signs that Steere measured as data points, almost every patient symptom, no matter how disabling or objective, was put in the minor group. All these, Steere theorized, were either post-infectious immune reactions or, more likely, unrelated to Lyme disease at all.

Once Steere divided the late manifestations into two groups, he was able to see his data in a new light. It was indisputable that when treatment with tetracycline was extended to twenty days, not a single rash patient with early disease went on to develop the "major" complications of Lyme disease, though minor complications were as abundant as ever, occurring in almost half.

Yale could declare twenty days of tetracycline a cure all they wanted. Patients who had Lyme disease, yet stayed sick after the treatment, and experts who read the fine print in Steere's new study, were distressed. The so-called minor late complications were far more disabling to many Lyme patients than the major ones, and rarely resolved with time.

As far as Carl Brenner is concerned, it was Steere's shifting definition of "treatment success" that set the stage for the later battle between academic researchers and clinicians in the field. "A patient with persistent headaches, pain and fatigue will, quite naturally, resent being characterized by his physician as a treatment success," he notes.

Why make such changes, then? Brenner thinks the Yale team had unwittingly violated one of the most important tenets of science by failing to eliminate experimenter bias and expectation from their experiments. At first the Yale scientists thought Lyme was caused by a virus incapable of responding to antibiotics, and reported high rates of treatment failure with many late manifestations of the disease. Later, after the spirochete was discovered, response to antibiotics was expected, and the researchers began reporting treatment success. But the only way they could manage to find consistent "success" where they had previously reported "failure" was to literally lower the bar for what they called a cure.

Steere's new distinction, Brenner felt, "created a massive dissonance between the researchers' so-called 'objective' findings and their patients 'subjective' experience. For the first time, the two groups were at odds over what constituted a positive result." In short, the change drove an impassable wedge between patients and the experts defining their disease.

So tortured was the logic that even scientists at Stony Brook, working with their own population of Lyme patients out on Long Island, were upset. When treated patients sustained intractable headache, disabling mental confusion, and profound fatigue, that was therapeutic failure in their book, not success. As the patients pouring into their new Lyme Disease Clinic began systematically failing treatment regimens recommended in Steere's publications, the doctors at Stony Brook determined that more had to be done.

Raymond Dattwyler, a clinical immunologist with an edgy aside for everything, was recruited by Stony Brook in the early 1980s from Harvard's Massachusetts General Hospital. Right from the start, the patients he saw were markedly different than those described by Yale; in fact he'd never seen the kind of chronic, refractory Lyme arthritis patient described by Steere. Instead, Dattwyler observed systemic infection driving neurological symptoms—the so-called minor problems of chronic headache, memory loss, and fatigue as well as "peripheral neuropathy," a condition marked by measurable damage to nerves outside the spinal cord and brain.

Ben Luft arrived at Stony Brook in 1984, having come from Stanford with a specialty in AIDS. A deep thinker with outside-the-box ideas he was adept at executing, Luft was just cautious enough when he spoke, just conservative enough in dress, to give the appearance of the company man when he was anything but. Once on Long Island, the tall, burly Luft, already a skeptic of dogma after serving on the AIDS frontline, also started seeing what were clearly Lyme patients who defied Yale's concept of the disease.

"At the time," recalls Luft, "the field was dominated by rheumatologists. I was an infectious disease person, and as such, I had a particular training and approach." Instead of focusing on immune reactions triggered by the infection, Luft was more prone to focus on the impact of the living organism, the spirochete itself. Instead of tracking the natural history of untreated disease, Luft had an interest in treating the infection aggressively enough to prevent it from progressing at all. The rheumatologists, it was apparent to him, had taken a different path, "gearing their treatments to the minimalist approach." This stood in stark contrast to Luft's scientific training in infectious disease, where most modern experts believed in a bit of overkill, the concept being that no pathogen— and no patient—be left behind.

Given the limits of testing, Yale couldn't *possibly* prove their treated patients were infection-free. Yet one line of investigation could shed some light on the situation: pharmacokinetics, a science devoted to the objective measurement of specific drug activity against specific pathogens in the test tube (in vitro) and in the body (in vivo).

To get the ball rolling, Luft reviewed research on the treatment of another spirochetal illness, syphilis, conducted at the dawn of the antimicrobial age. Back in the 1940s, researchers had been perplexed by the inability of a short course of penicillin to cure syphilis and entertained the notion that penicillin resistance was the cause. That theory was dispelled by Harry Eagle of Johns Hopkins University, who demonstrated that the syphilis spirochete, *Treponema pallidum,* divided slowly. Penicillin worked by preventing cell-wall synthesis in actively growing cells, and thus could do its job only while the organism was dividing. Penicillin had to be sustained at a killing dose for the entire time the division was taking place, about thirteen hours, or the organisms would survive.

Since *B. burgdorferi,* too, was a spirochete, Luft reasoned that the rate of division might be a factor here, as well. Indeed it was. Like *T. pallidum, B. burgdorferi* divided very slowly, requiring about eight hours for the process from beginning to end. If the dosage of antibiotics targeting this process fell below killing levels—"minimum inhibitory concentration," or MIC—at any point during the process, the organisms would survive and the infection would be sustained.

Over the next few years, in an effort to see if they could increase the number of patients who got well, the Stony Brook team altered the formula, changing the medications, pushing the doses higher, and stretching out treatment for longer periods of time: Using amoxicillin, they found they could achieve remission only if the body was saturated with the medicine at all times. With doxycycline, which worked by killing spirochetes directly whether dividing or not, they found they could achieve abatement of symptoms by spiking the dose high for a condensed period each day even if blood levels fell for part of the time as well. Their greatest achievement was the move to ceftriaxone (brand name Rocephin), an intravenous antibiotic that was a hundred times more active than penicillin in killing *B. burgdorferi* in the test tube and more effective with patients, too. As a result it became dominant in treatment for those with later stages of Lyme disease, and the drug of choice.

The Stony Brook crew did far better than the Yale group when it came to treating Lyme disease at virtually any stage. With extra weeks of treatment at higher dose, some 95 percent of early patients (those who came in with just the rash) recovered without going on to develop the devastating "minor late manifestations" reported by Steere. Stony Brook treatments were far more effective in the later stages, too. But when patients went untreated for a year or more after infection had taken hold, a disturbing number—some 15 or 20 percent in all—failed the treatment and stayed sick.

When patients meeting Stony Brook's expanded disease definition failed Stony Brook's new, more aggressive treatments, there was nothing more the doctors at Stony Brook could do. Like the Yale doctors, after all, they were university scientists whose treatments had to be backed by objective evidence of the most rigorous kind. They had tried to refine their diagnostic prowess and ramp up their treatments as far as their studies allowed, but eventually they exhausted their largesse. In fact, after a month or two of antibiotic therapy, Dattwyler felt that risk outweighed benefit for the group; for every patient additional antibiotic might help, he calculated, far more patients would get yeast infections, antibiotic-resistant infections, infections from the IV tubing, or even lose a gallbladder to the drugs.

Such fears were beside the point to patients with lives crushed by Lyme disease. For them, there was one more option. They could leave the bounded universe of evidence-based medicine, with all its strictures, and take a walk on the wild side. They could go east, to the Hamptons and the office of Joseph Burrascano, M.D.

15

❖

How the Lyme World
Split in Two

Arriving in East Hampton at the start of the eighties, his doctor credentials freshly minted, Joe Burrascano imagined himself maturing into a Marcus Welby kind of figure, "the sort of physician who takes care of children, and then the children of those children." In a moment of exuberance, he had even ordered for his new office waiting room a wall-sized mural of Hawaii, his favorite vacation spot; patients waiting their turn could enjoy the image of palm trees and surf, as if they were on vacation themselves.

Even in those early days, Joe Burrascano was aware of the local interest in ticks. He knew about Jorge Benach's investigation into Rocky Mountain spotted fever on nearby Shelter Island. From the moment he opened his practice he was puzzled by the stream of strange patients with inexplicable neurological symptoms. And then, like the rest of the medical community on Eastern Long Island, he learned that Willy Burgdorfer had used Shelter Island ticks and the blood of Shelter Island patients to explain the new disease called Lyme.

The nature of the problem really hit home for him after he got to know another doctor, Alan MacDonald, the Southampton Hospital pathologist. MacDonald explained that the system of straightforward magnification used in the ordinary light microscope was inadequate for biological specimens like spirochetes, which lacked contrast. Instead, to visualize spirochetes he was using another tool: a darkfield microscope purchased from Nikon for $40,000, in those days, a fortune. Using the souped-up scope, he displayed his specimens against a stark black background, scanning the field for spirochetes.

The tall, lanky MacDonald had a big scruffy beard and, except for a tie, looked like a Greenwich Village hippie. Naturally gregarious, he loved nothing more than regaling colleagues with jokes, often sprinkled with Yiddishisms. MacDonald felt excited to be at the epicenter of an emerging infectious disease, and had been thrilled when contacted by Jorge Benach, by then officially at Stony Brook, to track down Lyme.

Benach was eager to "play catch-up" with the crew at Yale and thought MacDonald could help. As a pathologist, it would be MacDonald's job to test for the new disease and identify the organisms under his fancy scope. Not only did MacDonald have the Nikon, he had "real Shelter Island spirochetes, gratis of Jorge." He obtained the recipe for Alan Barbour's famous growth medium, BSK, direct from Montana. "My material was home-grown, but state of the art," MacDonald says today. Soon he was culturing gallon-size vats of spirochetes in his Southampton lab.

As quickly as he could, MacDonald began testing patients for Lyme disease. First he took spirochetes from his personal stash and spread them on glass slides. Then he added a patient's blood. If the patient had been infected and the blood had antibodies to *Borrelia*, it would stick to the spirochetes on the slide. To measure the "stickiness," MacDonald treated each slide with chemicals that fluoresced when reacting with human blood, creating a soft, ethereal glow. If the slide fluoresced, then the patient was "positive" for Lyme disease. To see just how positive—how concentrated—the infection was, MacDonald would dilute the patient's blood: first in half, then in half again, all the way up to maximum dilution of one part blood to 8,000 parts solution. This was the lowest concentration, or titer, at which the slide might still glow.

Stoked by his ability to vet the new disease, MacDonald purchased a high-quality camera to go with the microscope, and soon had pictures of the arthritis, Bell's palsy, or rash of each Lyme patient who took his test. He collected "carousel after carousel of clinical slides" and, following his extroverted nature, created an educational exhibit, lecturing widely about Lyme to physician groups, rotary clubs, and more.

But then something happened to change MacDonald's future in Lyme forever. With a specialty in neonatal pathology, MacDonald happened to see a few Southampton babies who had, unfortunately, died in childbirth. "They were sent to me for autopsies as a matter of course because

I was the pathologist," he explains. He knew that syphilis, another spiro-chetal infection, had once been the most common cause of adverse out-come in pregnancy, frequently the explanation for a stillbirth. Syphilis wasn't as common anymore, but could the scenario be replaying in Lyme?

Whenever a dead baby arrived in pathology, MacDonald made sure to run some tissue, including placental tissue, through his "immunofluo-rescent" test. He was hardly surprised when some of it fluoresced with the same extraterrestrial glow as had the Lyme patients' blood. Then he took things further. Reading the worldwide literature on syphilis in En-glish, French, and German, he came to understand what Burgdorfer before him had pointed out: Spirochetes could uncoil and take on strange mor-phological forms—truncated strings, hooks, and rings; balls surrounded by tough, protective shells, known as cysts; and even granular arrange-ments that appeared like the dots and dashes of Morse code. Staining the fetal tissue with silver and viewing it under the darkfield, MacDonald didn't see many ordinary coiled spirochetes, but the odd shapes were abundant.

Could these forms be spirochetes?

To find out, he treated the tissue with special "monoclonal antibodies," molecules produced in the lab to bind to specific proteins, in this case, those of *Borrelia burgdorferi,* and nothing else. It turned out that when-ever the monoclonal antibodies made tissue glow, MacDonald was also able to see the odd forms under his darkfield scope. These were indeed the spirochetes, MacDonald guessed, but in altered form. The cysts, espe-cially, tantalized him: Could the hardened walls be protecting the *Borrelia* under adverse conditions (like antibiotic treatment) only to dissolve when the adversity was gone, permitting the patient to relapse?

By 1985, MacDonald had amassed what he deemed the world's largest autopsy collection of fetal death from Lyme disease and as a con-sequence, his slide show changed. No longer was his carousel stocked with pictures of swollen knees and rashes. Instead, when he boarded a plane for Vienna and the Second International Symposium on Lyme Dis-ease and Related Disorders in September of that year, he had a hundred slides of fetal tissue that had fluoresced with special dye or revealed strange forms under the darkfield, all of them suggestive, to him, of bor-relial infection in the womb.

At the conference MacDonald took no more than fifteen minutes to show his dead-baby slides, including slices of placenta, heart, liver, kid-ney, and brain. Each image hit the academic audience like a shot to the head. For scientists studying knees and rashes while trying to combat what they saw as patient hysteria, the suggestion that Lyme disease was a baby killer was blasphemy. Researchers like Steere and Dattwyler were incredulous. Studying the strange, truncated forms, even Jorge Benach wondered whether, rather than spirochetes, they could be mere artifacts—biological detritus, including cell parts, created by the staining process itself.

But MacDonald came away from the conference more convinced than ever that he was on to something. Listening to the speakers, he couldn't help but note repeated reference to "tertiary Lyme disease"—Lyme in the brain. From all his reading he knew that tertiary syphilis could cause dementia and all manner of neuropsychiatic disease. Could Lyme do the same?

"I couldn't wait to get a cab back to the airport. I wanted to get started," MacDonald recalls. In flight, he drew up a hit list of all the major neurological diseases where Lyme could play a role: Alzheimer's, stroke, Parkinson's, ALS.

Back at Southampton Hospital, he contacted Dr. George Glenner, founder of the well-known National Alzheimer's Disease Brain Bank at the University of California, San Diego, School of Medicine. Before long, MacDonald had become an affiliated Brain Bank investigator, and four intact Alzheimer's brains frozen on dry ice arrived by courier mail. He thawed the brains and took from each hemisphere the hippocampus—the horn-shaped centers of memory where Alzheimer's strikes first. These he put in vats of pure BSK culturing medium sent from Montana. After a month, he reports, the vats were swarming with spirochetes. When those spirochetes were coated on a glass slide and combined with either Lyme patient's blood or the special monoclonal antibody, the entire complex glowed—something that could happen only if the spirochetes were *B. burgdorferi*. "I grew spirochetes right out of the Alzheimer's brains," MacDonald says.

If Lyme in the womb was controversial, culturing *B. burgdorferi* from Alzheimer's brains appeared fantastical to scientists in the mainstream. If correct, the finding would imply that at least some Alzheimer's was actually Lyme disease—an extraordinary suggestion that amounted to outright heresy. Unfazed, MacDonald sent his report in to the *Journal of the American Medical Association* (*JAMA*) for publication. But it was quashed after a reviewer (MacDonald says he has reason to believe it was Steere) said he had never heard of spirochetes in Alzheimer's brains and suggested the culture had been contaminated. In the end MacDonald changed the label "Alzheimer's" to "dementia," and *JAMA* published his report in the form of a letter in October 1986.

In the Hamptons, it was Burrascano, not MacDonald, who actually treated patients. Hearing of MacDonald's results at a conference in 1987, it occurred to Burrascano that the bizarre, "lupus-like" symptoms he'd been observing might be due to Lyme disease. Shortly thereafter Burrascano recalled the patients with strange neurological symptoms. "Some were very pleasant little old ladies who were so confused they couldn't talk a complete sentence. Every week they were in with another strange ailment," he explains. Burrascano drew their blood and sent it off to MacDonald, who reported finding spirochetes in eighty-seven patients in all.

With MacDonald's guidance, Burrascano diagnosed the patients with Lyme disease, but he didn't know how to treat them. He had read the treatment studies from Yale, but like the Stony Brook researchers, found these guidelines left too many patients ill. So, working with the NYU dermatologist Bernard Berger, he decided to take a clue from early syphilis, which often required longer treatment at a higher dose. Burrascano and Berger pushed the outside of the envelope, treating Lyme disease patients for thirty days, but those patients stayed sick, too.

After attending a talk by Willy Burgdorfer, Burrascano lengthened the treatment further. "Willy had noticed that the ability to culture the spirochetes varied in a monthly cycle, and proposed that Lyme *Borrelia,* like relapsing fever, might wax and wane." Burrascano was seeing the waxing and waning of symptoms in his patients as well. Based on this observation, he decided to bracket the cycle with antibiotics, expanding his initial treatment timeline to six weeks. This step, too, he reports, increased the chance for success, with more patients able to kick not just the "major" manifestations of the disease, but the devastating "minor" ones, too.

It was around this time that researchers from Stony Brook contacted him. They needed patients for a study, and wondered if he could help out. "Sure," said Burrascano, more than happy to comply. The study was a comparison between treatment with twenty-one days of either amoxicillin (with another drug, probenecid) or doxycycline for early Lyme disease. After researchers analyzed the results, Ray Dattwyler informed Burrascano that both treatments were excellent. Yet sometime after this communication, Burrascano noticed that patients he had sent to participate were relapsing. He called Dattwyler on the phone and told him that the patients needed more treatment, that the cultures (Alan MacDonald's cultures) were turning positive.

As far as Burrascano is concerned, the episode marked the end of his relationship with Stony Brook and the start of all his professional battles to come. "It seemed as if I dug a knife into Raymond Dattwyler's heart the day I told him the patients were relapsing," Burrascano says.

Up until that point, the criticism from mainstream researchers had been directed primarily at MacDonald. But from that point forward, Burrascano, too, was labeled a quack. One story held that he had installed a spirochete-shaped swimming pool in his backyard.

If Burrascano was a pariah, his chronically ill patients were suspect, too. "I had a large group of Lyme patients who were getting better with long-term treatment, but I needed to prove it," he says. So in 1988, in the aftermath of his disagreement with Stony Brook, Joe Burrascano closed his East Hampton office for a week, placing each employee in a private exam room with instructions to analyze a stack of charts, 733 in all. Results of the analysis contradicted assessments from Stony Brook and Yale: A patient with uncomplicated Lyme disease who had been sick for less than a year required, on average, four months of oral antibiotic treatment to get well, according to Burrascano's data. If the case was especially complex, or if the patient had gone undiagnosed and untreated for over a year, longer treatment was required.

"Much longer treatment," Burrascano found. Using oral antibiotics at doses exceeding those provided at Yale and even Stony Brook, 17 percent of these late-stage patients got well in the first month and remained so. Another 20 percent got well in the second month. There would be a plateau between the fourth and sixth month, at which point 67 percent of the patients, in total, recovered.

"But that would be it," Burrascano says. If a patient remained ill six months after commencement of treatment, only intravenous antibiotics would do the trick. "First we did three weeks of Rocephin, and then four weeks, and then six weeks," Burrascano says. "At the end of the treatment, virtually every patient was negative on Alan MacDonald's culture. But one month later, they all started to relapse; when they did, Alan MacDonald used the darkfield to confirm the cause as Lyme.

"One patient was an elderly woman I'd known for years," says Burrascano. "She started to get sick when she was about seventy-two, at first in a vague, neurological way. But she eventually developed full-blown Alzheimer's disease. This was a woman who used to take care of her whole family, was celebrated for her great meatball recipe, among other things. Yet now she couldn't take care of herself. She had to be fed and dressed and cleaned, and was virtually a vegetable. On a hunch I sent her blood to MacDonald. She was negative on the conventional tests, but in his culture she was positive. So I admitted her to the hospital and put her on intravenous Rocephin. I remember very distinctly walking down the hall in the ward where she was—and the delight of seeing her walk down the hall, too. This was a woman who had been bedridden and couldn't speak. 'What are you doing?' I asked her. She said, 'I'm going to the refrigerator to get my yogurt.' It floored me. After ten days on Rocephin, a woman whose Alzheimer's had seemed so advanced she was a virtual vegetable, could walk and remember to get her yogurt, too.

"She got a month of Rocephin in the hospital and we released her," says Burrascano. "She was almost 100 percent normal so she went back to driving and taking care of the family. The following year the 'Alzheimer's' seemed to return so we put her right back in the hospital and gave her antibiotics again. Once more she recovered completely— but with a personality change." She was mentally intact, could drive and take care of her family, and even balance a checkbook. But now she appeared to have a clarity and attunement to her inner life that she'd previously lacked. Her husband had been abusing her for years, she told friends. This time around, imbued with heightened motivation and energy, she divorced him and picked up and moved to Texas.

Patients appeared to benefit, but it all came to a crashing halt for Burrascano a few months later, when MacDonald, in the aftermath of a divorce, decided to start a new life, too. He halted his Lyme research and, following in the footsteps of the cured "Alzheimer's" patient, ultimately moved to Texas himself.

While Alan MacDonald had left the Lymelands for safer ground, Joe Burrascano and his chronically ill patients lumbered on. His clinical study of the 733 patients, conducted in 1988, stood in stark contrast to findings at Yale and Stony Brook. Burrascano understood that no one treatment was a panacea for all patients, yet he was often willing to try something new if he deemed it safe. In the end, he felt, his study supported his empirical style of treatment: By customizing therapy for each individual patient, Joe Burrascano was able to help many of those in the intractable 20 percent get well.

But despite the urgency of the results, there was a fatal flaw: It had all been confirmed by Alan MacDonald's diagnostic techniques, widely dismissed by the mainstream. With MacDonald no longer present to defend the results or reproduce them, the study was unpublishable in any medical journal refereed through the process of peer review. He could do more research in the future, Burrascano knew, but for now these particular data and this group of patients would march forward in Lyme's shadow land— figures in chiaroscuro, motioning wildly on the cave wall of proof that might have been and delivery that might have come.

Convinced he had hit upon essential truths nonetheless, Burrascano— by now infamous for treating chronic Lyme patients—decided to write up his findings. So it was that Joseph Burrascano, the country doctor from East Hampton, incorporated the results of his doomed study and his expanding clinical experience into his *Diagnostic Hints and Treatment Guidelines for Lyme Disease.* Each year he updated the guidelines, photocopied them at his own expense, and sent them by U.S. mail to physicians calling for advice.

By 1990, Joe Burrascano's dream of becoming the Marcus Welby of East Hampton had been shattered for good. In its place he had acquired the fractured legacy of the absent pathologist, Alan MacDonald, and a practice of chronically ill patients, long since rejected by mainstream practitioners and now clamoring (beneath a fading panorama of Hawaii) for his help.

16

⁘

Lost in the Ruins:
The Infestation of the Suburbs

Before I realized our environment was making us sick, I viewed the natural beauty around me as a gentle, beneficent luxury, a reward for my success. After I understood how tick-borne disease had derailed our lives, it was as if, like Willy Burgdorfer, I had swirled a pencil through the sand, changing my perspective and evoking the resident evil beneath. Before Lyme, I threw parties on my forty-foot deck, going out at dusk to barbeque skewers of mushrooms and steak, all the while dazzled by another red sunset beyond the pines. After Lyme, I woke up at dawn and, venturing out on my forty-foot deck, saw twenty deer grazing in my yard. I'd clang my pots loud, making them bolt and run. Before Lyme I hiked deep into the woods, smelling the cool moist breath of pine needles and moss. After Lyme I hesitated even stepping on the grass in Chappaqua without high socks and boots, my suburban version of the Hazmat suit. What had once seemed pristine now felt toxic and ruined.

Eventually I understood it wasn't only my perspective that had altered, but the ecosystem itself. The night I recognized the magnitude of the change I was driving with my husband and sons outside Ithaca, New York, on a much-needed getaway to Niagara Falls. They were asleep, and I was at the wheel. It was shortly after midnight and, although I was on a highway, I traveled slowly to navigate in fog. Whenever the road rose, the fog seemed to lift and I could see clearly. Whenever the road dipped, the fog deepened so that I could see only a few feet ahead.

I was already steeped in a sense of the surreal when a huge brown buck hurtled through the fog toward our car.

I was in a dip of the road and the fog was dense, but I could see enough to grasp that the buck, at warp speed, would strike the window near Mark's head. So I swerved blindly into the fog. My gamble worked. Instead of crashing through the car's side window the buck exploded onto the hood, then ricocheted across the highway as the headlights illuminated a gentle rain of blood.

All this jolted my family to wakefulness and though the danger was past, they started to scream. No, we did not collide with an SUV, I explained. It was a deer, bigger and faster than anything we'd seen in Chappaqua, by now hundreds of miles to the south. With the engine grinding, we made our way to town.

In the morning we stepped out of the motel room to take a look. The entire front and side of our bulky Dodge Caravan had been demolished. The hood was smashed in so far the van was snub-nosed. And pieces of the deer—not just skin and hair, but bits of limbs, entrails, and organs—stuck out of the car's crevices. Other parts of the deer had been pulverized and coated the vehicle with a thick, beige sludge. We got the Caravan to a body shop, and expected the mechanics to cringe at the carnage. But they had seen it all before. "We get these every day," the shop owner said.

The folks at the rental car place, where we went for a vehicle to tide us over while the Caravan was in repair, were equally nonchalant: "A lot of people rent because their car gets smashed up by a deer," the clerk said, making conversation. "They're back an hour later when another deer totals the rental car, and they need an exchange."

The explosion of deer throughout America's suburbs represents environmental mismanagement on a continental scale, but it wasn't always this way. The last time the continent was in balance, the Indians were in charge. Sculpting the land over millennia, they created spacious parklike arenas for roaming herds of antelope, buffalo, and deer—along with their natural predators, the wolves, panthers, and bears. The Indians' primary tool in terra-forming North America to create this exquisite balance was fire, which burned the underbrush and stimulated the growth of grazing grass. The grass fed the animals, including the deer, that the Indians caught in the hunt. With natural predators keeping the deer and other species in check, balance was maintained.

The balance was threatened when the Europeans arrived. In 1620, when the Pilgrims landed at Plymouth Rock, they planted their wheat in a cornfield the Indians had abandoned the year before. A year later the Pilgrims celebrated Thanksgiving and judged that life was good. Yet abandonment of the fields represented, for the Indians, a tragic end. The cornfield had been abandoned because the Indians were sick with diseases brought by the Europeans—measles, chicken pox, and the mumps—to which they had never before been exposed.

After thousands of years in equilibrium, the continent was about to slide into chaos, and for the Indians, its longtime guardians, two factors were at work. First was disease, decimating entire families and tribes. Second was the arrival of iron, useful for making tools. The Indians had to barter for the iron, and the currency came from leathers and furs acquired on the hunt. The more the Indians hunted, not just for food but for extras, the further they stepped outside their ethic of sustainability and the sparser the animal populations became. Aware that they had betrayed the environment but unaware of microbes, they reasoned that the animals themselves had placed a curse on them, accounting for the plague of disease. With entire communities wiped out, they took revenge on the animals, by 1650 obliterating much of the large game remaining in the eastern part of the United States.

Along with the obliteration of big game came the deforestation that occurred as Europeans farmed. The process of deforestation was completed with the arrival of the railroads, which required wood for ties, and the growth of the iron industry, which razed great tracts of land in its incessant search for coal.

By 1800, much of the East Coast was denuded of trees. Yet there was one exclusive domain in the eastern United States where forests and wildlife remained timeless and lush: islands isolated enough to escape the Indians' intensive management and the ecological scourge that came next. The most notable were the Elizabethan Islands, including Martha's Vineyard and Nantucket off the coast of Massachusetts, Block Island off the coast of Rhode Island, and Shelter Island and Plum Island off the coast of New York.

For hundreds of years the Elizabethan Islands had been owned by the Forbes family, the Brahmins of Massachusetts. Throughout the centuries of destruction, the Forbes had protected these islands. In the 1800s and early 1900s, when most people were deprived of contact with nature, the Forbes and their privileged friends—Teddy Roosevelt, Ulysses S. Grant, and Daniel Webster, to name a few—basked in the forest primeval and hunted in the only place there was anything left to shoot.

Just when it seemed as if the Elizabethan Islands might be the last refuge of nature, the pendulum swung again. With the building of the Erie Canal and the completion of the railroads came access to the superior farmland of the western plains. People slowly abandoned the farms of the East. At the same time, new technologies reduced the demand for coal, eliminating the deforestation that went along with it. Slowly the forests returned. In 1860, just 27 percent of Connecticut was forested. By 1910, forest covered 45 percent of the state and, in 1965, 63 percent was covered by a canopy of trees. Of course, the new landscape looked nothing like the continental parks the Indians had sustained. Instead, the state of Connecticut and the rest of the reforested Northeast began to resemble the unruly wilderness of the islands off the coast.

By the time I traveled the northeastern roadways in the 1970s en route to college and then graduate school in upstate New York and Massachusetts, forest surrounded me, but deer were still sparse. Residents of the newly forested lands had missed the deer and shipped them in from Nantucket, Martha's Vineyard, and other Elizabethan Islands. But the explosion in numbers would require more human error, and take more time.

As the seventies gave way to the eighties, as cities emptied into suburbs and then exurbs, Americans increasingly built their homes at the edge of the expanding forests. With natural predators gone, deer and other species that thrived at the forest's edge proliferated in close proximity to our homes. The deer population multiplied every year, until, by the 1990s, a paradigm shift had occurred. It was a new world. Driving the Lymelands from Westchester County in New York to Cape Girardeau in Missouri, I saw the new order everywhere: the large splatters of blood covering multiple lanes of a highway, the deer splayed on the shoulder or, if especially recent, straddling the center of the road.

The human icon for the shift was the yellow diamond-shaped traffic sign with the happy leaping deer. Today, virtually ubiquitous along suburban roads throughout much of the United States, the sign communicates the danger we pose to the unwitting deer, but not the hazard we face ourselves. The signs do not explain that there will be more roadkill, deer and human, because the large bucks, graceful does, and clusters of spindly fawns no longer hang back in the woods.

The white-tailed deer (species name *Odocoileus virginianus*) now live among us: more than 250,000 in Maryland; about 800,000 in New York; in Pennsylvania, a whopping 1.3 million alone. Nationwide, the deer population has increased from about 500,000 in the early 1900s to some 30 million today. Like mice, they are "edge species," thriving best on the rich nutrients of low brush and fertilized lawn so generously provided by our suburbs, but requiring, as well, the cover of the dense woods they abut. Where woods are continuous, few deer are found—but where woods are fragmented, in our suburbs, in my Chappaqua neighborhood, deer abound.

For a resident of Chappaqua, the ultimate deer environment, it was possible to get up close, and I did just once. The deer I sidled up to harbored ticks by the hundreds in the comfortable folds of its head and neck, and especially about the ears. It was from deer and other large mammals that most adult ticks obtained a blood meal, and thus the ability to lay eggs en masse.

In a very real sense, Lyme is a disaster of our own design. The new American concept of carving suburbs from forest has provided deer with an ideal habitat—possibly the best deer habitat in the history of time. The same woods contained the smaller mammals, the mice, chipmunks, and shrews that harbored the spirochetes themselves, keeping a reservoir of infection alive. Looking around me, at the woods and cul-de-sacs of Chappaqua, I realized its planners had created a Lyme incubator. With its fragmented forest and well-stocked gardens and yards, with its abundant wildlife and systematic denial (not even a warning sign could be found in the town's many parks), Chappaqua was a haven for *Borrelia* and a hazard to us.

By the time I killed a buck outside Ithaca, New York, the creation of the Lymelands was complete.

PART TWO

THE LYME DIASPORA

Everybody must get stoned.

—Bob Dylan

17

⁂

Mutts Like Us:
Lyme Tests and Tribulations

Chappaqua, New York, 2000

Mark and I were so concerned about Jason that we'd barely paid attention to our own faltering health. Yet after Jason began improving with antibiotics in the summer of 2000, we had to agree: We probably suffered from less advanced, but still draining versions of the same disease. Though I never took a day off from work, I had functioned for years through an avalanche of impediments. By 1994, a migraine with nausea had become my steady companion. I had intermittently sore and swollen knees, and the buzzing in my left hand was so intense my fingers sometimes formed a claw. My eyes, testing at 20/20 for most of my life, had begun a sudden, precipitous decline. Often my mother would ask me why I didn't get prescription glasses, but I refused: Since my vision fluctuated so dramatically from day to day in the course of its downward spiral, I preferred the series of off-the-shelf eyeglasses in a range of magnifications I purchased from Rite Aid. In that way, at little expense, I could use the "prescription" that suited me most at any given time.

Most disturbing was a strange inability to focus and think. I was under a publishing contract to write a book with the psychiatrist Thomas Verny on new findings in brain science. It was ironic: As I endeavored to write about the brain, my own brain was shrouded in fog. As days turned to months and I got little done, Verny grew increasingly concerned. I told him that Jason was sick, but I did not explain that I, myself, could not comprehend most of the material he had sent along for inclusion in our book.

Mark, meanwhile, was teetering at the brink of professional disaster. He'd spent twenty years writing for national magazines and health foundations in New York City, yet now was so blocked he was in danger of losing his job as editor in chief of the newsletter *Bottom Line Health*. His memory, previously detailed and precise, had become so spotty he had trouble following the train of a simple story. His physical symptoms were blatant: An ace amateur tennis player, he used to run and pivot his way through the weekends, but now his balance was so poor he continually walked into walls and cabinets, smashed his elbows going through doorways, and tripped on his way up or down stairs. Inexplicably, he had to urinate throughout the night, making it hard for him to sleep for more than an hour at a time. He was strangely irritable and quick to anger. His neck often crackled so loudly that, getting up close to him, it sounded like popcorn microwaving in his head. He said that it felt like carbonated water was bubbling inside.

The two of us still cared for our kids, still worked and paid the bills—we were pictures of robust health compared to Jason, but we were still sick. We were also at a terrible disadvantage: We both lacked the absolute "proof" of Lyme disease in the form of a rash or CDC-positive blood tests that our family physicians at the Mount Kisco Medical Group required before they would actually treat.

In the end, we sought treatment from a nurse practitioner working out of a storefront office across from Chappaqua's favorite watering hole, Starbucks, right on the main drag. When you thought about it, she was as natural to Chappaqua as its medical massage parlors, as native as Lyme disease itself. A fixture in town, her daughter went to the public school and her SUV, sporting the personal license plate TICK BITE, broadcast its ominous message to the ranches and colonials along the peaceful country roads. Considered a skilled practitioner by the reckoning of the Lyme patient community, our nurse had a small clientele sent from a handful of Westchester M.D.s, physicians who rejected the mainstream mantra on Lyme but would not assume the professional risk of treating beyond the guidelines themselves. We were lucky we landed on her stoop. She treated us skillfully yet cautiously. And most important, despite our equivocal test results, she understood that we were sick.

While Jason's test for Lyme disease had been off-the-charts positive at a standard commercial lab, Mark and I had more modest results. Equivocal antibody patterns, interpreted by most neighborhood doctors as "negative" for Lyme disease, often constituted the best level of lab evidence a Lyme patient could muster, no matter how sick he felt and how real the disease. Some of the most conservative researchers I interviewed would later tell me that in a place so infested, a place like Chappaqua, these partial results on top of disease signs were potent indicators of infection. If subsequent tests showed rising antibody levels or increasing numbers of bands, the experts told me, that was evidence of infection, even if patients didn't meet the CDC cutoff. Moreover, since the standard tests were indirect, measuring antibody reaction to infection instead of infection itself, they couldn't prove the organism was still present. So it was the physician's clinical judgment that mattered most.

But Westchester county doctors, unnerved by the controversy, would have none of it. Instead, most of them deferred to the absolute decree of "positive" or "negative" stamped on a lab sheet by large commercial facilities like LabCorp or Quest. The tests screened for the specific antibody pattern required by the CDC for surveillance; patients who failed to mount the complete response were rubber-stamped "negative," or sometimes, "equivocal," and routinely sent packing.

For patients like us—Lyme's mutts—equivocal blood test results, summarily dismissed, could mean a life sentence. You could wander the diagnostic desert with headache, foggy thinking, profound fatigue, and debilitating pain, the sensation of an electric current through your arms and cotton in your brain, yet be told you lacked evidence for any organic ill. How easy it was to wash their hands of us, tell us we were stressed, just imagining our illness, how simple to insist our blood work discounted us from any treatment for Lyme.

Few people understood how misleading these commercial Lyme disease tests could be. By the summer of 2000, when Mark and I sought diagnosis, labs used a two-step method to analyze antibodies formed against spirochetes in human blood. The first step was an inexpensive, purportedly sensitive *screening* test to see if Lyme was even possible. Only if you passed this first test could you go on to the second step, a more costly, far more specific *confirmatory* test aimed at weeding out the many "false positives" said to be found by the screen.

The tests could miss patients at any stage of disease. First of all, large numbers of patients couldn't mount a measurable antibody response for up to six weeks after a tick bite. Stony Brook scientists, moreover, found that patients exposed to antibiotic right after a tick bite could have their immune response so blunted they might elude detection forever, no matter how much the spirochete had spread. In other patients antibodies stuck to proteins (or antigens) from the spirochete in so-called immune complexes. Antibodies bound in complexes couldn't attach to the test substrate, causing many such patients to go undiagnosed. Other times, common strains of the spirochete simply lacked all the proteins the test screened for.

And in patients with neurological forms of Lyme disease, immune response was sometimes quieter, at risk for slipping through the cracks. The Stony Brook researchers shed light on the problem while studying the potential of what was, at the time, a new antibiotic, Zithromax, shown to be highly effective against the spirochete in the test tube. To test Zithromax for treatment in humans, Ben Luft and team split 246 Lyme rash patients into two groups. The first group was treated with three weeks of the old standby, amoxicillin. The second group was treated with a week of the newer Zithromax (plus two weeks of placebo so that no one would know which treatment arm they were in).

The study documented what doctors have long since accepted: 20 days of amoxicillin will cure most (but not all) early Lyme. Seven days of Zithromax, by contrast, proved a poor treatment, overall. Six months after the study's end, just 4 percent of the amoxicillin patients had relapsed or failed the treatment, while four times as many—16 percent—of those treated with Zithromax remained ill.

The real bounty from Luft's Zithromax study came from a side question: Would the strength of a given patient's individual immune response have any impact on cure? As it turned out, it did.

It was hard to ask the question with the amoxicillin group, of course, because the antibiotic worked so well that virtually every patient was cured.

But in the Zithromax group, with an abundance of treatment failures, the scientists were able to tell how individual immune response played a role. As it turned out, the treatment failures overwhelmingly were those with immune responses so low that they literally failed the blood test for Lyme disease. This suggested, says Luft, that "a strong, early immune response plays a role in limiting the disease, but also, that it is precisely those without a strong immune response—the seronegative patients who do not test positive on ELISAs and Western Blots—that may be most sick."

For all these reasons, in each step of the testing process, real Lyme patients were missed. Take the screening test: Called ELISA (for enzyme-linked immunoabsorbent assay), this test consisted of ruptured spirochetes that had been coated on a plate. Infected patients generated antibodies to the spirochete, the concept went, so when their blood washed over the plate, naturally it would stick. An enzyme that made human blood change color was added to the plate, and the more intense the color, presumably the worse the Lyme.

Presumably was the operative word. Patients with other infections—syphilis, mononucleosis, even AIDS—could light the Lyme ELISA, sending a false alarm. But when it came to Lyme disease, ELISA tests on the market actually *lacked* sensitivity. The problem was undisputed, documented beyond doubt in the medical peer review. In fact, even patients with advanced disease and high levels of antibody failed the Lyme ELISA between 9 and 69 percent of the time depending on the laboratory used. Stony Brook researchers said that patients with high levels of Lyme antibody, including those who later passed the far more specific confirmatory test, failed the screening test some 30 percent of the time.

As hard as it was to register a positive on the screen, *I* did. My ELISA, conducted at Stony Brook, was sky-high, four times the level needed to pass me on to the second stage of testing, the confirmatory Western blot.

Yet the Western blot, too, missed many patients with Lyme. In this test the spirochete's proteins were separated by weight and spread out on paper, with the lighter proteins at bottom and the heavier ones up top. If you'd been infected and had generated antibodies to Lyme, then a horizontal line, or "band," would form wherever a given antibody and the protein it targeted matched up on the sheet. A couple of weeks after a tick bite you needed two of three specific bands to pass the Western blot for Lyme. (This was called the immunoglobin M, or IgM, response.) A month or more after the bite, you had to register positive on five of ten designated bands. (This was the immunoglobin G, or IgG, response.)

I was out of luck. Presumably I'd been infected for years, yet my Western blot had only *four* of the requisite bands, indicating four antibodies to the spirochete. They were good for nothing. "Not Lyme," the local doctor said, leaving me to deal with my migraines and traveling joint aches, my clawed fingers and tingling arms and mind-numbing fatigue as if, at age forty-five, these were the normal consequences of age.

If I was a mixed breed, Mark was a mongrel. He failed ELISA utterly. Allowed to do a Western blot anyway, he came up with two paltry bands. Never mind that he'd lost his talent for words, not to mention his balance. "It's a psychological problem," a doctor at the Mount Kisco Medical Group told him to account for the dizziness and fog. If Mark was tipping over and walking into walls, if his neck crackled like Rice Krispies, well, maybe some talk therapy would tone him down and set him straight.

It was only years later, when Mark was tested at Stony Brook, that we learned he had the stuck-together immune complexes, explaining his poor results and supporting his diagnosis of Lyme disease. But Lyme patients didn't need immune complexes to fail the Western blot. The CDC-approved pattern had been derived from a single strain of the spirochete, while there were hundreds of *B. burgdorferi* strains with varied protein coats worldwide. Because the spirochete's coat could vary from strain to strain, so could the resulting antibodies and banding patterns, not to mention disease presentation, leaving untold numbers of patients out of the diagnostic loop.

Adding insult to injury, two critical antibodies produced by many late-stage Lyme patients (including one so specific its target protein was the active ingredient of a new Lyme vaccine) weren't included in the CDC's list of approved bands. The CDC said that the bands, while true markers of infection, were discounted simply because those who tested positive were positive without them—so why bother putting them in? Critics insisted the bands were important evidence for late-stage patients like me, and suggested they'd been removed to clear the way for LYMErix, the controversial Lyme vaccine made from OspA.

Insight comes from Phillip Baker, who went from director of the Lyme program at NIH to official spokesman for the mainstream viewpoint as director of the American Lyme Disease Association, or ALDF. Baker was not present in 1994 when the current Western blot pattern was chosen, *first* for the vaccine trials and months later for diagnosing the disease in the public at large. But he comments that the decision would surely have reduced confusion where the vaccine was concerned. "Antibodies against OspA would have presented problems in diagnosis when the LYMErix vaccine was being used. Since LYMErix was an OspA-based vaccine, all vaccinated people would have been OspA positive. Thus, one would not be able to distinguish a vaccinated from an infected individual based on that criteria," Baker says. (Since OspA and B were linked on the same DNA strip, removing one required removing the other in the manufacture of the Western blot.)

It turned out that I had OspA *and* OspB on my Stony Brook test. If only those bands had been tabulated as significant, I would have had six positive markers instead of four, putting me over the top. If only they'd been included, I, too, could have joined Jason on the elite list of real Lyme patients on record at the CDC.

How many true Lyme patients actually failed these imperfect tests? According to a critique from the International Lyme and Associated Diseases Society (ILADS), a group of physicians with less restrictive views, the CDC's two-tiered approach misses more than 40 percent of the patients. A year after the tick bite, 50 percent of patients with later stage disease routinely slip through the cracks.

But the ILADS doctors aren't the only critics. According to the peer-reviewed journal *Mayo Clinic Proceedings*, "The tests are prone to false-negative and false-positive results and can be misleading, especially early in the course of the disease. . . . Because serologic [blood] testing is not 100 percent sensitive or specific, some people with Lyme disease will not have confirmatory laboratory results."

The most comprehensive review of the tests comes from Johns Hopkins and a paper published in the *Journal of Clinical Microbiology* in 2005. Working with patients from Pennsylvania and Maryland, the Hopkins scientists studied state-of-the-art serology—ELISA and Western blot—along with polymerase chain reaction (PCR) tests for *B. burgdorferi* DNA. Not surprisingly, the Hopkins scientists found they could culture spirochetes from the erythema migrans rashes of early Lyme disease patients with a high degree of reliability. But they found other test methods wanting: For instance, when the standard, two-tier method recommended by the CDC was used on patients with other laboratory evidence of Lyme disease, it was positive between 45 and 77 percent of the time. For those patients proven to be culture positive—the incontrovertible gold standard for any diagnosis of Lyme—8 percent still tested negative on the blood tests. As for PCR tests searching blood for borrelial DNA, the Hopkins researchers report these are so poor that they rarely pick up otherwise-confirmed Lyme disease at all. The researchers concluded that the best diagnostic results come from using all the tests, in aggregate, because "no single test . . . achieves a high rate of diagnostic sensitivity."

Even Andrew Levin, founder and president of Immunetics, the Cambridge, Massachusetts, company that manufactures the Western blots used by commercial labs, has his doubts. Suspecting the CDC pattern was overly rigid and prone to miss cases, he'd obtained samples of validated patient blood and had them analyzed by a computer program built with help from scientists at the Massachusetts Institute of Technology. Using a small NIH grant to develop his system, Levin showed the presence of several antibody patterns, of which the CDC's was just one—and not the best one, at that. "If the two-tier criteria had been the best possible criteria," notes Levin, the computer program "would have taken us to it. But it did not. A number of other patterns emerged as the statistical front runners, instead."

Surveying the limitations of the tests, Stony Brook scientists suggested the best way to diagnose Lyme disease might be to look not at a single test, but at changes in *sequential* tests over time. They saw signs of positivity in rising antibody levels over subsequent ELISAs or the flowering of bands on Western blots conducted over months. But it was the rare pediatrician or family practitioner who understood these concepts and could follow suit. Instead, it was the CDC formula that stuck.

It was this fuzzy universe that enveloped Mark and me as we trekked each week to downtown Chappaqua and the treating nurse we called "Tick Bite." A small, feisty, dark-haired woman who was a ringer for Sally Field, Tick Bite had gotten her Lyme training in the offices of Kenneth Liegner and Charles Ray Jones. She'd acquired the esoteric skills of the LLMD over several years and had then moved out on her own. Sifting through our test results and ordering others, she found ample evidence in us for Lyme: It wasn't just our residence at the heart of the epidemic in Chappaqua and our constant exposure to ticks, but also our symptoms that informed her. The mainstream doctors had said Mark's confusion and my fatigue, Mark's dizziness and my migraine, had nothing to do with Lyme disease, but Tick Bite disagreed.

Slowly, and in steps, she treated us. For Mark the prescription was doxycycline, just two small pills a day. I was given amoxicillin at a dose Tick Bite deemed high enough to reach my brain.

At first we just got worse. It was the die-off of the spirochete coursing through our blood, causing the temporary immune riot that experts called a Herxheimer, Tick Bite said. My herx was so severe that after a few days of antibiotic I took to bed; every joint ached, my left hand formed a claw that couldn't unclench, and the current cranked up so high it felt like every nerve ending was electrified to the root. I felt the sensation of "cotton" pushing out of my extremities, especially my hands and my head. My migraine flared so that it felt like a drill in my brain, revving a tidal wave of nausea in my gut. I tried to stand up, but my muscles were too weak. Like Jason, I was bent. It lasted almost a week.

Then the illness subsided and I started to improve. Slowly the cotton thinned and the drill in my brain quieted, my claw straightened out, and I could get out of bed and walk. Several weeks after starting the antibiotic amoxicillin (supplemented, after a while, with Zithromax) I experienced a dramatic, life-altering change. One morning I woke up with a lightness of being I could not at first pinpoint. Part of me was missing, but what was it? Then I knew: the headache itself. Along with the nausea, it was completely gone for the first time in years.

A week or so afterward, I tossed my Rite Aid glasses—all the magnifications, even the low ones—into the trash. I was, once more, at 20/20, able to see into the distance and read the print in the phone book and the *New York Times*. One day I picked up the neuroscience articles my coauthor had sent for inclusion in our book on the brain. Though I had been unable to comprehend these articles the year before, I now read through them swiftly, cogently, and with ease.

To be sure, I was still sick. The migraine would come back. My hand was still stiff. My joints still hurt. I was exhausted, and I still buzzed. But a layer of the illness was gone. As if peeling the rot off an onion, Tick Bite had exposed a healthier layer beneath. She had made a dent.

. Mark, too, turned a corner as the weeks wore on. Though it was already too late for him to salvage his job, he slowly emerged from his stupor. He stopped slurring his words and stumbling over objects; he regained his ability to read. Even the rapid-fire glibness of his speech and his enormous vocabulary started to come back one piece at a time.

Mark and I would never have traced our symptoms to tick-borne disease had we not taken a detour through renegade medicine on behalf of our sick son. Jason was our small sacrifice, our loss leader: Had his rash been less gigantic or his Western blot less reactive, he, too, would have been consigned to Lyme's outback, relegated to wander its wilderness without explanation or a clue. Without Jason's stunning fight for diagnosis despite such overwhelming evidence, *textbook caliber evidence,* we might never have realized how high the cards were stacked against Lyme patients. Without that realization, we may never have defied our doctors or sought diagnoses, treatments, and productive lives of our own. For those who failed the tests and treatments or suffered only the devastating "minor" symptoms, for those infected with other tick-borne diseases, the burden of a mystery illness could be lifelong. With our controversial diagnoses and visits to Tick Bite we had joined a diaspora, a group beyond definition and off the grid, wandering the ruins of Lyme.

18

❖

Patients Dispossessed

As difficult as it was for validated patients like Jason, those without their Lyme bona fides—mutts like Mark and me—endured a special form of hell. Most of us had arrived at the Lyme diagnosis after years, by process of elimination, as we searched for clues to our declining health. Unable to obtain the diagnosis from one of the university centers or even a neighborhood physician, we went to the Lyme doctors: Joe Burrascano in the Hamptons, say, or Ken Liegner in Armonk. These doctors were willing to diagnose clinically based on evidence of exposure and subjective symptoms, including the devastating "minor manifestations" of pain, fatigue, and confusion so meticulously documented (but then dismissed as undiagnostic for Lyme disease) by Allen Steere.

The patients who failed the standard tests and therapies and then crossed the line did not buy into the theory that they suffered from some bizarre mass hysteria sweeping the nation's suburbs, or that they relished illness as an escape from their jobs, their marriages, and their kids. Most of them healthy until the day they were bitten by a tick, these typical suburbanites had been raised on antiwar protests and the flowering of rock and roll. Their collective memory included the shooting of John F. Kennedy, the travesty of Watergate, and the explosion of a space shuttle.

Their innocence long since shattered, they maintained a healthy skepticism of authority, and a more recent distaste for the new, monolithic

face of medicine embodied by managed care. As insurance companies rejected their claims and refused to cover their treatment, they couldn't help
but wonder whether the "evidence" these companies accepted (or not) had
to do with the actual facts of the illness or just its cost. In short, they were
not about to accept the prognosis of "untreatable" or the diagnosis of
"deluded" at the behest of some doctor—especially not if the doctor consulted for insurers at hefty fees, as so many of the academicians specializing in Lyme disease did. Instead, to the ire of the experts whose vision of
the disease they defied, the patients rebelled against them. Saddled with
hopeless diagnoses, a bizarre set of symptoms, and accusations that they
were nuts, Lyme patients who failed to recover after short-term standard
therapy felt they had no choice but to seek treatments outside the box.

Among the hardest hit and most vocal of the families were the Forschners of Stamford, Connecticut, Karen and Tom. A glimmer of all their
troubles emerged during Karen's pregnancy, when her joints started to
swell and doctors diagnosed arthritis. By the time she gave birth in
1985, she was on crutches. She would never walk normally, doctors said,
unless she happened to be suffering from a strange new disease called
Lyme. To test the possibility, she was offered two weeks of antibiotic.
The arthritis disappeared and Karen seemed to get well.

But the Forschner baby, Jamie, was out of luck. Even compared to some
of the sickest of the Lyme patients, his case was extreme. By six weeks of
age he suffered eye tremors and vomiting. At six months he was blind, and
doctors thought he might be deaf. At eighteen months he had surgery to
realign his stomach but the surgery failed, so he was fed through a tube.
By the time little Jamie was two, his care was so challenging that the
Forschners were advised to institutionalize him for his own good.

Desperate, Karen began searching the medical literature and discovered Alan MacDonald's work on transplacental transmission of Lyme
disease. Jamie was tested for Lyme disease, and with the test coming up
positive, antibiotics were prescribed. At first his recovery seemed near
miraculous: His vomiting stopped and he gained weight. His vision returned. He began to eat by mouth and even talk. But because Lyme was
considered so curable, every time Jamie seemed to be getting better the
antibiotic was stopped and he relapsed.

In seeking extended antibiotic treatment for their boy, the Forschners
had, without at first realizing it, stumbled into the line of fire: From transmission in the womb to long-term antibiotics and relapse after therapy to

widespread neurological damage, Jamie embodied the bitterest, most hotly contested elements of the fight over Lyme disease.

"I was told my son would get treated and the disease process would stop." Instead, Karen explains, "When Jamie's relapses were in process, even his throat would collapse, and he spent time on life support. Over time he was on life support many times. When Jamie received treatment he would recover. His vision returned. His speech started. He started to feed by mouth. His vomiting stopped. He gained weight. His lips could kiss and his arms could hug. But, despite the dramatic and documented improvements, over the years local doctors and health officials would interfere repeatedly with our son's retreatment because Lyme was 'easily curable.'

"When we asked the pediatrician for a three-month prescription of amoxicillin to give our son to prevent a relapse, we were told that amoxicillin was dangerous and there was no proof the Lyme bacteria could survive the short-term intravenous medicine he had been given while on life support," she says. But "two weeks later, we were back to the pediatrician for a potential ear infection. The same pediatrician prescribed the now-safe antibiotic amoxicillin to prevent an ear infection that had not yet started. And the prescription was issued in the same dose we had requested for Lyme disease, for a total of four months."

In a race against time to save Jamie's life, Karen and Tom attended the 1987 International Conference on Lyme Disease at the Marriott Marquis in New York City. Karen even posted signs around the Times Square conference center: "Mother with Lyme, three cats, dog, baby dying of Lyme. Please help."

Instead of finding a group of researchers working together to solve the Lyme dilemma the Forschners found just the opposite: The "Steeres" and "MacDonalds" of the Lyme world at each other's throats. It was a "polarized, noncooperative group," Karen Forschner recalls. That was putting it mildly.

Amid all the chaos, Karen and Tom managed to connect. The doctors who felt their research was being suppressed by power players couldn't help but see, in the Forschner family, a human face for the fight. Other diseases had advocacy organizations where patients had a voice, and Lyme needed that, too. Who better to give voice to the problem than a dying baby, a blue-eyed, blond-haired toddler with the face of an angel, and his mother, a well-spoken young woman, also a blue-eyed blonde, so prim and presentable she might have stepped out of a bandbox. "They asked for my help," Karen Forschner recalls.

Following through with the network of experts they met at the conference, Karen and Tom Forschner, both with backgrounds in finance, founded their organization, the Lyme Borreliosis Foundation (later renamed the Lyme Disease Foundation) in 1988. It didn't take long for Karen and Jamie, together with the new foundation, to find a spotlight in the media. "Media people saw our child as a great example for some sort of TV blurb," said Karen Forschner. "What we saw was a child who was courageous and might indeed help other people learn a little bit about this disease, and maybe, God forbid, yeah, maybe he might be able to get some funding from the government, so there would be answers before he would die." When Dan Rather put Jamie on television not as a profile in courage, but as "every parent's worst nightmare," the Forschners were appalled.

For Jamie, the worst of the nightmare was yet to come. Now famous, at least in the world of Lyme disease, the Forschners found doctors they didn't even know fighting over Jamie's treatment or whether he had Lyme at all. The doctors weren't fighting over the fate of one little boy, in reality, but over the meaning of the evidence and the very essence of the disease. For instance, electron microscope pictures from the NIH had captured spirochete-like structures in Jamie's tissue after repeated courses of treatment. The Forschners and many of the LLMDs said this proved that persistent infection continued to ravage Jamie's body. But skeptics would not accept that the images depicted actual spirochetes. It certainly wasn't sufficient proof for Jamie's pediatricians, said Karen, especially not after they "talked to the state health department and an academic expert who recommended no retreatment at all."

The Forschners waited over a year for a new NIH test that they hoped would provide more definite evidence of active Lyme disease and thus, enable retreatment with antibiotics. But it all took too long. Jamie's last relapse resulted in seizures and "within 24 hours he was put on life support," Karen Forschner says. "The day he was declared out of the woods, he died." By now immersed in the day-to-day work of the fledgling Lyme Disease Foundation, Karen Forschner was determined that Jamie did not die in vain. She hoped an autopsy would prove the phenomenon of congenital Lyme disease that scientists and officials at the CDC claimed could not be real.

"There was no tissue bank to send his remains to, so I had the unpleasant task of calling researchers around the country," Karen Forschner says. "I loved this little boy, and would have died for him. Instead I was faced with the devastating job of dividing up his body parts for scientists. Our lifetime savings were gone. Our jobs were gone. Our baby was gone . . . if public policy had been prevention oriented instead of anti-antibiotic hysteria oriented, my son would be alive today."

The Forschners' tragic story and Karen Forschner's chutzpah had finally put Lyme disease on the map. The TV news program *20/20* featured the story. *Family Circle* named Karen "Woman of the Year." And newspapers around the country carried stories about the disease. Lyme patients hardest hit appeared on TV with Geraldo and Sally Jessy Raphael.

Yet to many scientists, the publicity was a fiasco. As patients around the country heard the Forschners' story, they, too, thought they had Lyme disease and started support groups. Some doctors in these regions agreed with the patients, diagnosing them even without positive blood tests, and then treating them long-term.

But these new patients and their physicians were living in a fantasyland, not a Lymeland, according to the CDC and experts like Steere. There was no Lyme disease in Missouri, in Texas, in Florida, they said. How could there be when these regions had yielded neither evidence of the Lyme spirochete nor any sign of the Lyme tick, by then identified by Harvard as *Ixodes dammini*? The experts blamed the publicity for inciting hysteria in and out of the Lyme zone. In a consult letter, Steere suggested that one patient requesting more treatment might suffer "an addiction" to antibiotic, even though no such category of abuse had ever been recorded in the past. "She will require withdrawal, which will be difficult," he wrote of her case.

The most outspoken of the skeptics publicly charged that Jamie Forschner had never had Lyme disease. Lyme hysteria, they said, was far more dangerous and threatening than actual Lyme disease.

19

❖

The Scourge of "Lime" Disease

Leonard Sigal is a small, wiry, bearded man with an abundance of energy and intelligence, a quickness to anger, and the conviction that when it comes to Lyme, he knows the score. For more than two decades, he's been an outspoken critic of long-term treatment and diagnosing Lyme at all "when symptoms appear vague."

His involvement goes back almost to the start, when he signed on as rheumatology fellow at Yale under the mentorship of Allen Steere. "I saw lots of patients with Lyme disease, lots of incredibly cooperative and wonderful people. They dragged themselves down from Old Lyme on I-95 so we could study them," he recalls.

Sigal left Yale in 1984, joining the faculty at Syracuse Medical School in upstate New York. While Lyme disease has since spread to the region, "there was none to speak of back then," says Sigal. And so, as the Lyme brouhaha raged elsewhere, Sigal was blissfully unaware.

It was in 1988 that he arrived at the Robert Wood Johnson Medical School in New Jersey. "I was hired to focus on lupus," he says, "but once I got down here I realized there was this controversy about Lyme disease. There was this craziness going on in the community. So I set up a Lyme disease referral practice.

"I saw lots of people with standard Lyme disease, and others who did not have Lyme disease but honestly thought they might," says Sigal. "There were physicians who said 'I don't know if this is Lyme disease or not, what do you think?' Then I saw those who were being abused. These were people who had been on intravenous antibiotics for weeks, months, years, but who had no real evidence that they ever had Lyme disease."

Here Sigal stops to explain. He agrees one need not test positive according to the two-step CDC criteria to have serological evidence for Lyme disease. He knows, he says, that early, incomplete antibiotic treatment can abrogate the immune response. And, like most of the academic scientists I interviewed, he says that given exposure and objective symptoms, a couple of highly specific bands on a Western blot can certainly constitute evidence for infection—enough evidence, he says, for him to treat for a month.

"There are certain circumstances where empirical treatment is probably warranted," Sigal says. "I have treated people in whom I thought it was vaguely possible they might have Lyme disease but I wasn't sure. I treated them not because I wanted to see if they got better and therefore I could make a diagnosis. I treated them because if there was the slightest possibility that this person with cognitive dysfunction had Lyme disease I cannot condemn them to the inexorable fate they would experience without at least one trial of antibiotics. I couldn't do that. I've treated lots of people who don't have Lyme disease, absolutely, but it wasn't an empirical trial to see if they got better in order to make the diagnosis, it was in order to be three thousand percent sure that they have not been denied every possible treatment imaginable."

Sigal even thinks it's possible that some patients could be chronically, persistently infected with the Lyme disease spirochete, despite antibiotic treatment. "Is it possible that there might be some patients who have a form of Lyme disease, which—because of the peculiarity of the organism or the peculiarity of their own immune response—never truly goes away, leaving them with chronic, low-level symptoms? Sure, it's possible," he says. "I don't have any evidence to that effect and I don't know the mechanism, but it is certainly possible."

Yet as far as he was concerned, some of the patients who came to him had no evidence of Lyme disease whatsoever. "*Gornisht mit gornisht*," he says emphatically in Yiddish. "None. They once saw a tick, and that was it. Their blood tests were negative—without a single specific band—and they had never had a known tick bite or an erythema migrans rash." Of course, many patients never see the tick or manifest the rash. "But these people had nothing," Sigal says. "They never had seventh nerve [Bell's] palsy, they never had meningitis, they never had carditis, they never had true arthritis, they never had anything objective. They had aches and pains and headaches, and they just felt rotten, but despite lack of evidence they were diagnosed as having Lyme disease by the same doctors over and over again. Then they were treated, indefinitely, with antibiotics."

Sigal said that what he saw enraged him. "I think it's called righteous indignation. Some people got better and then they got worse again. Some got a little bit better but never got well. Others got better and worse over and over again. They just didn't feel well and they continued not to feel well, but they didn't have Lyme disease."

According to Sigal, the problem extended beyond mere long-term treatment. "It's the misdiagnosis of Lyme disease," he says. "It's the mismanagement and the lack of attention to what they really have. And then it is the insinuation into that patient's head of the belief that he or she has a chronic infection that will never go away. It is the psychological burden— the psychological aberration induced by the suggestion that these patients are chronically ill, maybe forever—that causes them to assume a sick role they can never escape. That's a terrible thing to do to a patient.

"By the time I see some of these patients they are so badly abused over the course of years that I have no idea what they were like premorbidly," Sigal says, adding that a small minority of them seem emotionally disturbed. "One potential reason for why they're not well is that they're crazy, to use a term. Let's live with it. Let's work with it. Such individuals walk in with a predisposing desire to find an explanation for why they don't feel quite right. I call it societal misfit syndrome. They don't feel comfortable with what's being required of them. As a result, they are looking for an explanation and an excuse for their dysfunction, and maybe they find it in Lyme disease. Part of the problem is that some physicians may have imparted a message to these patients that they're not sick. That's when such patients got annoyed, angry, venomous. How dare you accuse me of not being sick—I am clearly unwell."

Most of the time, Sigal believes, the patient doesn't start out emotionally disturbed, but rather is made that way by the chronic Lyme diagnosis itself. "Being chronically ill will make you 'crazy,' " he says. "You have to be really careful about these things before you consign people to chronic illness for the rest of their lives. If someone goes to his grave twenty-five years from now believing he had Lyme disease when he never really had Lyme disease at all, he's had twenty-five years of being convinced he has a chronic infection that will badly debilitate him. And the belief itself will badly debilitate him, even though he never had Lyme disease."

He places the blame squarely on the Lyme doctors, though he doesn't mention names. "The patients are just going with what they've been told," Sigal says. "There are physicians out there who tell them they are ill. There are clinicians out there who tell them, 'You have Lyme disease and you will experience such and such. Here, read this.' Then they read it, and they know what they're supposed to be experiencing, so they experience it.

"At first the patient just isn't feeling well, and the doctor diagnoses them with Lyme disease. Okay, the patient might think, that's cool, the symptoms fit. But then, when the patient doesn't feel better with antibiotics, he's told he'll have Lyme disease forever, and needs lots more antibiotics for a long, long time. 'God, Doc, are you telling me you can't cure this, that I'm stuck with these spirochetes crawling around in my head?' If I really believed that about myself," says Sigal, "I don't think I'd be a happy camper at all. I would be very upset, extraordinarily stressed out, and I wouldn't be surprised if whatever symptoms I had were remarkably worsened. And probably joined by new symptoms. Let's not look at the psychopathology of the patient as the sole issue here. There is also the power of suggestion of the demigod who is the diagnosing doctor.

"I told myself, this cannot be allowed to pass," Sigal explains, his face reddening and his voice rising as he speaks. "As far as I am concerned, if a physician sees something that is wrong and he does nothing about it, then he is a coward, and my parents didn't raise no coward. So I got involved."

One of his first steps, all the way back in 1990, was conducting and publishing a study that would help set Lyme's direction for years. Taking the first hundred patients to walk through his clinic doors, he determined that just thirty-seven met the CDC's definition of Lyme disease—either the EM rash or one of the late major signs and positive test. Instead of Lyme disease, he felt, many of the patients had something else: a pain syndrome of unknown origin called fibromyalgia.

Yet anyone familiar with the history of chronic illness understood that, in replacing one controversial diagnosis with another, Leonard Sigal had gone out on a limb. The American College of Rheumatology had just recently endorsed fibromyalgia as a diagnostic entity, defining it as widespread pain in combination with tenderness at eleven or more so-called tender points. The syndrome wouldn't be accepted by the World Health Organization until 1992 in what was known as the Copenhagen Declaration. Those writing the declaration at the second World Congress on Myofascial Pain and Fibromyalgia, held in Copenhagen, agreed to broaden the definition to include widespread pain or aching, persistent fatigue, generalized stiffness, and nonrefreshing sleep—to many Lyme patients, precisely the experience of Lyme disease.

It was all the more confusing because Allen Steere was now reporting that Lyme disease triggered not just fibromyalgia, but a second new mystery illness—chronic fatigue syndrome—often referred to disparagingly as "yuppie flu." Chronic fatigue syndrome had made its notorious entry on the world stage a mere three years after Willy Burgdorfer found the spirochete causing Lyme disease and two years after AIDS was given its name, in 1984. Just like Lyme patients, those diagnosed with CFS came down with a crushing, disabling, inexplicable "flu" from which they could not recover. The patients, often unable to continue in work or school, presented with a spectrum of objective signs, including tiny brain lesions, elevated cell count in cerebrospinal fluid, and short-term memory loss—just like some Lyme patients. They experienced headache, sensitivity to light, widespread pain, and a devastating, overwhelming fatigue, exactly like patients with chronic Lyme. Although doctors treating chronic fatigue patients fought for respect, the patients nonetheless found themselves cast as hypochondriacs, malingerers, and neurotics by the press, by the medical community, and even by the government agency charged with helping them, the CDC.

In truth, when it came to clinical presentation, there was often little to distinguish fibromyalgia and chronic fatigue syndrome from the "minor" late symptoms of Lyme disease. From the muscular pain to the cognitive impairments to the fatigue, these illnesses could seem virtually the same. Some academic scientists based the division between Lyme disease and one of the newer syndromes not on the signs and symptoms or even the lab tests, but on the fulcrum of treatment itself. Prior to treatment a symptomatic patient testing positive on a Western blot would be diagnosed with Lyme disease; if the same patient failed that treatment, he or she was said to have "post-Lyme syndrome," chronic fatigue syndrome, or fibromyalgia. Instead of antibiotic treatment, the standard of care was now aspirin, aerobic exercise, and antidepressants; such patients were routinely sent for psychiatric help.

The problem with all this, of course, was that many doctors outside the furor of the Lyme debate considered the new diagnoses of chronic fatigue syndrome and fibromyalgia more outrageous and more likely to represent some kind of mass hysteria or psychiatric plague than Lyme disease.

Inside the Lyme world, academic rheumatologists increasingly deferred to fibromyalgia as the stern statesman of reality—an incontrovertible category of ill while casting doubt on the legitimacy of many Lyme patients. In fact, in the wake of Leonard Sigal's call to arms, the sickest of the Lyme patients had become objects of derision and the butt of jokes. Writing in the prestigious *Annals of Internal Medicine* in 1991, humor columnist

Ludwig A. Lettau, M.D., clarified the stance. His article, purportedly written by a doctor from the "Centers for Fatigue Control (CFC)," described the foibles of a disease called *Lime*. "The growing national epidemic of Lime disease [paralleled] increased public awareness and knowledge of Lyme disease," Lettau wrote. "Cases have now been reported from all fifty states, but the national surveillance program has been hampered by persistent confusion between the two diseases, with clinicians frequently reporting a case of Lime disease as Lyme disease." Lettau noted that attack rates of "Lime disease" were "highest in adults of upper middle to upper socio-economic class, with a female-to-male sex ratio of 3:1 (in contrast to the more balanced age and sex distribution of Lyme disease). . . . Recent case-control studies of clusters of Lime disease have shown a weak to moderate association with previous attendance at cocktail parties serving lime-garnished mixed drinks, but very strong associations with recent exposure to media stories on Lyme disease."

Outside the Lyme zone, meanwhile, critics were coming to see not "Lime disease," but fibromyalgia as the poster child for delusion, yet another in history's long line of labels for chronic exhaustion and pain, including hysteria, muscular rheumatism, and neurasthenia, diagnoses of centuries past.

By the mid-1990s, fibromyalgia support groups (like chronic fatigue support groups and Lyme disease support groups) were springing up everywhere, and physicians, especially rheumatologists, had made the fibromyalgia diagnosis millions of times in the United States alone. Many of those ushered into this new diagnostic territory were patients previously diagnosed with Lyme disease. In fact, as the definition of Lyme disease narrowed to include just the rash or "major late manifestations" and as the scourge of "Lime disease" got more press, the definition of fibromyalgia broadened, enabling it to pick up the slack.

As the fibromyalgia umbrella opened wide, providing diagnostic cover, skepticism from the medical community soared. Sigal said that doctor demigods immersed in a belief system had hypnotized patients into acceptance of chronic Lyme disease. Yet the same charges were made against doctors diagnosing fibromyalgia, doctors like Leonard Sigal. It wasn't the patients alone who had conjured the sociological phenomenon of fibromyalgia, said Dutch researchers Ingvar Hazemeijer and Hans Rasker, but the "therapeutic domain"—the comprehensive medical environment, with the ringmaster the diagnosing physician himself. The authors, a psychiatrist and rheumatologist, respectively, published their paper in the journal *Rheumatology* in 2003. "The only certainty about fibromyalgia is that it is still being diagnosed," the doctors said. As far as they were concerned, fibromyalgia was not an entity that could be "described or explained." Rather, it was the "subjective experience of pain and fatigue" filtered through the prism of organized medicine. If fibromyalgia was a belief system, the true believers were the M.D.s.

In point of fact, one could always find a doctor to anoint a diagnosis. Leonard Sigal diagnosed fibromyalgia. Allen Steere diagnosed chronic fatigue syndrome. Joe Burrascano diagnosed chronic Lyme disease. To each physician, the diagnosis he supported was the one deemed real. But it was relative, all of it. One physician's reality was another physician's joke. All you had to do was listen to the chatter—or read the peer-reviewed literature—to realize that doctors endorsing fibromyalgia had shifted the Lyme patients not from the surreal to the real but from one belief system to the next. These scientists said their guiding light was evidence-based medicine, but with the evidence so controversial, so kaleidoscopic, and especially so flexible, it was natural to wonder where the evidence left off and the power of belief kicked in—not just for the patients, but for the doctors themselves. With no known cause (or on-ramp) and no known cure (or exit) the fibromyalgia freeway had become, for those actually suffering borreliosis or some other infection, a Sartre-esque highway to hell.

To Lyme patients who'd taken that detour, Leonard Sigal was seen as public enemy number one. On the Internet newsgroup sci.med.diseases.lyme, patients called him "Lenny the Weasel Sigal." One patient posted, "When the truth comes out about Lyme and other spirochetal and borrelial disease, Lenny is going to have scrambled, fried, Benedict, over easy, poached, and every other known form of egg plastered all over his face!" Some patients wished his family would be bitten by ticks and stricken with chronic, incurable Lyme disease. Others wrote letters to the state of New Jersey demanding that he be fired.

Yet Sigal would not relent. "People got angry at me," he says. "I wrote articles. They got angry at me. I testified in court. They got angry at me. I gave lectures. They got angry at me. It's okay, I'm tough."

For many years (until he finally took a job in big pharma) Leonard Sigal took on the Lyme patients regularly, and they railed right back. Unlike Steere, who shied away from public brawls with the angry multitudes, Sigal was willing to brave the outrage to get his point across. As the Lyme war spread, he remained a point of reference. Always at the ready with a sound bite for the newspaper or the evening news, he was standard-bearer for what the mainstream considered the logical, scientific, utterly rational view of Lyme disease, and its most passionate voice.

20

❖❖❖

Peeling the Onion

Just as energetic as Leonard Sigal, just as passionate, just as quick to anger, and just as convinced he is right, Kenneth Liegner of Armonk, New York, has a different lens. A brilliant critical care physician with interests from politics to jazz, Liegner is meticulous almost to the point of obsession—taping and transcribing every patient visit and storing parts of each blood and spinal fluid sample in a line of freezers kept purring by a generator of their own. The specimens, collected over the course of twenty years, await the day that new, more sensitive tests might emerge, revealing once and for all the diseases his patients have.

Ken Liegner arrived on the Lyme scene the same year as Sigal, in 1988. He, too, saw a specific group of patients, comprised, for the most part, of those who didn't get well. In fact, just as Sigal had refugee patients from doctors like Liegner, Liegner had refugee patients from Sigal. And Liegner's experience seemed the opposite of Sigal's, as if they inhabited matter and antimatter versions of the same world.

As time passed, Ken Liegner found that more and more local doctors were diagnosing patients with fibromyalgia, chronic fatigue syndrome, depression, or multiple sclerosis without what he considered appropriate evidence—and without performing the requisite differential diagnosis for Lyme disease as an alternate, more treatable, cause of their ills. As a result, Liegner says, patients were streaming into his office having been allowed to decline and become chronically ill, sometimes desperately so, with untreated Lyme disease. Some of the patients were so debilitated by the time they got to him they could no longer work or conduct normal lives. Others were so neurologically impaired they were on the verge of being institutionalized. Liegner subsequently diagnosed many of these patients with Lyme disease, treated them with antibiotics, sometimes for months or longer, and found that most dramatically improved. While he could return most patients to health, a sizable minority remained sick—often, he felt, because the delay in treatment had led to permanent damage that remained even after the infection was brought under control. Like Leonard Sigal, he, too, was enraged over the state of affairs.

Ken Liegner had always bucked the trend and bristled at the status quo. When he entered medicine in the 1980s, his personal notion of doctoring stood in stark contrast to the emergent medicine of the day. While the rising HMO culture sought to standardize medicine and mass-produce everything from diagnoses to treatments, Liegner dreamed of finding patients with the most complicated cases possible and helping them get well. While doctors were being asked to become cogs in a machine, Liegner wanted to be a medical Sherlock Holmes.

Toward that end, the young Ken Liegner did everything he could to broaden his medical horizon: He studied anatomic pathology and learned to do autopsies. He worked in critical care medicine, including a stint in the "the knife and gun club" at the Washington Hospital Center in D.C., where multiple trauma, open heart surgery, and drug overdoses were his daily fare. Yet with a young son, Kenneth Liegner soon found the demands of the job grueling—hardly conducive to parenting—and decided to come back home, to New York, and open a practice of his own. So he took out a loan and purchased a house, a large yellow ranch, on a beautiful country road in the northern Westchester village of Armonk, just a couple of miles west of the Connecticut state line. He hung out a shingle and waited for the world.

With a lone practice on an obscure country road, Liegner found business slow. Yet operating on the premise of "build it and they will come," the practice eventually attracted patients: They were neighbors and the friends of neighbors as well as people Liegner met moonlighting at local hospitals just to make ends meet. When Liegner was asked to give a talk at the local library, he decided his topic would be Lyme disease. He prepared by reading the worldwide literature of the time, and addressed a crowd of three hundred people on what he had learned.

Word got around that a doctor up in Armonk knew a thing or two about Lyme disease, and slowly some locals began making appointments after being bitten by ticks. Now, with a larger number of Lyme disease patients to follow, Liegner found that plenty of patients recovered after a single course of treatment, especially with IV Rocephin, but others remained ill or continually relapsed. For some patients, Liegner found, it didn't matter how long he treated—a month, or two, or five—whenever the antibiotic was pulled, all the symptoms came back.

One relapsing patient was a young man who'd made a fortune on Wall Street. Now living on a luxurious estate, he spent his days playing tennis and scuba diving. Liegner first encountered him in the emergency room, where he came in with a host of odd complaints: swollen groin, swollen lymph nodes, hip pain, and a rash. Liegner prescribed a short course of antibiotic therapy and the patient seemed to recover. Yet a few weeks later the patient was back, this time at the Armonk office. All the symptoms, including the rash, had returned. "It was very dramatic to see the rash fade and come bounding right back," Liegner recalls. Finally the patient tested positive for Lyme disease and Liegner prescribed six weeks of IV Rocephin. This time recovery was sustained.

Liegner found his experience shared by another doctor when, in 1990, he attended the Lyme Disease Foundation meeting in Orlando, Florida, near SeaWorld. It would be his first meeting with Paul Lavoie, the San Francisco physician who had studied the cluster of Lyme cases in the Coast Range near Ukiah and treated patients like Phyllis Mervine. Liegner found himself discussing the quandary. "Antibiotics can't just be open-ended," Liegner said. "You have to stop treating patients at some point."

"Why?" Lavoie had asked him. Lavoie explained that he saw Lyme disease in the context of syphilis—a progressive, neurodegenerative disease that inhabited the brain and could require rounds of antibiotic, sometimes in combination and at very high dose. Treating Lyme disease, Lavoie believed, was like peeling an onion: You had to strip infection away slowly, a layer at a time. With every peeling, the patient would first sink deeper into disease as the organisms died off (an extended Herxheimer) and then rise up to the next level as damaged tissue healed. Lavoie thought different layers of the illness required different treatments; so when Lavoie's patients hit a plateau on one antibiotic, he upped the dose or changed the antibiotic altogether. The peel could take years—or, for those longest-infected or most immune-compromised, Lavoie believed, forever.

The conversation would replay in Liegner's mind over the next few years, as his clinical experience veered ever more widely from the tidy studies of Leonard Sigal and Allen Steere. "I would see these patients with these odd symptoms that might be Lyme disease," he says, "and I would treat them and they would get better and I would stop treating them and they would relapse."

A case in point was a shop owner who lived in a woodsy area of Westchester near the Kensico Reservoir. He'd reported to his personal doctor with a Lyme rash and was duly tested for Lyme disease. As would be expected so early in the course of infection, the test came back negative; but instead of retesting, his doctor interpreted the results as definitive, and declined to treat at all. As time went on the patient developed symptoms associated with Lyme disease, especially mental confusion. His tests remained negative, but based on his exposure and the description of the rash, an infectious disease specialist—in fact, Peter Welch, the same local doctor who had first diagnosed our son Jason—treated him with four weeks of Rocephin.

Nine months later, when the patient found his way to Liegner, his knees were swollen and he was so mentally confused his employees were taking advantage of him. His family was on the verge of committing him to a psychiatric hospital. Ordering a brain scan, Liegner found the patient had diminished blood flow. Then a Western blot lit up with *B. burgdorferi* antibodies, though *still* not enough to satisfy the standards of the CDC. Liegner nonetheless treated him aggressively with nine months of IV Rocephin followed by more months on oral antibiotics.

"He greatly improved," Liegner says. Yet each time Liegner took him off the antibiotic, he "fell apart." So Liegner continued antibiotic therapy in open-ended fashion, as suggested by Paul Lavoie. The patient was kept on the antibiotic amoxicillin, and developed a fully diagnostic Western blot only after he had been treated for years.

Another patient developed such a severe case of Lyme meningitis that he was hospitalized near his home in upstate New York and treated with a few weeks of IV Rocephin. He improved but quickly relapsed. Eventually local doctors transferred him to Westchester Medical Center in Valhalla, known for treating Lyme disease. A spinal tap done there showed he still had meningitis, so doctors treated him with ten more days of Rocephin. But when he *still* failed to respond, the Valhalla doctors insisted he suffered not from Lyme disease but a psychiatric disorder. They issued papers transferring him to a psychiatric hospital. That's when the patient's mother stepped in, rejecting the idea that her son had suddenly, and for no apparent reason, developed a psychiatric illness so disabling he could barely think. She whisked him away from Westchester Medical before the transfer occurred and took him to see Liegner.

"He was the only patient I have ever put on Rocephin the day he walked into my office," Ken Liegner says. "He was so impaired he couldn't distinguish primary colors, and couldn't even recognize his mother." Liegner watched his patient slowly improve on Rocephin over the course of six months, and then decided to add the oral antibiotic, minocycline, a cousin to doxycycline. "That's when he really improved," Liegner says.

Spending his days treating such patients, Ken Liegner grew ever more perturbed. At night he often phoned his physician father, by then retired, to discuss the cases. In spare moments he pondered his untenable situation: Increasingly, the university physicians who set restrictive treatment guidelines were insisting the infection couldn't survive the standard course of antibiotic, and many had even gone so far as to deny the possibility of chronic Lyme disease as an entity at all. The Westchester Medical doctor who wanted to ship the upstate New York patient off to a psychiatric hospital—infectious disease specialist Gary Wormser—was a signatory to official treatment guidelines stating chronic Lyme did not exist.

Yet it was Liegner, not Wormser, who had to bear the burden of proof. Although Liegner had diagnosed patient after patient with chronic Lyme disease, although he had personally watched these patients improve with treatment and relapse without, he understood that his clinical observations amounted merely to anecdote. Science required more than that to validate a phenomenon as real. In order for a therapy to be codified in a treatment guideline, it demanded support from rigorous formal studies. It was virtually impossible to gather such evidence from a sizable group of Liegner patients, when one responded to Rocephin and another to minocycline and yet another to Zithromax, when one reported buzzing in the fingers and another, heart disease and yet another, encephalopathy, when one got well in two months while another took two years. With such a heterogeneous group of unpredictable patients responding so differently to such a diverse set of therapies, how could anyone devise a treatment study that would encompass them all?

Despite such limitations, Liegner continually searched among his patients for those cases and situations that might yield evidence, that is to say, biological, molecular proof that Lyme disease could be a relapsing-remitting illness, and that, in some individuals, the spirochete could survive the standard course of antibiotic therapy: That it could *persist*.

One patient he found particularly troubling but also especially illuminating was a former pediatric intensive care nurse named Vicki Logan,

who experienced a disturbance of her gait. Physicians she consulted prescribed physical therapy, but no one knew the cause. Dissatisfied with
the lack of a true diagnosis, and hearing of Liegner's detective work, she
made an appointment to see him in 1989.

Liegner knew that Logan had grown up in Golden's Bridge, a
Westchester town dense with deer and ticks. Finding nothing else to explain her condition after careful evaluation over the course of a year, he
decided to treat for Lyme disease in a trial, to see whether she might respond. So he admitted her to the hospital and treated her with twenty-
one days of intravenous antibiotic. The treatment did nothing to change
her clinical status—and spinal taps done before and after the treatment
showed the same, consistent level of meningitis. Just for good measure
he treated her with another four months of oral minocycline, but that
didn't make a difference, either. By then it was 1990 and, getting no results, Liegner backed off. Lyme appeared to be ruled out.

Getting progressively worse, Logan came back a year later hoping
that Liegner might finally figure out what was wrong. It so happened that
Liegner had, by then, begun working with the CDC. The CDC supplied
him with quantities of the special BSK medium developed in Montana for
culturing the spirochetes. Liegner, in turn, added Lyme patient blood or
spinal fluid to vials of the medium, shipping it back for study at the CDC
labs. Performing a spinal tap on Logan, he naturally added part of the
sample to one of the vials—maybe the CDC could shed some light?

Three weeks later, Liegner got a call from David Dennis, chief of the
Bacterial Zoonoses Branch of the CDC's Division of Vector-Borne Infectious Diseases, in Fort Collins, Colorado. Dennis knew Logan had already been treated aggressively and he was very excited. Despite the fact
that she had been too ill to go outdoors, risking new exposure to Lyme
disease, her spinal fluid had yielded a culture of *Borrelia*. Dennis was so
surprised he even asked Liegner whether he grew cultures of *Borrelia* in
his office; the unstated implication was that Liegner had spiked the
spinal fluid with spirochetes himself. "The question revealed how difficult it was for him to accept the possibility that infection could survive
the treatment," Liegner states.

The spirochetes in culture were later identified as *B. burgdorferi* by
the CDC. At the same time, Logan's blood had finally "seroconverted":
For the first time ever, her blood serum tested positive for antibodies to
the spirochete. As a culture-proven case of Lyme disease, Logan was able
to submit a unit of her blood to the CDC for future studies. She also
earned another distinction, becoming the first culture-proven case of

Lyme disease treatment failure in the United States. At last, Ken Liegner knew, there was at least one instance in which the spirochete *Borrelia burgdorferi* had survived aggressive treatment, in fact, months of treatment—there was at least one proven case of chronic persistent Lyme disease despite antibiotic treatment, and the evidence had been found by the CDC itself.

Evidence in hand, Liegner felt more confident about treating Vicki Logan for Lyme disease over the long haul. In fact, by 1993, he felt the strategy was her only chance. In the intervening years she'd been diagnosed with possible lupus and treated with steroids at the Mayo Clinic, becoming so ill in the aftermath that she had to be hospitalized at Northern Westchester. She was so debilitated she couldn't walk, hold up a cup, or even roll over in bed. Her memory was so poor that when you said something to her, five minutes later she would have no recollection of the conversation. "She was desperately ill," says Liegner. "She looked like she was going to die." So from May until October 1993, Kenneth Liegner treated Logan with 109 continuous days of IV Rocephin, the longest such treatment she had ever undergone. To his complete delight, she came back from the brink and truly began to get well.

But not even the clear improvement could stop others from getting in the way. Even as Logan began lifting cups and recalling conversations, Peter Welch, by then the hospital's vice president for Medical Affairs, called Liegner on the carpet. Kenneth Liegner was "obsessed" with the Lyme diagnosis, Welch charged, and had shown poor medical judgment every step of the way, in Logan's case, in particular. Liegner was preparing for the fight of a lifetime to continue Logan's treatment when fate shined down on him, and his patient as well. Among the signs of Logan's disease were "pericardial effusions," an increased amount of fluid inside the pericardium, the thin layer of tissue that forms a sac surrounding the heart. Liegner had sent some of the damaged tissue for a biopsy at NIH, and finally the agency reported back: It had been laced with spirochetes. "It's a complicated case," Welch demurred.

That same year Ken Liegner declared his position publicly in the *Journal of Clinical Microbiology*. His article, entitled "The Sensible Pursuit of Answers," provided chronic Lyme patients with an intellectual defense of their stance, pressing home two points: First, citing the Stony Brook findings, he pointed out that Lyme disease could be "seronegative," that is, it could fail to elicit a strong enough antibody response to meet the CDC's diagnostic bar on lab tests. Second, he believed that infection could be chronic—that is, it could persist after standard treatment occurred.

What scientists like Steere called "post-Lyme disease syndrome," Lyme anxiety, or fibromyalgia was often simply inadequately treated Lyme disease.

Just like Leonard Sigal, Kenneth Liegner saw Lyme disease in a psychosocial context, with aberrations emerging not from the patients but from other physicians. "In addressing the sociopathology of Lyme disease," said Liegner, whose mother was a psychoanalyst, "you have to explore why physicians behave as they do. It's just possible they are so blind they don't even realize they are wrong, but aside from that, if they acknowledge they are wrong, they are liable for medical neglect—for failure to diagnose and failure to treat. So they are doing the only thing they can—denying that chronic Lyme disease even exists."

From Liegner's perspective as a treating physician at the center of the debate, denial of chronic Lyme disease worked for the insurance companies, too. "They don't have to cover the costly treatment," he says, adding, "one could see the relationship between the doctors and the insurers as cozy. The doctors consulting for insurance companies are often the same ones who deny the existence of chronic Lyme disease in treatment guidelines and the same ones whose patients wind up in my office, misdiagnosed, mistreated, and horrendously sick year after year after year. If they didn't deny the existence of chronic Lyme disease, they would have no defense and would have to acknowledge they were lousy physicians." As far as Liegner was concerned, "chronic persistent denial of chronic persistent infection" was a social pathology as well as a medical epidemic, and the afflicted were the physicians themselves.

21

⁂

Family Therapy

Chappaqua, New York, 2001

The Horace Greeley High School psychologist had never seen a Lyme patient like Jason, at least that's what she said. Most of his health problems were due to anxiety, "and not just *his* anxiety, but *yours.*" Our family had channeled the illness from the depths of our own neuroses, she seemed to suggest. With her short wavy hair, practical shoes, and expert efficiency, she was not just a school psychologist but, unfortunately for us, a gatekeeper for dishing out help.

Following his Lyme diagnosis, Jason felt nauseous and went to the restroom to vomit during a test. It's no wonder, really—an antibiotic that he was on, doxycycline, is known for inducing nausea, and it had that effect on him. But that did not impress the psychologist, the watchdog on our case. After he finished retching, Jason called home in a panic. He'd emerged from the bathroom to find the psychologist waiting for him. If he did not want zeros, she told him, he would have to go back and finish that first test, and take a second, scheduled test as well. She diagnosed "test anxiety" while our doctor diagnosed Lyme.

She reiterated her skepticism some months later when Jason, still quite ill, felt too exhausted to make it to school for a stretch of time. She decided to pay him a visit at home. After sitting with him for a few minutes from a perch on our living room couch, she rose to leave. At our doorway, out of Jason's earshot, she looked me in the eye and delivered some parting advice: "Get him a good haircut." Then, as if choreographed for emphasis, she turned smartly on her heels, got into her car, and drove off.

During the entire time we dealt with Horace Greeley High School in Chappaqua, we found those in charge skeptical that Lyme could impact Jason's level of energy and focus in the way his doctors explained. It seemed as if no letter from a doctor, no appeal from a private psychologist, no expert article could change their minds. When I suggested that the Greeley psychologist attend a conference, she said she didn't have time. "I know all *about* Lyme disease," she explained. When Jason came back after the summer, ready to start anew, fatigue and fogginess continued to get in the way. "We've done enough for you already," an assistant principal, following the psychologist's lead, told us during a meeting, literally rolling his eyes.

For other diseases, disabilities, and disorders the Chappaqua school district could sometimes be understanding, but when it came to Lyme disease, the consensus seemed aligned with that of the Mount Kisco doctors up the road: It was impossible that Lyme disease could make a student this ill, this fuzzy. In fact, a few years later, when David became sick with Lyme disease and needed extra help, I brought a note on his diagnosis from our Lyme practitioner.

"So, you're saying he has Lyme disease," queried the district's coordinator for special ed. All I could do was recall my experience of just a few years before.

"*I'm* not saying he has Lyme disease," I said more than once during that meeting. "That's *her* opinion, not mine, I just brought the note for your files. All *I'm* saying is that he's exhausted and anxious, and needs help."

In this case Chappaqua was generous—but it had taken me years to learn the district ropes. It seemed to me that if you wanted special help, the "L" word could only hurt.

In Jason's case, I hadn't yet learned the drill. By fall of 2001, it was clear that Horace Greeley High School would be of little help: Our boy was too sick to get there at 7:30 in the morning, too wiped out to take every test, or get to every class. Yet because Greeley had "done enough" for us the year before, because they appeared not to *believe* in Lyme disease, helpful accommodations were unavailable and Jason was poised to fail.

It was after Thanksgiving that Jason left the toxic skepticism of the Chappaqua school system for the nurturing kindness of Harvey, a prep school in Katonah to the north. Harvey was expensive, but worth every cent. There, teachers and administrators actively educated in the implications of Lyme disease gave Jason what he needed most, the profound gift of credibility—they simply believed he felt sick. Rather than burden him with the weight of chronic illness as Leonard Sigal (and the Greeley psychologist) feared might happen by treating the disease as real, Harvey's validation of Jason's personal experience helped him heal. Vested with trust, he continued to regain his health through 2001. It was Dr. Jones's treatment combined with the caring of the Harvey School that finally allowed Jason to turn the corner from a person who was sick to one who, while still sometimes symptomatic, lived life as if essentially well. The high point of 2001 was learning that Jason had won a spot on Harvey's junior varsity basketball team, the Cavaliers. How happy I was as the new year approached to picture Jason as one of those cocky, frisky boys in the maroon-and-white jerseys, a number emblazoned on his back.

22

⋄⋄⋄

Bicycle Boy and
Other Lymebrains

The first time I met a group of severely disabled Lyme disease patients I spent hours listening to their stories, some of them heartbreaking, and mourned, with them, their lives of frustration and pain. A month later, when I met the same patients again, several could not recall me. At first I was insulted. Had I been that forgettable, my empathy that banal?

Then I realized something I had never fully grasped despite my research, despite my own Lyme disease. Unless you have personally encountered the shadow land of the most afflicted patients—a world eclipsed by strange lapses of memory, broken speech, and the struggle to follow the simplest train of thought—you cannot begin to fathom the dense, disabling fog that may accompany the disease.

To this day, popular perception holds that Lyme disease is an affliction of knees, characterized by swollen joints and an inability to serve in tennis or descend a flight of stairs. Musculoskeletal symptoms can be a hallmark of Lyme disease, but the early rheumatologists had recognized just one part of the elephant—it would take more time, and a broad array of specialists, for the widening picture to emerge.

Some of those early patients, selected for studies because of their remitting-relapsing arthritis, recalled the appearance of an expanding red rash before the arthritis had begun. Taking the cue, the Yale scientists looked for patients with the rash—early Lyme—and began studying them *prospectively*, at the *true* onset of disease. They found that only some of these untreated patients went on to develop arthritis. In others, the rash gave way to headaches and stiff necks (meningitis); facial drooping, choking, or visual loss like I suffered (attack of the cranial nerves); or terrible shooting pains throughout the torso and limbs. When these devastating signs appeared together, often the diagnosis was Lyme.

At Stony Brook, meanwhile, the neurologist John Halperin studied a far less devastating but more common "peripheral neuropathy," a kind of numbness or "pins and needles" feeling in the extremities. Could the intermittent numbness and tingling in one patient's fingers derive from the same dysfunction as the stabbing pain in another patient's torso and legs? By 1990, using the tool of electromyography (EMG) to study nerve cells, Halperin found that these symptoms, though diverse, were all due to the same thing: damaged nerve cells and, more specifically, abnormalities in the axon, the long, slender part of the cell that propagates nerve impulses along. The neurons were being "picked off" one at a time, in scattered clumps, as if snipers were at work. If the disease took out a big chunk in one place, you might get shooting pain. If it took out tiny, scattered groups of nerves you could get numbness in the toes or a weakness when you walked. Halperin's study, published in the journal *Brain,* concluded that the underlying pattern of nerve cell abnormality was the same no matter what the complaint. "All of them really had the same disease," he said. "It was just variations on a theme."

Other times Lyme caused psychiatric disease. One of the first to have this insight was Andrew Pachner, a Yale neurologist who moonlighted at psychiatric hospitals. On one such gig he was asked to evaluate a twelve-year-old boy who, prior to admission, had pedaled his stationary bicycle barely stopping to sleep or eat. Before the start of this behavior, the boy had been an excellent, hardworking student with a talent for soccer. But his soccer days were disrupted when he developed painful, swollen knees and was diagnosed with Lyme arthritis. The child was treated with doxycycline and seemed to get well. When his obsessive pedaling began some years later, his prior Lyme disease was already a distant memory, and no one saw the relationship between the two.

Except for Pachner: Given what he knew about syphilis, he wondered whether Lyme disease and the obsessive cycling might be linked. In a leap of insight, he moved the boy to Yale and began infusing him with 20 million units of penicillin for fourteen days. It was like a miracle. Literally within days the child started to improve, interacting with staff and eating food. Two weeks later he returned home and went back to school. When Pachner saw him a few months after that he had even returned to soccer. He seemed cured.

In 1989, writing for the *Archives of Neurology,* Andrew Pachner, by then at the Georgetown University School of Medicine, described six cases of central nervous system Lyme disease, of which his "bicycle boy" was just one. Another patient, a twenty-one-year-old man, had violent outbursts and wild laughing, attributed to a herpes virus thought to infect his brain. But he tested positive for Lyme disease and, treated with antibiotics, was finally cured. A six-year-old girl, so afflicted with vertigo that she staggered, tested positive for Lyme and was treated; she, too, got well.

The German neurologist Rudolph Ackermann found that the sickest of these neuroborreliosis patients suffered an inflammation of the brain and spinal cord called encephalomyelitis, also seen in syphilis. When the condition involved the spine it resembled multiple sclerosis and when it involved the brain, particularly the cerebral cortex, it could produce psychoses or seizures. The condition was progressive and degenerative without treatment, but even after antibiotic therapy, most of the patients retained the symptoms, though to a lesser degree.

From the devastating syndrome described by Ackermann to the odd presentations reported by Pachner, neuroborreliosis appeared almost protean, and, like syphilis, could be mistaken for a host of other ills. Syphilis had long been known as "the great imitator" among doctors. Now Pachner declared that Lyme disease was "the new great imitator." His statement seemed to unleash a torrent of bizarre reports flowing into the medical journals. A group from Stanford described a twenty-five-year-old woman with hallucinations, hypersexuality, nightmares, and a rash. Scientists from Germany found Lyme could cause Tourette's syndrome, catatonia, and even schizophrenia. Several teams have reported Lyme disease masquerading as—or even triggering—Parkinson's disease. And on the heels of Alan MacDonald's past work, there have been more studies suggesting a link between Lyme disease and Alzheimer's. In what would be a breakthrough of enormous scope—if borne out in other studies—neuropathologist Judit Miklossy of the University of Lausanne in Switzerland reported that she had isolated spirochetes from the blood, cerebrospinal fluid, and brain tissue of fourteen

Alzheimer's patients upon autopsy, essentially replicating MacDonald's work of a decade before. More than two dozen published papers associate neuroborreliosis with stroke, and others document that Lyme disease may cause seizures.

Perhaps most tantalizing is the work done on ALS starting years before Dave Martz ever got sick. In 1987, for instance, a Wisconsin team found that four of fifty-four patients diagnosed with ALS also tested positive for Lyme disease—and since ALS is fatal, decided that treatment with antibiotics wouldn't hurt. Following the treatment, one of the four patients was stabilized, the progression of her symptoms halted for good. Intrigued by the report, Halperin did a formal follow-up, testing nineteen ALS patients from the hyperendemic area of Suffolk County, New York. Of these, nine had Lyme antibodies and the Stony Brook doctors, like their Wisconsin colleagues, treated them with antibiotics. Three patients, those with abnormalities primarily in the lower part of the body, improved. But three of the sickest patients declined dramatically following treatment, which seemed to hasten their death. Though the Stony Brook scientists couldn't say for sure what was going on, they affirmed the statistical significance between ALS and Lyme disease, and theorized that in those who deteriorated, the cause might be the flood of dying spirochetes, that is, a classic herx.

If one were to describe all the terrifying and macabre presentations of neuroborreliosis, they would fill a book. But even added together they are rare compared to the most common neurological problem—the confusional state known as encephalopathy, or, as Lyme patients call it, "brain fog." Patients reported the experience: a disorienting lapse of memory, an inability to concentrate, difficulty in falling asleep, and profound fatigue.

Lyme encephalopathy was hardly controversial. John Halperin's colleagues at Stony Brook objectively measured deficits in spatial orientation, short-term memory, concentration, and mathematical and construction ability. Halperin himself used magnetic resonance imaging to scan patients' brains. In one study he found white-matter lesions, much like those seen in multiple sclerosis, in the brains of seven out of seventeen encephalopathic Lyme disease patients. The lesions represented brain damage. Following treatment he rescanned six patients, and found the lesions resolved in three. Even when the lesions resolved, symptoms sometimes did not.

As scary as brain lesions might sound, the academic description of these impairments as "mild" created dissonance between scientists like

Halperin and patients on the ground. Sure, Lyme patients were not usually as impaired as those with bullets in their brains, but the mental fog, the deficits in language and organization, the psychiatric leftovers of anxiety, depression, and OCD, could still disrupt lives. Adults lost houses, marriages, and jobs and were compromised as parents. Children lost their childhoods when cognitive or emotional disabilities forced them to be home-schooled, sometimes for years. The impact was major, but mainstream experts continued to characterize such symptoms as "minor," "nonspecific," and "vague."

The professionals able, finally, to traverse the space between the dismissive labels and the excruciating patient experience were the psychiatrists. If neurologists and rheumatologists deemed psychiatric symptoms "subjective," the psychiatrists said, it was because, when it came to psychiatry, these physicians were unschooled.

One of the first to enter the fray was Brian Fallon, whose interest had been sparked in the late 1980s while helping a close relative overcome a serious case of Lyme disease. He had just finished his psychiatry residency and secured a gig as a fellow of the National Institute of Mental Health. He was stationed at the New York State Psychiatric Institute, adjacent to the Columbia University Medical Center complex in New York City. The young doctor, whose kempt, longish hair, neat beard, and energetic demeanor made him look like he'd marched off the album cover of *Abbey Road*, specialized in anxiety disorders, with a focus on hypochondria. But news of his interest in Lyme disease had traveled through the grapevine to Polly Murray. Some of her friends and neighbors had developed psychiatric disorders after having Lyme disease. Could Fallon follow up?

Fallon and his psychiatrist wife, Jennifer Nields, drove out to Lyme and spent the day in Polly Murray's living room surrounded by her watercolors, talking to her afflicted friends. One of the first things they decided as a result of that meeting was to impose formal discipline on the loosely knit reports of psychiatric symptoms made by neurologists and rheumatologists. Fallon was well aware of the single-case studies and series of anecdotes continually published in medical journals. Studying Lyme patients, the German researcher Kohler had even reported a staging of the psychiatric symptoms that paralleled progression in the neurological realm. In the first stage, mild depression could parallel a fibromyalgia-like illness. In the second stage, mood and personality disorders often emerged alongside meningitis or neuropathy. Finally, in stage three, with the onset of encephalomyelitis, the clinical picture might include psychosis or dementia.

Fallon felt that when it came to Lyme, none of these reports, even Kohler's, was solid enough to vest psychiatry with the same objective underpinnings found in rheumatology or neurology. Part of the problem was a misperception about what psychiatrists did and what psychiatry was. Psychiatrists often started their work in the murky, subjective outback of a patient's psyche. But the scientists among them, like Fallon, were charged with the mission of anchoring thought, feeling, and experience in the firmament of objective data. Neurologists and rheumatologists often dismissed the psychiatric symptoms of Lyme disease as subjective, but they did so without applying the rigorous methodology that psychiatric research entailed.

And that's where Fallon hoped his contribution would matter most. His labor paid off. Conducting structured clinical interviews with people from southeastern Connecticut who had histories of Lyme disease, he learned that depression or panic could worsen after the start of antibiotic treatment, suggesting a kind of psychiatric Herxheimer reaction that resulted as infection died off. Speaking to the patients, he found that neuropsychiatric Lyme disease and regular psychiatric disease appeared much the same. This was of particular concern since so many patients failed to notice a rash or register positive on standard tests, making it likely that the true cause of their psychiatric condition—Lyme disease—would be missed.

The patients were in psychiatric trouble, to say the least. Surveying 193 patients testing positive for Lyme, Fallon found that 84 percent had mood problems; of those reporting depression, 90 percent had never had an episode prior to Lyme disease, which suggested the two were linked.

As for children with Lyme, Fallon found they resembled accident victims with head injuries. Like adults, they had trouble with short-term memory, word-finding, and concentration. Their performance IQ and spatial reasoning were particularly impaired. The children could still remember and learn—but they processed the information slowly and needed more time for tasks.

Lyme children entered in studies for impaired memory or processing speed, moreover, suffered anxiety, mood, and behavioral disorders at higher rates than healthy children as well. Especially notable was the increased risk for depression and suicidal thoughts. The findings were important because children with Lyme disease could be "misdiagnosed as having a primary psychiatric problem," while the root issue—infection with the spirochete B. burgdorferi—might never be addressed.

It was a dilemma that transcended Lyme disease. Time and again, Fallon, an expert in hypochondria, had seen frustrated doctors dismiss medically ill patients as psychiatric due to their own inability to diagnose the disease. In Lyme the mistake was especially damaging, he said, "since a delay in treatment could turn a curable, acute infection into a chronic, treatment-refractory disease."

The solution, Fallon the scientist knew, was to gather objective evidence of physical damage to the brain. Working with radiologists at Columbia, he found one useful tool was the SPECT (single photon emission computed tomography) scan, which generated a moving picture of the brain. A radioactive "tracer" solution was delivered intravenously, and was thereafter tracked to measure blood flow through the brain. Even when MRI scans appeared normal in Lyme disease patients, SPECT could show something amiss. In symptomatic Lyme patients, decreased blood flow, known as hypoperfusion, could often be documented in the center of thought and higher functioning, the cerebral cortex. After treatment, many of the patients showed improvement on SPECT.

In 2009, Fallon found more objective proof of damage in Lyme brains. This time using a scan known as positron emission tomography, or PET, he measured glucose metabolism in Lyme patients who were treated but reported continued impairment of memory nonetheless. No matter how he varied the circumstances, Fallon reported, the patients were functionally impaired—not globally, but in specific regions in the temporal, parietal, and limbic areas of the brain.

With so much documented damage, it was only natural for Fallon to bring in a brain trauma expert, neuropsychologist Leo J. Shea III, assistant director of the Brain Injury Day Treatment Program at NYU's Rusk Institute of Rehabilitation Medicine in New York. Sure he would evaluate a Lyme disease patient, Shea agreed, and perhaps offer the same kind of remediation he used to treat head injury patients, too. But as Shea began working with the Lyme patient sent by Fallon—the first of some 1,200 he would study and help over time—he found a form of brain dysfunction unlike any he had ever seen.

Indeed, in traumatic brain injury the patient experiences an insult and then progressively gets better, Shea explains. "There is an upward swing, a linear and progressive path towards improvement—but with Lyme it was an undulating course." Soon Shea had coined the term "Lyme undulation" to reflect the waxing and waning aspects of cognition, emotion, and behavior his patients would report. While clearly injured, Shea's brain trauma patients made steady progress as they learned and eventually mastered strategies for encoding information, compensating for deficits, and performing functional skills like reading, following maps, or arriving on time for appointments—but the Lyme patients were often too fatigued to benefit from the training, and made limited progress. "It was two steps forward and one step back," Shea states.

Many of the Lyme patients, in fact, walked through Shea's door with a second, often erroneous diagnosis—attention deficit disorder, or ADD. But Shea found they just didn't fit the mold. Sure they appeared to have trouble attending to tasks and concentrating, but unlike true ADD patients, they weren't getting up and walking around the room every half hour. Instead, they were "sticking in there for two or three hours, working with you," he states. While a patient with ADD might look around the room and start focusing on other things, the impaired Lyme patients tried mightily to stay on task. "It's just that the information wasn't getting in. At one session I would teach the patient compensatory strategies and he would say that he understood them and even show me that he understood it by performing an exercise," says Shea, "but then at the next session it was as if he never learned it at all."

Over the years Shea has documented in this unusual patient group not just memory impairments, but also slowed processing speed, impaired reading rate and comprehension, deficits in visual scanning, problems with multitasking, and difficulty with executive functioning like staying on task or effectively maintaining emotional balance. It was a maddening cognitive trap. "Lyme patients had difficulty learning because they could not remember what happened long enough to encode it; the information went by too fast or was too complex and they didn't have time to break it down into discrete elements so that they could remember it," Shea found. The effort was so tiring that anything learned might be lost without reinforcement. The person with ADD was bored and inattentive, but the Lyme patient was exhausted," Shea states. "He needs periodic breaks because he is so physically and mentally fatigued."

To help his Lyme patients, Shea first taught them to understand their illness—not just the pain and exhaustion, but also the waxing and waning of memory, focus, and processing speed. In the workplace, at home, and on the medical front, he told them, they had to explain the situation to others to prevent themselves from being labeled with a psychiatric instead of a physical illness.

Since Shea found it difficut to improve his patients' undulating memories or boost their waxing-waning processing speed, he opted to help them take advantage of those hours and days when symptoms abated.

He also helped them use written narration to hold facts together so that context rather than raw memory got them through the day. One young man challenged to finish papers for a college literature course was taught to talk through his ideas first, and then to break each essay into tiny, manageable chunks so he wouldn't have to hold too much in his mind at once. A corporate executive was taught to prepare and then summarize only the key points of a presentation, calling on his employees to explain in full. "He preserved his image in front of other executives and looked like he had a tight, productive team," Shea explains. A lawyer was taught to e-mail his list of daily tasks to his BlackBerry so he could stay on task. From use of assistive technology to understanding and then compensating for limits, Shea helped the patients maximize their intelligence and navigate the world.

Taking note of all this work was Robert Bransfield, a psychiatrist with a practice in Red Bank, New Jersey, along the sleepy Navesink River, just inland from the glitz and neon of the Jersey shore. Tall and professorial, with a charm and humility so natural it catches you by surprise, Bransfield seems an unlikely rebel, but he says that experience with patients at the heart of the epidemic has left him little choice.

The first Lyme patient he brought back from the brink worked as an assistant to a veterinarian, making her risk for exposure especially high. Late in the summer of her twenty-second year, she developed the classic symptoms of Lyme disease and was treated with oral antibiotics. When they didn't make a dent in her condition, her doctor placed her on intravenous Rocephin and she appeared to get well. But almost two years later, she came down with a new set of symptoms, this time psychiatric. Not only was she irritable and anxious, she also began to check things obsessively and eventually descended into a deep depression. Her psychiatric symptoms were so numerous, in fact, it was impossible to label her as having just a single disorder. She developed mania with rapid mood swings, from grandiosity to sudden tearfulness; paranoid delusions; auditory hallucinations; verbal aggressiveness; and violent impulses. She also suffered cognitive dysfunction, including trouble in spelling, writing, and verbal fluency. Despite hospitalization and treatment with "every psychotropic imaginable," says Bransfield, the patient declined, her depression becoming so severe that she tried to kill herself.

"This was very different from run-of-the-mill bipolar disorder," Bransfield said. "She kept getting worse, and she had physical symptoms, too. It forced the question: Could it be a reoccurrence of Lyme disease? She was so depressed I believed suicide was inevitable, so with no other option in sight, I began seeking a physician willing to treat her with antibiotics for Lyme disease. No one was willing to take the responsibility, so I wrote the order for intravenous Rocephin myself. It was a lifesaving decision. The patient responded to the treatment and today remains mentally and physically well."

Bransfield described the case in the medical journal *Psychosomatics* in 1995, and it didn't take long for other Lyme disease patients to beat a path to his door.

As a result of the influx, Bransfield reports he's found a connection between Lyme disease and aggression in a small but significant group. He had one Lyme disease patient who'd become so paranoid that he assaulted five police officers in an episode of rage, and Bransfield admitted him to the hospital's psychiatric unit. During the hospital stay the patient made his way to the river behind the facility to watch fireworks on the Fourth of July and was so startled by the sound that he jumped into the river. A fourteen-year-old boy in Bransfield's study repeatedly attempted to choke his mother to death, destroy his house, knock over furniture, and kick and punch holes through the walls and doors. A woman, age forty, became so enraged when a garbage truck cut her off on the road that she followed it back to the station, honking her horn and screaming all the way. In fact, she "was so crazed," she reported, that she felt like choking the driver to death. Bransfield says that in each and every case, the aggression resolved when these patients were treated for Lyme disease.

Hoping to spread the word, he's even testified in court when he believes defendants have been adversely influenced by Lyme disease to commit a crime. In 2001, he spoke out on behalf of a young man, age twenty-two, who attacked his neighbor with a medieval ax. It was partially treated, late-stage Lyme disease with brain involvement, including seizures that caused loss of memory and episodes of missing time, which led to the violence, Bransfield said. Despite his testimony, the young man was found guilty. Bransfield has had more success testifying for a few women arrested for shoplifting. "These cases involved encephalopathy," Bransfield says. "The women were in such a fog they'd be holding something they hadn't paid for, without even realizing it, and would walk right out of the store. When the guards stopped them they were so confused they weren't able to explain what had gone on."

Bransfield has also been following another thread—the theory that Lyme disease and autism are somehow linked. The idea derives in part from observation: Women with Lyme disease seem to be having more than their share of autistic offspring, he reports, and when children with autism get Lyme disease, their autism gets worse. Bransfield says that ten of the fifteen top Lyme states—including Connecticut, Rhode Island, New Jersey, and Pennsylvania—are also most endemic for autism. And he and his colleagues say they've found compelling evidence in studies of blood. In one study he references, 22 percent of autistic subjects tested positive for Lyme disease. In another, it was 20 to 30 percent. Other infections, especially mycoplasma, may be involved, he adds—and even if the infections themselves don't hurt the fetus, he proposes, immune molecules produced by an infected mother just might. As the theory gains traction, families with autistic children have formed organizations and held conferences, testing their children for Lyme disease and seeing if treatment can help. Is Lyme disease causing the autism? "Not exactly," Bransfield believes. Instead, the children are already immunologically vulnerable, and a multitude of triggers, be it Lyme borreliosis or a chemical sensitivity, might set them off. To see if the theory holds, Brian Fallon has launched an epidemiological study comparing the rate of autism in two heavily Lyme-endemic areas in New Jersey and Connecticut to areas where Lyme is rare.

Bransfield's colleague, Virginia Sherr, a psychiatrist from Holland, Pennsylvania, meanwhile, says the prevalence of tick-borne disease has transformed the face of her practice—and not because Lyme disease patients sought her out. "I find that many patients walking in off the street are infected, but unaware," Sherr states. "They don't know what has happened to cause their depression, confusion, obsession, anxiety, tendency to lose things, or other complaints." When Sherr suspects Lyme or a coinfection, she has no compunction about sending blood out for laboratory tests. "When tick-borne disease is the cause, it's only with antibiotic therapy that psychiatric symptoms resolve."

Sherr inhabits a reality different from that of the Steeres and Sigals of the world. "Doctors can destroy patients by telling them that a true, physical disease is all in the head," Sherr says, "and suicide is a possible result." In the hyperendemic area of Bucks County, she sees a new case of Lyme encephalopathy every week and, sometimes, almost every day. "I am a psychiatrist. These are not people who are referred to me because they have Lyme disease—they are sent because they have panic attacks, hallucinations, obsessive compulsive disorder, depression. They are in agony—not only neuropsychiatric pain, but physical pain as well. They have never been hypochondriacal in their lives, but that is how they have been labeled before they come to me. They are encephalopathic, but they have been told they are not by physicians who wouldn't know a case of encephalopathy if they fell over it. They are physically sick, but are blamed for their illness by doctors who say things like, 'You belong to a cult if you think you have Lyme disease,' or 'You look okay to me.'"

One of the most dangerous trends she's found is the impetus by some doctors to accuse mothers of Lyme children with Munchausen Syndrome by Proxy: the crime of causing or fabricating their children's disease to gain attention for themselves. "So many children sick from complex diseases like Lyme have been forcibly removed from mothers who insist the children are ill," Sherr says. "The mothers may be vilified, publicly shamed, or even jailed. Many such cases," she adds, "involve unrecognized Lyme borreliosis that mothers insist is valid despite negative tests."

Doctors like Sherr remain light-years apart from Sigal, who has gone on record saying that some of those diagnosed with Lyme disease may have psychiatric disorders instead. Fallon explains the divide: "Those first describing Lyme disease in the early literature were trained in rheumatology and dermatology. The 'objective signs' they recognized— palpably swollen joints, antibody production, and an erythema migrans rash—derived from the specialty-specific training they had. Later, neurologists added their specialized 'signs' to the mix: cranial nerve palsy, gross meningitis, and measurably damaged nerves. By these standards, virtually one hundred percent of those treated for Lyme disease are cured, but that ignores the fact that a huge number of patients still have cognitive problems, fatigue, pain, and mood swings. Because those symptoms weren't objectified early in the history of the disease, by the specific specialties first involved, many doctors still think they don't count. As psychiatrists we are used to dealing with diseases that can't be objectified with the tools of rheumatology, even the tools of neurology, but they do count. If someone has schizophrenia, that counts. If someone has severe bipolar disorder, there's no blood test for that, but to psychiatrists, that counts. Because Lyme disease was originally researched by rheumatologists and later on by neurologists, there was a lack of appreciation for these other ways of defining illness and objectifying signs and symptoms of disease."

One did not need to be a scientist or doctor to observe the obvious: If John Halperin offered no relief for their illness, patients trucked off to Fallon. If Fallon didn't have an answer, back they bounced to Halperin or Steere. To scientists and clinicians, Lyme disease was laden with history, territoriality, and points of view. On the other hand, new patients came to the scene fresh. Because patients stayed with doctors based on treatment outcome—and because outcome varied so widely depending upon whom you talked to—it was impossible to say that John Halperin and Robert Bransfield were seeing the same kind of patient. Even if the precipitating infections had once been identical, was it now the same disease?

23

A Devastating Realization

Framingham, Massachusetts, 2002

Sheila and Russ Statlender decided they had just one option: going back to the beginning and, rather than relying on others, figuring it out for themselves. They had both trained in the sciences, after all, with Sheila a clinical psychologist who had research experience and Russ a physician. They gathered copies of the medical records from their pediatrician, and spent weeks reviewing every office visit, laboratory result, and consult note from the many specialists who'd seen each of their three children since the night of the fateful fire in the impossibly distant year of 1996. They organized hundreds of pages, and set up shop in their home office, right by another window with yet another view of the deer preserve, to read the litany of their fall from grace and the archive of their pain. By degrees detached, cold, rude, and skeptical, the entries appeared, in aggregate, to be a jumble of half thoughts, dismissive conjectures, and missed connections. "It's amazing how many consult notes were missing from their charts, given the number of specialists the kids had seen," Sheila says.

They also began poring over the medical literature—not some journalist's rendition of it or some physician's interpretation of it, but the actual, original research articles published in the peer review since Lyme disease had been recognized in Connecticut more than twenty-five years before. Often Sheila, with a more flexible schedule, would gather the documents by day, and Russ, finally home from the hospital, would review the offerings at night. They studied, as well, whatever information was available on the official Web sites of the NIH, the CDC, and the Massachusetts Department of Health. Striving to avoid the politics of the fight over Lyme disease, they read the material for scientific input alone.

"We started reading carefully, with open minds but a great deal of skepticism regarding Lyme disease. We'd taken the children down so many false paths, and spent so much time dragging them to doctors who couldn't help them; we didn't want to be fooled again," Sheila says.

Yet as they read the medical records and the journal articles, the deer preserve in their line of sight, their jaws dropped. Time and again, they found, doctors had used the ELISA and Western blot to rule out Lyme disease in their children—while it was plain as day that many of the world's top experts, even the National Institutes of Health Web site, said the tests were unreliable and could generate not only false positives, but also false negatives—a lot of them—thereby missing a lot of patients. During the early years their children were tested with ELISA, for instance, while major studies said it could miss a third of patients screened. As for the Western blot, the Statlenders learned it had been derived statistically and somewhat arbitrarily, the exact band formula for "positive" the subject of constant, furious debate. Bands had been taken out of the test, making it harder to pass. And the criteria had actually been established for purposes of surveillance, not diagnosis—by definition a far more conservative bar. Russ wondered why it was being applied to patient care.

"It was one thing that ELISA had been used routinely as the screening device for Lyme, and that two of our three kids had Lyme ruled out simply by checking it off on a lab slip. But to read about the madness with the Western blot—how certain irrelevant bands came to be included in the reporting, and other highly species-specific bands were excluded— well, it struck us as sheer stupidity, to be frank," Sheila says.

"I don't believe it," Russ muttered repeatedly, astonished at each new page he turned and every journal article he took in. The uncertainties and approximations that had determined his children's fate were nearly beyond belief.

"It dawned on us slowly, and then hit us like a ton of bricks: None of our three kids, in all those years of illness and a multitude of medical appointments at some of the best centers in the world, had ever been adequately worked up for Lyme disease," Sheila says. "I looked out the window with new eyes and thought, 'Oh my god, it was out there all along.' " With Russ's family on the Cape, and Sheila's in Connecticut, the children had had multiple opportunities for exposure in many locations. They could have been reexposed repeatedly, Sheila and Russ agreed.

"It was heart-wrenching," says Sheila. Seth had been sick for six years at that point and Amy for at least five—without an explanation or a clue. They had virtually fallen off the face of the Earth—nearly forgotten by busy friends and largely ignored by their schools. All three once-talented athletes, none of the Statlender children now were able to run, jump, or score goals. Amy, about to go up and balance on her toes after years of ballet lessons, had stopped dancing for good. Instead, they spent many days in pain or suffering from bone-crushing fatigue. Now Eric, their youngest, was falling into the illness. Sheila and Russ surveyed their surroundings: a spacious, light-drenched home on three acres of lawn bordered by more than fourteen acres of forest—their very own deer- and mammal-filled woods.

"It was one of those moments when you just feel sickened," says Statlender. "We knew we'd been had."

24

Longing for Lyme

Colorado Springs, Colorado, 2003

As Dave Martz lay dying, an idea serpentined around his mind and would not loosen its grip: Despite the absolute diagnosis and the insistence of the doctors, including a world expert, that he was dying of ALS, despite his own vow to face things head-on and reject the lure of denial, Martz couldn't shake the notion that possibly, just maybe, he actually had Lyme disease.

He'd had plentiful exposure, starting from the time he was young: numerous fishing trips to endemic parts of Minnesota and Canada, a summer at a tick-infested church camp in Wisconsin. And his ALS was so atypical, with its joint involvement and pain, so *Lyme-like*.

Even after he failed a test trial of oral antibiotics, Martz wondered whether Lyme was at the root of his ills.

"Not a chance," said his doctors, who could see the seduction of the Lyme diagnosis to a dying man like Martz. The new great imitator, said to mimic any disease under the sun, was preferable to a death sentence. Who wouldn't rather have Lyme disease, generally considered treatable, than a one-way ticket to the great beyond?

25

A Nantucket Burning:
I'm Diagnosed with Babesiosis

Chappaqua, New York, 2001

It was sometime after the new year when, feeling better but hardly well, I drove a mile down my hill for a latte at Starbucks and my appointment with Tick Bite. She greeted me with a smile, waving a paper in my face. She seemed so pleased she was literally aglow. A few weeks before, dissatisfied with a plateau in my treatment response, my returning migraines and fatigue, she'd drawn blood and sent it to Quest Lab for a *Babesia* test. "When Lyme disease patients don't get well," Tick Bite told me, "coinfection with babesiosis can be the cause." Now the results had come back, and as with my Lyme ELISA, antibodies were four times the cutoff for positive—sky-high.

The pieces were falling into place. With my spiking headache and continued exhaustion, babesiosis certainly made sense for me. A decade earlier, in 1990, I'd spent a couple of weeks as a science-writing fellow at the Marine Biological Laboratory at Woods Hole, Massachusetts, right across the water from Nantucket Island, where human babesiosis had been studied more than fifteen years before.

It was during the early seventies, before Lyme was even recognized, that Andrew Spielman, a tropical medicine expert at the Harvard School of Public Health, was asked to investigate what locals called Nantucket fever. At the time, only two patients were known. The first was a wealthy Nantucket woman who came down with a disabling mystery illness marked by extreme anemia, fatigue, and fever that local doctors could not explain. So she chartered a plane to Rutgers University in New Jersey. Rutgers doctors examined her blood under a microscope, diagnosed her with malaria, and placed her on the standard treatment, chloroquine. When the treatment didn't work, they grew alarmed because drug-resistant malaria is, after all, a threat to public health. A slide of blood was shipped off to the CDC, where experts identified not malaria but another similar agent that also inhabits red blood cells— *Babesia microti*, a cousin of *Babesia* ssp., known to cause cattle epidemics that wiped out entire herds. With the identification of her infection, the woman was finally treated correctly and got well.

When a second case of babesiosis appeared on Nantucket Island a few years later, physicians again were stymied. But the second patient happened to be friends with the first, and finally, with doctors throwing up their hands, it fell to the first patient to diagnose the disease in the second. Her lay diagnosis was correct, and the second patient was treated and recovered as well.

That's when Spielman entered the fray. Would he care to find the cause of these cases in the environment? Observing the cycles of infection year after year, he finally tracked *Babesia* through the ecosystem, discovering that it lived in the blood of mice and spread from one mammal to the next through the bite of an *Ixodes* tick. Larva and nymphal (baby and adolescent) ticks ate by sucking the blood of mice and other small mammals like shrews and chipmunks. But adult ticks, far bigger in size, generally required larger mammals like deer for a blood meal. It was only in geographic areas with an abundance of large mammals that *Ixodes* ticks could mature to adulthood and reproduce substantially enough for the disease to be widespread.

When the spirochete *B. burgdorferi* was identified by Willy Burgdorfer as the cause of Lyme disease in 1981, Spielman realized that the newly discovered illness involved the same tick and same natural cycle he'd already charted for human babesiosis on Nantucket Island and beyond. For Spielman, the connection between the two infections—Lyme and babesiosis—was immediately clear. Every year since his first discoveries on Nantucket, after all, new *Babesia* patients had been diagnosed. And some of them had exhibited not just the malarialike headache and fever spikes typical of babesiosis, but also a confounding circular red rash and strange pains that migrated from joint to joint—symptoms classically associated with Lyme disease. "There was a woman who lived opposite our field station who had migratory arthritis and the expanding rash and—babesiosis. She obviously had Lyme as well, but no one had the organism, and restrictive case definitions came into play," Spielman recalled, "because in the beginning, the differential diagnosis for Lyme disease included a travel history to Lyme, Connecticut!"

Eventually Spielman realized that both infections were spreading at different but proportional rates. With each infection requiring a treatment ineffective for the other, the coinfected patients of Nantucket Island provided important clues to the spectrum of disease. Sometimes physicians just needed to treat babesiosis for an intractably sick "Lyme" patient to get well. Even as babesiosis extended its range and came to rival Lyme disease as a cause of illness, the lessons of Nantucket's coinfected patients would fall on deaf ears.

Indeed, few Lyme disease patients were ever tested for, or had even heard of, babesiosis; and though the two epidemics had been spawned in tandem from the start and could be equally debilitating, few primary care doctors in endemic areas like Chappaqua ran the babesiosis test. "We don't test for that," our Mount Kisco pediatrician explained at the time. The internist who tried to treat my headaches—classic for babesiosis— never mentioned the possibility that infection, either Lyme or babesiosis, might be a cause.

Yet in retrospect I believe the *Babesia* diagnosis was my missing link. Most science-writing fellows at Woods Hole had stayed in residence halls near the lab, but with a family in tow I was given a gorgeous rustic cabin in the woods. Way before my arrival, *Babesia microti* had begun its migration west and south, first over Cape Cod and then down the Long Island Sound, fast on the heels of Lyme disease toward Connecticut, Westchester, and the points beyond. In 1990, still traveling incognito toward New York State, *Babesia microti* was already rife in the forested enclaves of Woods Hole.

It wasn't just my exposure that fit with the Quest results, but the mystery illness I'd suffered after returning from Cape Cod. Doctors could never explain the strange spikes of fever to 105 degrees Fahrenheit that hit me in hallucinogenic waves for more than a week that summer, or the gullies of sleep so black that, except for the nightmares, I thought I might be dead. When the fever broke and I noticed the sweating, it seemed just a consequence of summer. It was after the sweat leveled off that the headache-without-end licked its first noxious path through my brain.

This was classic acute babesiosis. Without treatment the acute infection had flared and apparently smoldered, Tick Bite theorized. Then it had synergized in concert with the Lyme. She had a treatment to push the *Babesia* back. Like Jason before me I now added Mepron to my arsenal of antibiotics. The thick gold sludge, known for treating malaria, made me retch and want to vomit. But I held it down. Some six weeks later, the drill in my head stopped whirring and the nausea and dizziness I'd lived with for years receded like a tide pulled back to sea. I still wasn't better, not entirely, but Tick Bite had peeled another layer off the onion and extinguished another set of symptoms from my disease.

26

Photo Safari

Colorado Springs, Colorado, and Kenya, Africa, 2003

As he grew sicker, babesiosis signaled itself to Dave Martz, too—though it would be months before he realized what it was. It started with the notion of an African photo safari; while he could still walk on his own, the idea of capturing big game on film had special appeal.

As daring as the trip sounded to others, Dee felt it might cheer them up. So, tapping the connections of friends, she finally contacted Gary Clarke, the former director of the Topeka Zoo and safari-leader extraordinaire. She explained that Dave was dying, and asked what Clarke could do for them. Amazingly, Clarke offered to take Dee and Dave on an individual, two-week photo safari of the big-game preserves in Kenya, from the open plains of the Maasai Mara in a hot-air balloon to the northern Samburo preserve, all for the same fee they'd pay if they went with a group of fifteen. "I would enjoy spending two weeks just getting to know you," the compassionate tour leader told Dee over the phone. The plan was to travel in a chauffeured Land Rover with a sizable moon roof—all the better for photographing those lions and rhinos—and to sleep in lodges or under the stars, in tents.

Preparing for the trip, Martz, like all safari travelers, started taking Lariam, a medication routinely used for preventing (as well as treating) malaria, a cousin to babesiosis. Although he didn't at first make the connection between the medicine and his increased energy, to his utter surprise he started feeling stronger than he had been before. On safari, things only improved, so much so that, touring the African bush, he was able to participate in *all* the game trips. He was up at 7:30 each A.M., riding and standing in the Land Rover, his head sticking out through the wide-open gape of the moon roof. He spent hours photographing leopards and water buffalo, elephants and cheetahs, wildebeests and zebras in the soft morning glow. Then it was back to camp for lunch and rest, and out again for the afternoon. "We thought it was the excitement and adrenaline of the trip," says Martz, whose photos of fearsome lions and posturing chimps adorn his home to this day.

Yet the "adrenaline" seemed to last back in Colorado, at least for a while. Continuing the prophylactic Larium for two more months, per doctor's orders, Martz kept getting better. He had so much energy that he hit the lecture circuit, taking the fruit of his photo safari to local book clubs and even the Pikes Peak wildlife haven, the Cheyenne Mountain Zoo.

27

❖

Tick Menagerie:
The Coinfections of
Lyme Disease

From the time Willy Burgdorfer first sliced open those Shelter Island ticks in his Montana lab and began exploring under the microscope, he observed a glut of microbes. He traced just one of them——*B. burgdorferi,* the spirochete named after him—to the disease Steere studied in Connecticut. But right from the start he suspected that in other situations or other patients, different organisms could be involved. Sitting next to Burgdorfer in a sun-drenched conference room at the Rocky Mountain Laboratories, I watched him remove from his ancient briefcase a handwritten chart that had withstood the test of time. Yellowed and creased, the paper listed microbes, six in all. "These," he told me, "are what I found in the Shelter Island ticks." He would not give me a copy, but he let me look. I saw the spirochete *B. burgdorferi* on his chart, of course, but I also observed an organism, larger than a bacterium, called a nematode worm. (The worm's potential for disease, said Burgdorfer, was unknown.)

I took definite note, therefore, when Richard Ostfeld, an animal ecologist at the Institute for Ecosystem Studies, in the Dutchess County town of Millbrook, New York, told me he'd found nematode worms in deer ticks, too. I paid even more attention when the finding was confirmed in Connecticut by University of New Haven microbiologist Eva Sapi and announced at the school's Lyme symposium in 2007. Neither scientist knew what to make of the worms, nor that they'd been observed by others before.

Whether nematode worms living in ticks will ever be implicated in human disease has yet to be seen. But if they are, says Sapi, then treating that infection could make all the difference in the world for a subset of patients who remain sick. The take-home message is this: Ticks that carry the pathogen of Lyme disease harbor many other organisms, some known to cause serious human disease, others not traced to human infection or still undiscovered and unexplored.

Some of those coinfections—babesiosis, ehrlichiosis, and anaplasmosis—are no longer controversial. Though overshadowed by the uproar over Lyme disease they can be just as debilitating, and have been studied and documented for years. For patients who suffer these infections in combination with Lyme, illness can be especially severe. These infections don't respond to all the antibiotics used against Lyme disease, and so even when Lyme is treated and cured, *Babesia, Ehrlichia,* and *Anaplasma* can persist, keeping the patient ill. Patients who suffer more than one infection may have more symptoms and a longer course for the disease.

One of the first to understand the implications was Peter Krause, a professor of pediatric infectious disease at the University of Connecticut School of Medicine in Hartford. Krause became fascinated after writing a chapter on *Babesia* for a textbook, and asked the man who studied Nantucket fever, Andrew Spielman of Harvard, to team up in researching the disease. Together, they tracked the infection, publishing findings in the *New England Journal of Medicine* and the *Journal of the American Medical Association,* producing what amounted to the new chapter and verse on the disease whose pathogenesis and clinical course resembled that of malaria.

Clearly, *Babesia* was spreading. By the early nineties, two-thirds of Lyme patients on Long Island had *Babesia* antibodies. *Babesia* had risen so dramatically, Krause and Spielman reported in 2003, that in some areas it virtually rivaled Lyme. To reach their conclusion, they spent a decade testing and retesting 60 percent of the residents on Block Island, off the Rhode Island coast. Year after year, an ever-higher percent of the residents had *Babesia* antibodies until, by the middle of the nineties, *Babesia* and Lyme were literally neck and neck. Some critics said the numbers were so high because Block Island, off the mainland, was cut off. Yet when Krause and Spielman repeated the study on residents in mainland Connecticut, the numbers held.

Patients with Lyme and babesiosis together often felt sicker, and stayed sick longer, than those with just one disease. In one telling study, Krause found some 3 percent of patients treated for early Lyme were still fatigued six months later, compared to more than a third of those coin-fected with babesiosis and Lyme.

Yet one could have babesiosis without having Lyme disease, and it could be devastating on its own. It was fatal in 10 percent of patients, especially the elderly or those with immune problems. Untreated, *Babesia* could smolder, persisting without perceptible symptoms for months or even years. Smoldering *Babesia microti* created a worst-case scenario, leaving patients with such a high parasitic load that the illness, when it arrived, and generally it did, was especially disabling and profound. One man tested positive for *Babesia* yet remained asymptomatic for seventeen months, all the while refusing treatment. "He felt fine," explains Krause, "and he didn't like the idea of taking a drug." But eventually the man got so sick he had to be hospitalized. Following treatment in the hospital, he relapsed.

In fact, like *Borrelia burgdorferi, Babesia microti* is persistent, pro-grammed by evolution to live in mammals over the very long haul. Any-one who's ever had babesiosis may no longer donate blood—even after treatment—because while they may feel just fine, microbes may linger on. Increasingly more *Babesia* infections are spreading through the blood sup-ply, the American Red Cross said in 2006. "Recrudescence" is the word Peter Krause uses to describe what happens when, despite standard ther-apy (today, usually Mepron and Zithromax), babesiosis recurs. In the most severe cases of the disease, the treatment of choice is literally an ex-change transfusion. By replacing all of a patient's blood cells, the parasitic load can be lowered to the point where infection can finally be cleared.

Babesia is not just rife in Massachusetts and Connecticut, but has spread to Lyme zones nationwide. *B. microti* has been isolated from ticks in New Jersey and Maryland as well as those from Westchester and Dutchess Counties in New York. A new species, *Babesia duncani*, was first discovered in Northern California and Washington State, while one called MO-1 has been isolated from humans in the South. These alternate *Babesias* now infect Northeast patients too—but due to differences in the organism, cannot be detected on most serological tests for the disease.

Finally, new *Babesia* strains have been found worldwide—creating the same kind of complex scenario typical of Lyme. With international travel and the certainty that these organisms can spread through blood, babesio-sis can sometimes be easy to miss and its diagnosis complex.

Even as Krause and Spielman studied babesiosis, other researchers ze-roed in on a second group of coinfections, generally referred to as the

Ehrlichias, also transmitted by ticks and communicated in transfusions of blood. The first to make the leap here was Johan Bakken, M.D., on duty at St. Mary's Medical Center, in Duluth, Michigan, one day in 1990, when an elderly man arrived with a high fever and what seemed like a severe flu. Along with others on the staff of St. Mary's, Bakken suspected the presence of a bacterial infection and treated the patient with high-dose antibiotics. Despite the treatment the patient declined rapidly, and three days later he died. What had been wrong with him? The only clue, the physicians said, were berrylike clusters inside his white blood cells.

Bakken soon realized the "berries" were similar to those characteristic of ehrlichiosis, caused by a *Rickettsia*—a type of intracellular bacteria—recently discovered in the lone star tick and known to infect patients in the South. The only problem was that, as far as Bakken knew, the lone star tick wasn't seen as far up as Minnesota or northern Wisconsin, where the elderly man lived. After sending a sample of the man's blood to an expert in Texas, Bakken received confirmation of the seemingly impossible: The patient had indeed suffered ehrlichiosis. Weeks later, when a second severely ill patient presented with a flulike illness and berrylike clusters in the blood, Bakken treated with the antibiotic tetracycline, known to cure ehrlichiosis. This time, the patient's spiking fever plummeted overnight and the condition resolved.

Hoping to learn how his decidedly northern patients had contracted a disease thought endemic to the South, Bakken sent some blood down to Galveston, Texas, where a scientist named Stephen Dumler, now at Johns Hopkins, was put on the case. "Within five minutes of examining the samples," Dumler reports, "I was convinced it was something completely different from the human ehrlichiosis we had already identified." One important difference that Dumler ultimately documented had to do with the white blood cells. The disease first observed in the North, today called *Anaplasma phagocytophilum* after being reclassified by microbiologists, infected white blood cells known as granulocytes. It is frequently referred to as human granulocytic anaplasmosis, or HGA. The disease first observed in the South, caused by the microbe *Ehrlichia chaffeensis,* infected white blood cells called monocytes and is known as human monocytic ehrlichiosis, or HME. By 2000, a third southern species, *Ehrlichia ewingii,* was recognized as another source of human disease. All three organisms cause similar symptoms: fever, malaise, muscle pain, nausea, and sweats. There are also differences: HME is more likely to cause a rash. HGA is more likely to infect the nervous system and brain. Finally, both HME and HGA have been found in ticks from the North and the South.

When Lyme disease patients are treated with doxycycline—often considered the first-line drug—ehrlichiosis anaplasmosis, and related infections, will, de facto, be treated as well. But when doctors treat Lyme disease with amoxicillin or the intravenous antibiotic Rocephin, *Anaplasma* and the *Ehrlichias* will persist. Many an "incurable" Lyme patient has discovered the existence of a second, lurking disease—ehrlichiosis or anaplasmosis—only to be treated with doxycycline and, finally, get well. With ticks on the move, scientists say, all versions of these infections can infect patients in northern and southern parts of the United States.

Added to the triad of Lyme-babesiosis-ehrlichiosis are other microbes found in Lyme ticks; though controversial, these, too, are now considered possible agents of the disease broadly referred to on the street as Lyme. Frequently mentioned are the rod-shaped bacteria called *Bartonella henselae,* known as a cause of "cat scratch" disease and commonly transmitted by cats. More recently, forms of *Bartonella* have been reported in deer ticks. Some clinicians see *Bartonella* as a culprit when symptoms are particularly neuropsychiatric, and Lyme treatment does no good. In California, more than 20 percent of the *Ixodes pacificus* ticks that transmit Lyme disease are positive for *Bartonella,* more in fact than carry Lyme itself.

Calling up his clinical experience, Joe Burrascano of the Hamptons says he's seen a distinct *"Bartonella* syndrome": agitated irritability and insomnia; cognitive deficits and confusion; gastritis, including lower abdominal pain; red rashes that look like stretch marks; and, sometimes, sore soles. These afflicted patients, he adds, don't test positive for the kind of *Bartonella* found in ordinary cat scratch disease, nor do they respond to treatment for that disease, so he refers to the infection as a *"Bartonella-*like organism," or BLO. "The antibiotic of choice for BLO is Levaquin," which penetrates inside cells, says Burrascano, who insists that patients sick for years can get well in a month or so on modest doses of the drug.

If this sounds somehow *out there,* keep in mind: Even the CDC journal *Emerging Infectious Diseases* has mentioned the surprising genetic diversity and the investigation of novel forms of *Bartonella.* And in 2007, Bruno Chomel, a researcher at the University of California at Davis, reported alternate and novel species of the organism in Northern California foxes and dogs, especially older dogs, who presumably had been harboring the organisms for years. "Dogs are excellent sentinels for human infections," Chomel has said; infections often show up in canines before getting diagnosed in us. He's found a range of *Bartonella* in deer from California and Oklahoma, and notes that these *Bartonella* "could act as . . . agents" in human disease.

Another tick-borne suspect, *Mycoplasma,* sometimes treated with the drug Rifampin, has now been invoked as a cause of neuropsychiatric symptoms and chronic fatigue. In 2007, Eva Sapi reported that over 84 percent of the 150 Connecticut ticks she tested at her University of New Haven lab with graduate students were infected by three species of *Mycoplasma—pneumoniae, fermentans,* and *genitalium.* When patients don't respond to treatment for Lyme, they might respond to *Mycoplasma* treatments like Rifampin, some clinicians now believe. "This could be the missing link," Sapi states. The list goes on. In Massachusetts and Connecticut, researchers have found deer ticks with *Tuleremia,* a deadly agent of bioterrorism. In 2009, Harvard epidemiologist Sam Telford reported deer ticks transmit as well a rare but deadly new virus, known as tick-borne encephalitis, or TBE.

Because so many "Lyme patients" are positive for other organisms on a host of lab tests, some of them controversial, debate over their role rages on. Some doctors view *Bartonella* as a huge problem, "maybe bigger than Lyme," says Joe Burrascano. Others like Brian Fallon say the jury on *Bartonella* is out. "Seventy percent of the patients we test are positive for *Bartonella,* even the healthy ones," he comments. "I don't know what it means."

Still, when Lyme patients stay ill despite weeks or months of treatment, many doctors peeling the layers of chronic illness may try to treat for *Bartonella, Mycoplasma,* or other infectious agents, many of them just theoretical or literally unknown. Lyme doctors treating empirically insist that when multiple infections are addressed, more patients get well.

Alone and in combination, microbes transmitted by ticks can make us ill, and for each known infection, another tick-borne pathogen may be awaiting discovery in the wings. In the farscape of emerging infectious disease, the tick is the final frontier. The ultimate germ generator, it is the ideal wet lab for microorganisms to mix and remix in infinite formats, spewing a kaleidoscopic ouvre of novel bacteria and viruses, some of them pathogens the world has never seen. As long as we live in suburbs abutting the woods we'll be in the path of the tick tornado and its toxic output—and it could be decades or even centuries before science transcends nature's gusto for evolving new germs. No one would think of trekking through Africa without prophylaxis for malaria, yet we take a similar risk every day by venturing, without worry, through our own backyards.

The archaeologist of my family's illnesses, I sifted through the years: Perhaps we'd first gotten sick at Woods Hole with a mix of infections that make up the Lyme soup. As a catchphrase, a concept, as *slang,* the word *Lyme* would do fine; it wasn't Allen Steere's Lyme, the straightforward disease of swollen knees and five of ten bands. How could it be with other microbes in the mix? With infections smoldering but symptoms under the radar, our family had traveled to Montauk and the Hamptons, to a campground in Dutchess County, to a bed-and-breakfast in Bucks County, to Martha's Vineyard and a dozen towns on Cape Cod, to beaches and parks up and down the Jersey shore. Then the disastrous move to Chappaqua and our decade-long residence in the woods. Had we *arrived* with tick-borne infections—possibly a stew of them? Perhaps constant reexposure in Chappaqua had heightened and multiplied the illness like oil peaks a tan.

Already, three infections—Lyme, *Babesia,* and *Anaplasma*—had been diagnosed in my family, but the scientists I interviewed said the ticks were sewers, and who knew what lurked beneath?

28

❖

Hole in the Donut:
The Fight over Southern Lyme

Coinfections like *Babesia* and *Anaplasma* have finally gained acceptance, but the argument over Lyme and other spirochetes rages on, especially in the South. The reality of Southern Lyme, central to the Lyme war in a way few have grasped, challenges the boundaries and defies the rules. For if Southern Lyme is real, then we'll have to rethink everything: the diagnostic tests, the spirochetes, the ticks. The nuances of the fight are rooted as much in the embattled South as in the Northeast and out west, where the disease was first defined.

In a sense, the uproar over a southern version of Lyme disease was preordained from the moment a northerner—Andrew Spielman of Harvard—tracked *Babesia microti* and *Borrelia burgdorferi* across the Nantucket landscape from ticks to mice to us. By unraveling the interplay between microbes, ticks, and mammals, the brilliant, swashbuckling Spielman had mapped Lyme's geography. It was Spielman who found the ecological niches where Lyme hunkered down, stealthily waiting to strike, Spielman who sleuthed its trajectory from the Elizabethan Islands off Massachusetts to the yards and playgrounds of New York State.

But Spielman's Lyme maps were filtered through a personal lens. Just as Steere had claimed a new disease and Burgdorfer a novel microbe, Spielman now claimed a brand-new tick, a creature so mercurial and extraordinary it was the pinnacle of his career. His disease maps restricted human babesiosis and then Lyme disease to the places the tick could be found.

The twists of this strange saga wind through the back roads of entomology: the study of bugs. Indeed, in the early days of the research everyone, including Spielman, had assumed that the tick spreading human babesiosis (and therefore, Lyme) was the common, hard-shelled *Ixodes scapularis,* found from the northernmost border of the continent to its southern horn. Yet observing the tick's life cycle over the course of years, Spielman eventually saw something that startled him: Sure, the adults were ringers for *I. scapularis,* but the larvae, he reported, resembled offspring of a separate species, the mouse tick, *Ixodes muris.*

"How could an adult of one species give rise to larvae of another? That was shocking," Spielman said. That's when it hit him: The tick in question had to be something different from either one, something never before recognized, something unique. So in 1979, he announced the discovery of a *new* tick species, *Ixodes dammini,* named after Gustave Dammin, the Brigham and Women's Hospital pathologist who aided him with his work. By the early eighties, Spielman was issuing a decree: It was his spanking *new* tick, *I. dammini* alone, that transmitted *Babesia* and Lyme disease to humans; without the proven presence of *I. dammini* in a given region, there could be no Lyme.

The effect of this decree was profound: In mapping Lyme's misery so tightly to his new tick, Spielman had de facto restricted the geographic areas where Lyme could be diagnosed. Soon, the influential Spielman—with backup from Allen Steere—was describing two specific and very limited Lyme zones circumscribed by *dammini:* One had started at the Elizabethan Islands like Nantucket, Martha's Vineyard, and Block Island and spread, generally on the backs of birds, through Connecticut, New York, New Jersey, and Pennsylvania—and then down the East Coast to Maryland, but not beyond. The other Lyme zone, where the tick was also found, started in Wisconsin, spreading through Minnesota, Nebraska, and Illinois.

Lyme out West was described several years later by entomologist Robert Lane of the University of California at Berkeley, who heard Burgdorfer discuss his great discovery in 1982 and was enthralled. Already working with tick-borne Rocky Mountain spotted fever, Colorado tick fever, and *Tularemia* in his neck of the California woods, Lane offered his pioneering colleague heartfelt congratulations.

Soon Burgdorfer was suggesting that Lane himself track Lyme disease out West.

"I would love to," Lane said.

That spring Bob Lane started collecting ticks in northwestern California in hopes of isolating the Lyme disease agent. With Burgdorfer's expert help, he soon discovered a microbe nearly identical to the one causing Lyme disease in the Northeast.

But the vector, that is to say, the tick, transmitting the disease, was not Spielman's *dammini*, nor even *scapularis*. Instead, it was a thoroughly Western relative: *Ixodes pacificus*, the western black-legged tick, a vicious human-biter that transmitted *Anaplasma* as well.

The California scene differed from the Northeast situation on a number of fronts. For one thing, Lane and colleagues found that the dusky-footed wood rat and the western gray squirrel, not the white-footed mouse, served as the primary reservoir hosts for the Lyme disease spirochete on the ground. The western Lyme strains and species were often different, and far more varied, than those reported in places like Connecticut or Long Island. (Indeed, five different species of Lyme disease spirochetes have been identified from California to date, Bob Lane says.) And adult *pacificus* ticks usually were infected with Lyme spirochetes just one or two percent of the time—a far cry from the high infection rates of 60 percent reported by Burgdorfer in the Northeast.

That low infection rate proved a source of unending confusion in the late 1980s, as Lane, along with the late rheumatologist Paul Lavoie and the University of California at Davis veterinarian John Madigan, began studying Phyllis Mervine and her afflicted neighbors in the Coast Range, where 25 percent or more could have the disease.

"We had no way to explain it," said Lane. "It didn't make sense that you could have such a high prevalence of people testing positive for Lyme disease and have such a small percentage of infection in the adult ticks."

The mystery was solved when Lane and his colleague Jim Clover tracked the disease through the ecosystem, describing the complexity in a breakthrough paper in 1995. In a leap of insight supported by data, the duo had traced the high rate of infection to the nymph—the poppy-seed-sized juvenile tick with a prevalence of infection several times higher than that found in *pacificus* adults.

How could ticks shed infection as they aged? Lane found that nymphal ticks in nature tended to feed on the Western Fence Lizard, which sterilized the ticks' midguts, clearing them of infection. But if an infected nymphal tick bit a human instead of a lizard, it was capable of transmitting the infection.

While the disease was far more prevalent in Northern California, Southern California was endemic, too. And these findings appeared to extend to comparable habitats in the Pacific Northwest from Oregon to

Washington State, wherever the spirochete, the Western Fence Lizard, and the disease might co-exist.

All these findings, in aggregate, led some scientists to argue that Southern Lyme could not exist. "Separate identity is key to understanding the ecology and epidemiology of tick-borne diseases," Spielman said. "Southerners don't get Lyme disease. And it is immediately clear why that is so, if you understand that the South doesn't have the *Ixodes dammini* tick that spreads the disease."

The Spielman Lyme maps, with their rigid borders and all their restrictions, were embraced by America's academics and the mighty powers at the NIH and CDC. But that didn't stop Texans and Floridians, along with neighbors from Alabama and Tennessee and, of course, the Carolinas, from falling sick with the uncanny symptoms of Lyme disease—the rash, the malaise, the memory loss, the swollen knees. Without any other explanation for their illness, the patients were diagnosed with Lyme disease by their doctors. They were treated with antibiotics and improved or got well. When some of them pointed to spirochetal forms in local ticks, they were told that southern *scapularis* ticks fed exclusively on lizards, which killed the Lyme organism cold. Called delusional by titans from Harvard and Yale and ignored by their government, patients from the South grew miffed and then outright furious. Given their bull's-eye rashes and memory loss and swollen knees, in light of proven tick bites and response to antibiotic, how could they be so rudely dismissed as wrong?

It was amidst this dissonance that the war over southern Lyme erupted with nuclear force. Front and center in the battle royal was the country doctor Edwin J. Masters of Cape Girardeau, Missouri, who reveled in fighting for a cause. It was near the start of his career, in 1979, that Masters wrote to his U.S. congressman, an ultraliberal in a region of Midwest moderates, asking if he'd voted himself a raise. The congressman, Bill Burlison, wrote back claiming he couldn't remember how he voted on his pay raise, but if the doctor wanted to know so much, he could look it up himself. Incensed at the rudeness, Masters's father-in-law alerted the media. The exchange made TV news.

Burlison retaliated by reporting Masters to the Federal Election Commission for writing a political missive on medical clinic stationery (an illegal tax deduction). But Masters, a self-described "Eagle Scout and a stickler for every last detail," had proof in the form of canceled checks that he'd paid for the stationery himself. Backed by the evidence (and the

American Civil Liberties Union), Masters lashed back in anti-Burlison opinion pieces emblazoned on clinic letterhead and sent to newspapers throughout the state.

As election time neared, the drama increased: Whenever Burlison's opponent, conservative Republican Bill Emerson, couldn't attend a debate, Masters came in his stead. Once word got out, people crowded the debates not to see the candidates, but to watch the engaging Dr. Masters. A six-term incumbent, Burlison lost the election of 1980—and Masters's new friend, the freshman congressman Emerson, was swept in.

Despite his love of the brawl, Masters (who died of diabetes in 2009 at age 63) was your quintessential hail-fellow-well-met: If you wanted a congenial sports buddy or a friend to confide in, Masters was your man. Tall, affable, and classically handsome, with a swath of thick hair and a wide, friendly grin, he entered the fray when, as an amateur forester, he was asked to give a talk on Lyme at a forestry meeting in 1988. Because he'd never seen a case of Lyme disease, he prepared exhaustively, even borrowing slides from health departments in Minnesota and throughout the East. "I spent a year working on the talk," Masters said.

The lecture went fine, but when he returned home to Missouri he started recognizing what seemed like Lyme disease in his own patients. The first such patient was a farmer, age fifty-five, who'd been the picture of health for years. One day he came in, emotionally overwrought, and said, "I ache all over, knees and ankles, I can't think clearly and I need help getting out of the combine."

Masters knew his patient's hobby was fishing, and asked him whether, in the course of that activity, he'd ever been bitten by ticks. Of course he'd been bitten, the farmer responded, like anyone who fished. In possession of a good-sized collection of Lyme rash photos following the forestry talk, Masters took some out and asked the farmer to look at them. Had he ever noticed one of these?

"I had one of those last summer," the farmer said. He'd gone downhill ever since.

First, Masters tried to rule out any other cause for the illness. When he could find nothing else the matter with the farmer, who was headed for disability, Masters treated him with antibiotics. Not only did the farmer recover, but one year later he was so full of energy he expanded his operation by buying an adjacent farm.

Now that Masters knew what to look for, he started seeing Lyme in other Missouri patients, too. Not only did they have the typical erythema migrans rash but also swollen joints, meningitis, neuropathy, and other specific hallmarks of the disease. Masters sent their blood to a lab, and many tested positive on the ELISA, the standard Lyme disease test of the day.

Thus validated, Masters reported his cases to the Missouri Department of Health, but his reports were ignored. If he'd read just a couple of articles on Lyme disease, he might have backed off, but after a year of prepping for his forestry talk he couldn't believe he had it wrong. So he started documenting the cases as precisely as he could. Every erythema migrans rash warranted an entire roll of film, and he made sure to photograph a rash and face together so he wouldn't be accused of recycling the same rash again and again. In preparation for the day that better tests would come, he obtained a special refrigerator for his office and began to store samples of patient rashes and blood.

By 1990, Ed Masters was regularly diagnosing Missouri patients with Lyme based on presentation with the EM rash (which the CDC called diagnostic for the disease) and other objective signs. After sending his patients to specialists to rule out other health problems, he treated them with antibiotics, generally amoxicillin or doxycycline. Masters knew the Yale scientists were reporting a treatment failure rate between 10 and 15 percent for early Lyme disease and he "deemed that unacceptable. If I had an 85 to 90 percent success rate treating strep throat I would be drawn and quartered. So I treated patients at the longer end of the recommended scale—for about three or four weeks—assuming that I would then be at the higher end of the success curve as well." Intuitively he'd hit upon the treatment that scientists at Stony Brook would soon recommend for early Lyme disease, and his patients got well. "It was a new thing, but I was getting enough success that I was enormously encouraged," Masters said.

Masters's credibility was bolstered not just by the quantity of his data and his treatment success, but also by the work of the preeminent Missouri entomologist Dorothy Fier, a specialist in Rocky Mountain spotted fever at St. Louis University. Fier had visited Masters's personal tree farm and collected samples of the common lone star tick (species name *Amblyomma americanum*) notable for the distinctive white dot, or "lone star," on the backs of females, found not just in Missouri but throughout the Midwest, the South, and the Northeast all the way to Maine. A force to be reckoned with, the influential Fier found some kind of *Borrelia* in 2 percent of the lone star ticks she sampled, and came out in support of Masters's Missouri Lyme.

With the support of Fier and data on about 125 patients, thirty with well-documented erythema migrans rashes, Masters was publishing his findings and taking his show on the road. His reports garnered so much interest he was invited, in July 1990, to present his findings at the prestigious Fourth International Conference on Lyme Borreliosis, in Stockholm, Sweden, where experts from the United States and Europe studied his pictures and case histories and agreed they could see no difference between his patients and those with classic Lyme disease. Ben Luft of Stony Brook was so impressed he invited Masters to enter his patients in an upcoming NIH study on the antibiotic treatment of Lyme disease. By 1991, Masters had made such a stir that the *New York Times* was prompted to run a story about the "mystery" Lyme disease cases along the Mississippi River in Cape Girardeau. That's when the CDC *really* took note.

The CDC had long told doctors that the EM rash alone was diagnostic for the disease. Yet now they insisted the rule did not hold for Missouri, where neither *Ixodes dammini* nor *Ixodes pacificus* ticks could be found. Without the expected tick, CDC scientists said, they wanted a higher level of evidence: Namely, *B. burgdorferi* spirochetes would need to be cultured from biopsies of human rashes, from ticks, or from animal hosts, and that had not been done.

"I was living in two worlds," Masters said. "I would go to conferences and present to academic experts, and they would say, 'Hmmm, that's Lyme disease.' Then I would go back home to Missouri and the people from the CDC would tell me I was misdiagnosing all these patients. Diagnosis of Lyme disease based on the erythema migrans rash was controversial only in Missouri, and nowhere else in the world."

Through 1991, as his differences with the CDC became increasingly heated, Masters traveled to conferences equipped with a poster of his patients' erythema migrans rashes and a quote from William Harvey, the seventeenth-century physician and father of physiology who had been ostracized for years for daring to suggest that blood circulated. "I appeal to your own eyes as my witness and judge," William Harvey had said in 1651, just as Ed Masters appealed to his colleagues now. The EM rashes on Masters's poster were powerful visual evidence for some sort of borreliosis, Lyme disease proper or not. And Missouri rashes had been found to contain spirochetes by the pathologists Paul Duray and J. de Koning, who were widely recognized as top experts on such issues. Blood from Masters's patients had by now tested positive for Lyme disease by ELISA at numerous labs, including the University of Connecticut, the University of Minnesota, and the CDC itself.

Things came to a head during one of Masters's presentations, when a

CDC representative declared that none of it proved the phenomenon in question was Lyme disease.

"Why can't you accept this?" Masters countered. "The evidence is overwhelming."

"Because you haven't proven it's *Borrelia burgdorferi*," the CDC official said.

"Excuse me!" Masters bellowed in front of a crowd. "You're the CDC, the federally funded, taxpayer-supported research institute that's supposed to check this out, and you are telling me, a solo family physician finding these patients, that I haven't proven it's *Borrelia burgdorferi*? I think we need a little job clarification here. It's not my job to prove it or disprove it, it's yours!"

That's when the CDC invited Masters and a few of his colleagues, including Dorothy Fier and Denny Donnell, the Missouri state epidemiologist, to apply for a grant to study the matter. The group wrote a proposal for studying Masters's patients along with ticks captured in the vicinities where infection had likely occurred. Then Masters heard through the grapevine that the proposal had been rejected. Some time later the CDC called to say that while it lacked funds to outsource the study, they could conduct it with in-house researchers—in other words, scientists employed by the CDC itself. Masters could provide the patients and the ticks.

For two weeks in July 1991, CDC researchers occupied a space in Masters's office, interviewing his Lyme patients and reviewing their charts. Based on their interviews, the CDC scientists went to the areas where the patients said they had been bitten and collected ticks. Masters provided the CDC with blood and biopsy samples taken from the patients during their illness. Finally, the CDC took the ticks, the samples, and the data back to Fort Collins to conduct their analysis and write their report.

It was almost two years later, in May of 1993, that the CDC sent a final draft to Masters for input, and he was alarmed. The first thing that stood out was the CDC assertion that, according to "unpublished data," Missouri rashes differed from real Lyme rashes on the basis of "coloration, degree of homogeneity, sharpness of borders, and shape." The CDC also contended that EM lesions in Missouri were smaller, on average, than those observed on Lyme disease patients in Wisconsin, based on a twelve-patient study still in press.

Masters was flabbergasted. After all, he had shown his rash photos throughout the world, and the most expert dermatologists on the planet, from Sweden and Germany to Long Island, had said he had a "ringer."

As to lesion size, why, he wondered, had the CDC deferred to this small Wisconsin study over the work of the dermatologist Bernard Berger, an internationally recognized Lyme disease expert who had done the seminal studies on the rash? Berger's widely cited report on 196 patients showed that the average rash size of confirmed Lyme cases and Missouri Lyme cases were exactly the same.

Could some of the confusion be traced to careless error? Comparing his patient charts to CDC data, Masters found inexplicable mistakes. One patient with a rash stretching across his back was reported with a lesion just a quarter-inch in diameter. Two patients with obvious bull's-eye rashes were listed as having "no central clearing." And a patient whose chart contained a photograph of a rash across his abdomen had been reported as having no rash at all.

Another thing he found particularly galling was the assertion that his patients had developed rashes after unusually short periods of incubation—the amount of time it takes to go from tick bite to appearance of the rash. The statistic is important in establishing a pattern because in Lyme disease rashes appear an average of 7 days after the bite. Masters's patients fit in with an average of approximately 5.5 days, as determined by notes written in his charts at the time the rashes appeared. But when the CDC reinterviewed these same patients years later based on memories of the experience, an average of 3 days was recalled. The CDC decided to use the fuzzy memories of the patients, recalled years after the event, and discard the chart data, recorded at the time. Then they emphasized the discrepancy in their write-up as evidence that whatever was happening in Missouri was different from that observed in proven cases of Lyme disease.

"I called Fort Collins and a group of them were around the speaker phone. I went ballistic," Masters recalled. "I said, you are telling me that my rashes are visibly distinct from real Lyme, which means that you can tell by looking, that these are not real rashes? Then why are we doing the friggin' study? Hey, if you can tell by looking, I demand that you hold a press conference to teach us dumb yokels out here in the boonies how to do it." He was especially mad about reliance on the unpublished rash data from the tiny Wisconsin study. "I'm an author on this paper— and you say you have unpublished data? I have never seen it, I have never even heard of it, and if this data exists it is one of the most important keys to this puzzle. I want to see the data now."

The CDC team was virtually silent. Then, three days later, Masters received a new version of the article, with the material he'd challenged removed. But as Masters and his colleague Denny Donnell read through what would be several more drafts of the CDC manuscript, they knew they could never sign on. As Masters saw it, the CDC had "skewed everything, and had literally tossed out data, to make what we found in Missouri look like a rash-only illness, and as different from Lyme disease as could be."

Most misleading, he felt, were the arbitrary stop-and-start dates the CDC had imposed on the study after collection of data was complete. In most studies of this type, each patient is studied for the same amount of time as all the other participants. Start dates are based on the start of illness for each individual patient, and end dates are determined by adding a consistent amount of time—the same for each and every patient—onto that. But in the Missouri study, the CDC decided to cut all patients off on the *same date,* no matter when the illness had begun. Thus, some patients were followed for a couple of years, others for a couple of weeks. The disturbing part was that the stop dates placed patients with the most objective signs of illness, including carditis (inflammation of the heart) and arthritis, outside the study period and thus, beyond the scope of the report. To wit: Even though patients in the study had developed serious, late-stage signs considered classic for Lyme disease, the CDC paper referred, without qualification, to the "absence of documented early neurologic, cardiac, and arthritic complications." (An analogy would be the situation in which scientists studying HIV infection cut their study off after two weeks and so conclude the virus is not a cause of AIDS.)

Masters complained passionately about the cutoff dates to Phillip R. Lee, M.D., assistant secretary for health, who he hoped might intervene. One of the patients, he wrote to Lee, was a previously healthy young man who had developed carditis fourteen days after appearance of his rash, but five days after the arbitrary end of the study period. There was no reason to cut him off, said Masters, because it took another year before the manuscript was ready to submit. Similarly, three cases of arthritis were excluded from the "study period," and from the report. One patient's rash occurred before the CDC start date, "and what a shame," said Masters, "because he also had a positive Western blot and documented joint swelling in his knee." Two other patients developed arthritis after the stop-point. "One of those arthritis patients had symptoms emerge fifty-eight days after the onset of the rash, just thirty-four days after the study's arbitrarily determined end." Such omissions were "absurd," said Masters, given that onset of Lyme carditis occurs, on average, 4.8 weeks after the rash and Lyme arthritis may not develop for months.

There was more: The CDC had dismissed laboratory work, a wide swath of it, that indicated some kind of borreliosis in play. For instance, the report did not put much stock in the finding, by CDC scientists, of "motile spirochetes" in nearly 5 percent of the lone star nymphal ticks observed by darkfield microscopy. Nor did the CDC report that when spirochetes from the ticks were inoculated into mice, they later cultured spirochetes from the animals' ears. "Having seen these spirochetes myself, in both rash biopsies and ticks, I am not comfortable with the CDC's position that Missouri is the hole in the donut," Masters wrote to Lee, "and that somehow Missouri is a magical, 'Lyme-free' zone and that these observed Missouri spirochetes have nothing to do with human disease."

Finally, and this was the last straw to Masters, the CDC rejected dozens of positive blood tests performed at its own lab. While it was true that the CDC used more specific tests as years went on—methodologies unavailable when the study began—Masters could not understand how so many positive and equivocal results over so many samples were not considered suggestive of another, similar organism, even if not *B. burgdorferi* itself. Instead, positive results where no Lyme disease was deemed possible, as in Missouri, were just the sort of incentive the CDC had needed to tighten the valve. The CDC kept changing its blood tests from year to year and retesting the Missouri blood until samples once considered positive by the agency itself no longer passed the diagnostic bar for Lyme.

In a nutshell, the CDC insisted the illness in Missouri, whatever it was, had nothing to do with Lyme disease, while Masters insisted the evidence had been left on the cutting-room floor. When it came to Masters's insistence, Duane Gubler, head of the CDC's Vector-Borne Disease Division in Fort Collins, was especially clear: When you biopsied a Lyme rash in the Northeast, you cultured *B. burgdorferi*—not so with rashes from Missouri. If he couldn't culture *B. burgdorferi* from the rashes, then it wasn't causing the illness. If the Missouri rashes weren't caused by *B. burgdorferi*, then no amount of other evidence could convince Gubler to call the outbreak Lyme disease. Whatever data Masters felt had been left out, it could mean little compared to that. The Lyme maps drawn by Spielman, and later by Lane, officials held, were the only true maps to the disease.

Masters disagreed: By dismissing so much data, the CDC gave the impression that it had no evidence, whatsoever, for a *Lyme-like* borreliosis in the state, and that simply was not the case.

The dispute between Masters and Donnell and the CDC grew so heated that, though they were coauthors on the study, the agency wouldn't let them read the final draft unless they agreed to sign off in advance. "I had never heard of an author being prohibited from reading the final manuscript," said Masters. "This heavy-handed attempt to force us to indicate agreement without knowing the content resulted in our refusal to sign."

By the summer of 1994, Masters and Donnell had resigned from the CDC effort and struck out on their own. Working night and day, the Missouri researchers were able to execute two preemptive strikes—a detailed letter of objection to the *Journal of Infectious Diseases,* where the CDC would be submitting the manuscript, and an article of their own for the journal *Missouri Medicine.*

They were so efficient that their article in *Missouri Medicine* was actually published first. There, in July 1995, Masters and Donnell presented the results as they saw them: Missouri patients fulfilling the strict CDC surveillance definition for Lyme disease had been documented in significant number, and there was growing evidence that lone star ticks were infected with a still-unidentified spirochete.

When the CDC article came out in the *Journal of Infectious Diseases* a month later, cooler heads had prevailed. Whether due to further reflection from the authors or pressure from the editor who had reviewed Ed Masters's critique, the final, published article conceded the possibility that some lone star ticks were infected with a new spirochete, but, the CDC emphasized, likelihood was low. Instead, said officials, the rashes in Missouri—which they called STARI (for Southern Tick-Associated Rash Illness)—might be an allergy to tick saliva.

It would take a world-class entomologist to put it all together, explaining the flaws in the Spielman Lyme maps and the rationale for a southern version of the disease. That scientist was James H. Oliver Jr., Callaway Professor of Biology and director of the Institute of Arthropodology and Parasitology at Georgia Southern University. The first thing Oliver did was challenge Spielman's Lyme zones. As early as 1992, Oliver determined that mice through the Carolinas, Georgia, Florida, Alabama, and Mississippi tested positive for the Lyme disease spirochete, *B. burgdorferi,* generating as many reactive antibodies as mice from Connecticut. In 1993, he isolated *B. burgdorferi* spirochetes from black-legged *Ixodes scapularis* ticks on Sapelo Island, off the coast of Georgia.

Later that year, Oliver went for the jugular, showing that Spielman's *dammini* was merely a subset of the common species *Ixodes scapularis* and not a species of its own. To prove the relationship, Oliver mated

Spielman's ticks from Massachusetts with ticks from Georgia, showing that fertile offspring could result. Since the ability to mate and produce fertile offspring occurs only *within* a species, experts around the world lined up to support Oliver in his assertion that *dammini* and *scapularis* were one and the same. In one fell swoop, the species *Ixodes dammini* was wiped from the record books, and with it, the clear delineation of a "Lyme zone," long held up as a barricade against diagnosis, crumbled to dust.

Nothing is ever so simple, of course. Oliver later learned that northern *scapularis is* different from southern *scapularis,* as Spielman held, even if the two can procreate; less prone to bite humans than its northern cousin, southern *scapularis* is not a major cause of Lyme. Instead, southern Lyme is transmitted most often by the lone star tick, which carries a spirochete that is still unknown. But there's more: Oliver has ultimately found a range of new southern ticks transmitting a pastiche of *Borreliae.* And he's recently reported a unique southern strain of *B. burgdorferi* with outer surface proteins so unusual they are undetectable on blood tests used up north. The newest evidence shows that even the lone star tick can transmit classic, *Borrelia burgdorferi*–based Lyme.

Adding nuance and weight to the case for Southern Lyme is University of North Florida epidemiologist Kerry Clark. Fascinated with the study of tick-borne disease, Clark spent three years at the Wedge Plantation, a forty-seven-acre research station in South Carolina once devoted to growing rice but later a lab for vector-borne disease. "It was a wild place. It was studying out in nature and living in your lab, which was right in your backyard," Clark recalls.

The young scientist was told he'd find no Lyme disease in South Carolina, but he decided to see for himself. He went out into nature, collecting animals throughout the state and testing their tissues. Unlike the simple scenario described in the Northeast, Clark found the South was complex: Small mammals, including cotton mice and eastern wood rats, were loaded with *Borrelia* infection—levels rose as high as 80 percent in some species along the coast. Instead of the limited numbers of strains that Northeast scientists were reporting, Clark found a veritable menagerie of over 100 strains of *Borrelia burgdorferi,* some of them expressing unique patterns of the proteins screened for in standard human tests. He also found other species, including *Borrelia bissetti,* another potential human pathogen with multiple strains.

As for the vector, Clark found that two tick species, *Ixodes minor* and *Ixodes affinis,* helped keep the cycle of infection alive in nature, though they didn't transmit to humans. But ordinary *scapularis*, the same vector implicated in the Northeast epidemic, easily picked up infection from mammals on the ground and could spread disease to us. (He later found Lyme *Borrelia* in the lone star tick, too.)

By 2001, Clark was running a lab of his own at the University of North Florida, an institution in another state claiming to be a Lyme-free zone. He'd long attempted to culture spirochetes from tissues of local mammals using the standard medium cultured by Alan Barbour at Rocky Mountain Labs, getting positive results just 5 percent of the time. But using a technique known as polymerase chain reaction, or PCR, to analyze his mammals for species-specific DNA, Clark's positive findings surged. Depending on the gene target he used in his screen, he could find evidence of diverse strains of Lyme disease in some 80 percent of the rodents on the ground.

"When you move from the North to the South, the diversity in the natural ecology drives diversity in the Lyme *Borrelia* strains," says Clark. The standard culture medium "is selective for strains that will grow in that culture medium, uniquely," he explains. Even antibody and DNA analysis will fail to detect the organism "if there are too many mismatches between the target molecule and your test."

Indeed, Clark found that PCR could miss the motherlode of infection if scientists tested for the common outer surface protein (OSP) A, so specific to Lyme in the Northeast it had been used to make the vaccine. But in southern strains, Clark theorized that the OspA molecule had gone through so much change it eluded DNA testing. Instead, he found that another molecule—the flagellin gene, specific to Lyme *Borrelia*—was far more conserved from strain to strain, and made a better screening tool.

Demonstrating Lyme in the South has been an uphill battle for Clark despite his collaboration with the acclaimed Jim Oliver and his mountain of data, published in the *Proceedings of the National Academy of Sciences*, the *Journal of Parasitology*, the *Journal of Clinical Microbiology*, and other prestigious peer reviews.

One objection relates to lizards, the primary host for *scapularis* ticks down South. "It was widely assumed that our lizards sterilized ticks because that's what they found out West," states Clark. But the southern model veers. One Clark study shows that, California notwithstanding, Southern Lyme strains appear to cycle through multiple species of lizards without being killed and may still find their way to us.

Clark was pondering abandoning research of Southern Lyme when, in 2007, a student walked into his Florida lab: She'd been on a field trip west of Tallahassee and had "a large, beautiful erythema migrans rash." Though she didn't test positive on the standard ELISA, her blood glowed positive on Clark's flagellin PCR test. A few days later Clark went back to the park the student had visited, collecting ticks and ultimately sequencing their *Borrelial* DNA. The spirochetes Clark sequenced were virtually identical to each other, but highly divergent from typical northern strains.

Today Clark has matched the Tallahassee strain to one James Oliver found long ago—SCW30h, named for its collection site, the South Carolina Wedge Plantation where Clark began his Southern Lyme research years before. The new strain may be common, says Clark, who reports he has found its footprint in a significant percent of human patients—members of the Lyme diaspora—not just from Florida, but also from Maryland, New York, New Jersey, Pennsylvania, Missouri, Oklahoma, Arizona, New Mexico, Oregon, and Washington State.

As scientists learn more, they're finding that complexity may be the rule everywhere we see Lyme. For instance, Yale entomologist Durland Fish has found a new kind of *Borrelia* in ticks throughout New York, Connecticut, Rhode Island, and New Jersey. The new spirochete, still unnamed, accounts for 10 to 20 percent of all those bacteria previously thought to be *B. burgdorferi*, the proven agent of Lyme, according to Fish, who says it most closely matches a species from Japan. "If the new spirochete infects humans," he adds, "it could explain a lot about unexplained illness," including all the negative Lyme tests and lack of treatment response. Taking their lead from Oliver and Fish, Montana scientists are now investigating the possibility of a novel *Borrelia* that they think has adapted to the local wood tick, causing a bull's-eye rash, fever, and fatigue.

"Zones of borreliosis overlap with and extend way beyond the Lyme zone," says Joe Piesman, chief of the Bacterial Zoonoses Branch of the Vector-Borne Ecology Lab of the CDC. "Those arguing about all these things may not be as far apart as they think."

Indeed, no one was clearer on the differences between Lyme disease and its southern doppelganger than Ed Masters himself. "Lyme disease in the United States is now defined microbiologically as an infection caused exclusively by the spirochete *Borrelia burgdorferi sensu stricto* [strains like those originally cultured from northeast ticks] and is vectored by ticks of the *Ixodes* complex," he wrote in the august *Infectious Disease Clinics of North America* in 2008. "An enigma for the past twenty years has been the recognition and reporting of a condition in nonendemic states that is not primarily caused by *Borrelia burgdorferi sensu stricto* and is vectored by the lone star tick. . . . This Lyme disease mimic is now being recognized as a separate disease."

Working with more than a dozen scientific collaborators around the United States in the years before he died, Masters found that the southern illness peaks in June, compared to September for northeastern patients. Patients in the South are less symptomatic at the time of the rash, and when treated in timely fashion, recover at a faster rate; their arthritis, when it occurs, is less severe. After a three-year study comparing Missouri Lyme–like patients to New York Lyme patients, Masters even agreed the rashes could have group differences, though there was so much overlap you could not distinguish individual lesions by appearance alone. According to one study, the most classic of the bull's-eyes—the near-perfect round red circles with white centers—were four times more common in southern patients than northern ones.

Whether we are dealing with a Lyme-like illness or Lyme disease, "the patients deserve Lyme-like treatment," Ed Masters held. And, he added, northerners beware: The term "Southern" in the CDC's label of Southern Tick-Associated Rash Illness could be most misleading of all. The aggressive lone star tick has expanded its range relentlessly. Found up the East Coast as far north as Maine as well as throughout the Midwest, it carries Masters disease and a host of other illnesses—including the southern versions of babesiosis (strains that don't test positive on many standard tests) and ehrlichiosis—wherever it goes. "We believe that in areas where both *Amblyomma americanum* and *Ixodes scapularis* ticks are common, places like New York and New Jersey, some of the seronegative and culture-negative cases in Lyme studies might be due to Lyme-like illness," he said.

Regarding the spirochete at the root of Southern Lyme, Kerry Clark thinks the mystery may be solved, and goes beyond Ed Masters in giving the southern epidemic a name: Lyme disease. "I truly believe that in the South, the search for the elusive *Borrelia* that causes Lyme-like disease is a dead end, and that the idea of Southern Tick-Associated Rash Illness, or STARI, as a disease apart from Lyme is a myth," Clark states. "We don't have STARI, we only have Lyme."

The philosophical divide remains vast. Where Masters and Clark see "Missouri Lyme" as just one borreliosis on a spectrum, the CDC still contends that STARI is a rash-only illness—probably not infectious and surely unrelated to Lyme. "Until studies indicate otherwise, physicians who observe EM-like rashes in patients who do not have known endemic *B. burgdorferi* exposures should be highly circumspect of a diagnosis of Lyme disease or other infectious condition and should question the use of antimicrobials in its treatment," David Dennis, formerly of CDC and now a professor at Colorado State University in Fort Collins, wrote in *Clinical Infectious Disease* in 2005.

In 2009, a CDC study published in *Military Medicine* cast doubt on the presence of spirochetal disease in the South once more. The CDC researchers studied adults from Fort Campbell, Kentucky, bitten by the Lone Star tick. Each subject submitted the tick, and thirty-three completed a survey on their health. Of the thirty-three subjects, fourteen reported at least one symptom and two had an erythema migrans–like rash. In fact, the researchers said, they were "unable to identify any sequelae that distinguished the symptoms from Lyme disease." They nonetheless *rejected* the possibility of infection largely because patients lacked fever (hardly a requirement of Lyme diagnosis) and because the ticks lacked DNA from *Borrelia lonestari* (already dismissed by most scientists as a cause of Southern Lyme) or *Borrelia burgdorferi* outer surface protein A (undetectable in most Southern Lyme strains).

Year after year, Masters sought a unified field theory of borreliosis that included southern patients. Year after year, the CDC dismissed Lyme in the South.

We were sitting in Ed Masters's basement, a room so long it had the feel of a football stadium. The length worked well: Ed Masters's full and varied life, starting from his earliest days, was splashed in photographs and news stories across the walls. I saw Ed Masters, a strapping, athletic Dartmouth kid, holding a basketball. "I always liked to run with that ball," he said. I saw him on his wedding day, his beautiful wife, Jackie, dressed in white. I saw him as father to his kids. I saw his friends. Then there was the section devoted to his fight with the congressman, the one he chased from office a quarter of a century back: Reading the news clips on Ed Masters's wall, you got the story straight—the initial dispute, the weekly editorials written on medical clinic stationery, and finally, a congressman toppled from office, never to be heard from again. Masters noted how ironic life was, how everything that went around came around, in the end.

After all the years of struggle, many of the establishment academics offered him respect, and despite CDC intransigence, scientists had begun studying his disease—Masters disease—in earnest. Credibility had been hard-earned. For so many years, he'd been a tempting target. "With my data, nothing fit anymore—not the tick, not the microorganism, not the serology," he reflected. "One person told me, 'Masters, they were having a big old fine party, and you were the turd in the punch bowl. You spoiled it.'" And so he had.

Masters's findings challenged the CDC's Lyme concepts, and caused a serious disconnect. In Masters's version of Lyme, nothing was the same, from the spirochete to the tick to the region of the country itself. For scientists and government officials credited with discovering and defining the disease and now in the midst of developing diagnostic tests and vaccines for it, pushing Lyme beyond the paradigm was like swinging a wrecking ball through their work.

Yet as time went on, discrepancies between the textbook-perfect paradigm and the real world only deepened, pointing to a Lyme reality that is increasingly varied and complex. Until the agent of Masters disease is proven for sure, some patients will be suspect and diagnoses will slip through the cracks. Lyme *writ large,* with its coinfections and mimics, demands we do more research and keep open minds. "Absence of proof is not proof of absence," Ed Masters said.

29

❖

Restricting Diagnosis
and Keeping the Riffraff
Out of Lyme

The fight over Southern Lyme had profound repercussions throughout validated Lyme zones in California, the Midwest, and the
Northeast. As patients in states outside the so-called Lyme zone
began flocking to the diagnosis, officials became alarmed. Their response was to redouble efforts to keep "Lyme wannabes" outside the
vaunted gate—not just in the South, but the North and West as well.
With Ed Masters's patients testing positive for Lyme disease, the CDC
had changed the tests until Missouri blood failed. Yet the higher bar for
diagnosis meant that northern patients were failing Lyme tests in greater
number, too. Even patients with bull's-eye rashes and classic signs of the
disease, patients like Jason, were often out of luck.

In the Garden State of New Jersey, the flames of discontent were finally
whipped to inferno by a child's death. The tragedy, which was to alter the
face of the patient movement and push the Lyme war to new heights, un-
folded after ten-year-old Mandy Schmidt from Sayreville went pumpkin
picking and was bitten by a tick in the fall of 1988. A few weeks later she
developed a rash that her doctor diagnosed as "strep," though without a
lab confirmation. She seemed fine until April 1989, when, after returning
home from school, she developed a raging fever. She had a grand mal
seizure that evening, and by the time the paramedics arrived she was in a

coma. When she emerged from the coma, she had changed. "There was evidence of brain damage, and she got progressively worse," said Mandy's mother, Mary Schmidt. As Mandy declined, she manifested strange rashes just like the original rash, and her joints started to swell. This time, with no proof of any other cause for her illness, her parents began to think of Lyme disease. Community physicians signed onboard with the diagnosis and commenced to treat for Lyme, but to no avail. Mandy died on September 24, 1990. Lyme disease was listed as the official cause of death.

The death unleashed a firestorm of controversy in New Jersey, with skeptics insisting Lyme disease could not be at the root. Leonard Sigal, director of the Lyme clinic at Robert Wood Johnson University Hospital, was front and center in the effort to debunk the claims: "An unfortunate 12-year-old girl died of progressive neurologic dysfunction recently," he wrote to colleagues. "She had been evaluated by infectious disease, immunology, rheumatology, and neurology specialists at three hospitals, all of whom stated that there was no evidence of infection with *Borrelia burgdorferi*. Nonetheless, her physician states categorically that she died of Lyme disease (no autopsy done)." Sigal was especially incensed because Lyme patients had "used her demise to berate the Lyme disease academics," insisting that they took the disease lightly and were unresponsive to public need.

Outraged at Sigal's letter, New Jersey patients vowed to act. At the forefront in the effort to make a difference was Patricia Smith, today president of the national Lyme Disease Association, the largest of the patient advocacy groups in the United States. Back then, as the mother of a very sick teen in the shore community of Wall Township, her involvement in the Lyme situation was wrenching, and as personal as it gets.

In the beginning, the tall, auburn-haired, outspoken Pat Smith, an elementary school teacher by trade, had barely heard of Lyme disease. Her bright red house with the happy yellow shutters in the middle of the Jersey woods had the corny, feel-good look of a gingerbread cottage, and the last thing she expected to find out back was a disease.

When her youngest daughter, a sixth grader, began to tire quickly, Smith at first chalked it up to adolescence. Eventually, however, the problem was hard to ignore. A goalie on the local traveling team, the girl had a hefty game schedule on weekends. While other kids could play and then do a pajama party, Smith's daughter would play and then come home and go to bed. Eventually, following a Sunday game she would be so exhausted she could not even get up for school on Monday. "I just don't feel well," she said.

When her daughter started getting tendonitis in her forearms, Smith took the girl to a rheumatologist. A blood test confirmed his suspicion that the child had Lyme disease, so he treated her with oral antibiotics, and she seemed to get well. She continued on with soccer as well as baseball; she took piano lessons, joined the school band, and participated, fully, in the gifted and talented program of the Wall Township schools.

One day is etched into Pat Smith's memory: It is the day her daughter, presumably recovered, participated in a state soccer tournament in one of the new, indoor arenas. "It was very fast-paced, and it was the best game of her life," Smith recalls. "She came home, went to bed, and never got up."

The first thing Smith did, as the weeks passed, was to seek help at a local medical clinic. The doctor there tested her daughter for everything—except Lyme disease, the one thing he was sure it was not. But when other tests came back negative he ran a Lyme test at Smith's insistence. More weeks passed, and though Smith called the clinic almost every day, she was told they did not yet have the result. By now her daughter was sleeping eighteen hours a day, and when awake could tolerate neither light nor sound, and could barely drag herself the few feet from her bedroom to the living room couch. Finally, Smith insisted that either a doctor call her back or she would sue. That day, a physician called back to tell her that the test had, indeed, come back positive. Nonetheless, "intellectually, I don't believe your daughter has Lyme disease," he told Pat Smith. He didn't know what was wrong, but he wouldn't treat for Lyme.

"Intellectually, I don't care what you think, and if you won't treat her, I'll find someone who will," Smith replied. And so it was that Patricia Smith of Wall Township stepped deeper into the Lymelands. At first she took her daughter back to the rheumatologist; this time he treated her with IV Rocephin, and gradually she began to get well, with *gradually* the operative word. Still too exhausted to attend school through the seventh and eighth grades, the girl continued on home instruction. Yet improvement was continual, and it seemed as if she would be able to start her freshman year of high school, grade nine, with her peers.

A couple of days before the start of school a neighbor called and asked her to babysit. "She was thrilled to finally be doing something normal kids do," says Smith. But shortly after she arrived at the neighbor's house, she called home in a panic. The baby had a virus—something the neighbors had neglected to mention before she arrived.

"She came down with the virus, and it seemed to set off her immune system," says Smith. "Her Lyme symptoms returned." But with a difference—now, from time to time, she would feel strange episodes of anger for no apparent reason. The doctors said this could be preseizure activity, a harbinger of the seizure disorder they were seeing in some other Jersey Lyme patients. Doctors placed Smith's daughter on IV Claforan, but the intervention didn't work. Soon true seizures began— grand mal–like episodes of jerking and flailing for some thirty minutes three times a day, interspersed with periods of total exhaustion. Not knowing what else to do, the Smiths pulled their daughter off all antibiotics and waited. Three months after they had started, the seizures stopped. "They turned off like a faucet," recalls Smith. "One day she had three seizures, the next day two, the next day one, and then none. They were gone.

"For two weeks she was completely well," says Smith, "and we thought she was cured. We were thrilled."

Then one day, while sitting by the console playing Nintendo, Smith's daughter started to scream. "I have bugs, I have bugs," she yelled, clutching herself. At first Smith thought a fly might have gotten into her daughter's hair, and checked her. But nothing was found. As the hysteria increased, her husband came in, too. That's when the Smiths, together, realized their daughter was hallucinating. It was the first of many such episodes to come.

"This epoch lasted three years, from ninth through eleventh grades," Pat Smith says. "There were different manifestations. Sometimes there was an autistic state, where she could not communicate; she would just sit and stare and you could not reach her. Other times she would have a childish speech pattern, like a four- or five-year-old. Other times she would just stop cold in the middle of what she was doing and you could bring her out of it by touching her." She had psychotic episodes where she said "they" were coming to get her, though the Smiths never learned who "they" were. She had terrible nightmares: "She woke up screaming that she had six fingers, and I spent hours counting them for her, but it didn't help," Pat Smith says. "She would scream, 'I want my mom, I want my dad, I want to go home.' We would be right there with her and she would be in her room, in her bed, but she didn't know it. She was inconsolable." Smith's daughter was in the throes of such altered states between fifteen and eighteen hours a day.

Pat Smith herself was a prisoner. Doctors told her that if she did not put her daughter in the hospital, then she could never leave her side. "I could not go out and get the mail or the newspaper. I could not cook," Smith recalls. "From one second to the next, I never knew what she might do. One minute she would try to rip off her clothes and run out the door, the next minute she would appear totally normal—'waking up' without any realization that something untoward had gone on."

The truth of the matter is that the Smiths were afraid to place their daughter in the hospital in New Jersey—afraid that, with everything going on in connection with Lyme, and the controversy surrounding it, she would be labeled simply psychotic, and they would lose control of her medical care. Loss of control, even removal of parental rights, had happened to others in this situation: By 1990, tales of that nightmare scenario abounded in the towns and suburbs of New Jersey, reaching all the way to the south of the state, near Princeton and Trenton, and to the north, including the Bergen County communities abutting Manhattan. Leonard Sigal and a few other doctors had begun throwing around the term Munchausen Syndrome by Proxy (MBP) as the proper explanation for some of the sickest Lyme children and the mothers who dragged them to doctors, trying to get them well.

The hotly disputed Munchausen by Proxy diagnosis, by far more controversial than Lyme disease, has disturbed a bevy of psychologists and psychiatrists, who say evidence for the syndrome is lacking. While medical-related child abuse surely occurs, evidence for an actual *syndrome*—based on the theory that mothers fake children's illnesses just to get attention—consists of fuzzy, uncheckable anecdotes without a single controlled study ever published in the medical peer review. Still unproven to this day, the MBP hypothesis continues to raise expert hackles and has never been accepted as a formal diagnosis in the psychiatric bible, DSM-IV. That didn't stop some of the same university professors who insisted on absolute proof for Lyme diagnosis from bandying about the MBP label to explain why some children didn't get well.

The Smiths did not want to be caught up in that particular witch hunt. Yet they also understood they could not treat their daughter's bizarre episodes with the antibiotic regimens of the Lyme doctors, alone. So instead of putting her in a local hospital, they piled in a car and took her to a physician in Maryland.

That doctor spent a lot of time with the family. Then he pulled out a sheet of paper and asked them to read it. The disease described was uncannily familiar, from the zombielike fugue states to the childlike patter to attempts to run outdoors without clothes. "These were temporal lobe seizures," Smith now explains. Temporal lobe epilepsy, which may result from all kinds of brain damage (including an accident or infection) can often be treated only with surgery. But the doctor in Maryland was able to push the symptoms back with a variety of targeted drugs.

Within a couple of weeks, what the doctor had diagnosed as temporal lobe seizures precipitated by Lyme disease began to taper off. Over time, their daughter maintained normal consciousness for increasingly more hours, and was able to resume home instruction. Using a host of modalities, including acupuncture, to restore their daughter's balance and correct her sleep pattern, the Smiths were able to halt the seizures, for good.

Yet their daughter still had severe signs and symptoms of Lyme disease: arthritis, mental confusion and short-term memory problems, headaches, extreme fatigue. With the seizures under control, Pat Smith says, the antibiotics that seemed useless before now did their job, and her daughter finally started to journey toward health, for real.

All Pat Smith had to do was look around her to see she was hardly alone. Folks all over New Jersey were coming down with Lyme disease, but they weren't getting diagnosed. The sicker they got and the more neurological their presentation, the more doctors surmised they couldn't possibly have Lyme disease, the syndrome of swollen knees, so treatment was denied. Those doctors who recognized Lyme "outside the box" and dared to dispense more aggressive treatment were themselves targeted, their licenses at risk. Naturally this discouraged other physicians from getting involved. As a school board member, Smith was shocked at how many students diagnosed with Lyme disease were now out of school in Wall Township—and how high the home instruction budget had soared.

"This isn't right," Smith told herself, and placed a call to the U.S. representative of New Jersey's Fourth District, Chris Smith. "My district is loaded with Lyme disease," Chris Smith told Pat, asking if she would help him out. First on the agenda was a Washington meeting between Representative Smith, Lyme patient advocates, and officials from NIH and CDC. Given Pat's position on the school board, Chris Smith requested that she talk about the impact Lyme disease was having in the schools. "The hope," Pat Smith now explains, "was that we could get some federal monies to help. But I had no real data, so I got on the phone."

Pat Smith spent five days calling officials in nine school districts within two contiguous New Jersey counties—her own county of Monmouth, and Ocean County, to the south. The statistics were shocking, even to Pat Smith. The Jackson School District in Ocean County had more than 170 children with Lyme disease then on home instruction. Pat Smith's district of Wall Township had 54 Lyme students out on home instruction, raising the home instruction budget 88 percent as a result. Families caught in the grip could spend $100,000 on medical care for a single member.

On March 12, 1992, with a group of federal officials gathered in Chris Smith's D.C. office, Pat Smith handed out her small report. "I could see them flipping through it," she said, "and I thought it would end up in the circular file, but I was wrong."

Duane Gubler, the CDC's director of the Division of Vector-Borne Infectious Diseases, in Fort Collins, Colorado, was incredulous, to say the least. "This can't be right," he said to Pat Smith. "People can't be spending this much money on Lyme disease. These cases must be flukes."

"No," Pat Smith assured him, indeed, they were not.

She ended her presentation by talking about her daughter. First she described her before Lyme disease: the student, athlete, musician, friend. Then she said, "I would like you to meet my daughter today." Smith took out a plastic bag she had been storing under her seat and dumped dozens of bottles and boxes of pills across the long, polished conference table. "She takes fifty-four and a half pills a day for her Lyme disease," Pat Smith told officials in the room.

Duane Gubler, particularly, appeared moved, Pat Smith reports. "He got up and started asking me what each medication was for. Then he said, 'You have renewed my faith in trying to do something about this disease.'"

A week later Pat Smith got a call from the New Jersey Department of Health. "Who *are* you?" they asked. The long and the short of it was that the CDC had contacted the department about Pat Smith and her ad hoc school study. Now the CDC was sending real researchers to see just what was going on. It didn't take long for a contingent of CDC epidemiologists to roll into town. The team leader was David Dennis, the CDC's new head of Lyme disease and the same official who sparred regularly with Ed Masters over the reality of Southern Lyme.

"Either they thought there was some validity to my work, or they wanted to prove me wrong," Pat Smith reasoned. She put herself at their disposal, making introductions and assuring schools and parents the CDC was there to help.

Finally the CDC's report was ready and Wall Township scheduled a congressional Lyme Disease Forum for October 9, 1992. The planners had expected a few dozen people from nearby communities, but when the day arrived, the audience filled the meeting room to overflowing. Hundreds had come not just from New Jersey, but also New York, Connecticut, and Pennsylvania. The audience stood against the walls and sat on the floor. People came with wheelchairs, canes, and walkers. "Some appeared so sick it was extraordinary that they had been able to make the trip at all, and yet they thanked us for hosting this," Smith says. "Among the general population—even among those who had Lyme disease—there seemed to be very little known."

There were many speakers, including Pat's sick daughter, but the star attraction was David Dennis, who had come to announce the long-awaited results. Until Duane Gubler brought Pat Smith's school information back from Washington, Dennis told the crowd, he'd never considered how devastating Lyme disease could be to communities of people, let alone children. He was so surprised, he'd traveled to New Jersey this past June to oversee the CDC's investigation himself.

Of the sixty-five children studied, Dennis said, almost half met the CDC case definition for Lyme disease. Neurological problems were significant, with 90 percent experiencing memory impairment and 92 percent reporting headache and fatigue. Median reported duration of the illness was 363 days, and 80 percent of patients had been hospitalized at an average cost of $30,000. Some 90 percent of patients had been treated intravenously, at a cost of $63,000 per case. The average cost: $100,000 per patient. About a quarter of the patients in the study had fully recovered, and the rest had been in treatment for between two and four years. None of this included the social cost to the children: dramatic declines in grade point average, and lost extracurricular activities and time spent with peers. "This is the story of people's lives being disrupted," David Dennis said. The report showed "a compelling need to get the whole story," he added, and Monmouth was a good place to start. There was more to do: "We looked only at children requiring home instruction," said Dennis. But what about children not on home instruction? What about adults?

Finally, there was a segue Patricia Smith had not expected: CDC researchers had noticed that some of the children reported gallbladder problems, a well-known potential side effect of Rocephin. Now, Dennis explained, they wanted to determine the extent of the problem. Documenting the side effects of all this treatment was the next phase of the CDC's ongoing school report.

There was a vast silence in the room, and then a collective gasp.

Panelists at the podium spoke up first: "We know Rocephin causes gallbladder complications. We can use other antibiotics. Why waste money studying crap we already know when we haven't gotten to the bottom of the disease itself," Dr. Derrick DeSilva Jr. asked.

"It's just adding fuel to the fire," protested Ken Fordyce, head of the New Jersey Governor's Council on Lyme disease, explaining that the insurance companies would have yet another reason not to reimburse. The audience was so enraged that the room started filling with hisses and boos.

But Dennis stood his ground: Doctors had to know the downside of the treatments, he insisted, and a study of antibiotic side effects was the next logical step.

Before anyone could blink, the CDC was back in Jersey, this time not in the schools but at the hospital: the Jersey Shore Medical Center in Neptune, headquarters of Dorothy Pietrucha, the neurologist who treated the sickest children in the state. With a short blunt haircut and dark boxy suits, Pietrucha had the stern look of a boot camp commander, but to her patients, she was beloved. "They went in like gangbusters, pulling records without patient consent," Pat Smith says. "I was very disturbed, and parents who had cooperated with the CDC were outraged."

Even Pat Smith could not have predicted the fallout when the CDC published its gallbladder study in the *Journal of the American Medical Association* three months later, in February 1993. CDC epidemiologists had conducted a computerized search of hospital discharge data from Dorothy Pietrucha's institution, Jersey Shore, and found that 2 percent of the young patients on Rocephin had gallbladder complications, while just over 1 percent had gallbladders removed.

"The study hammered doctors who treated with intravenous antibiotics, calling them up for scrutiny by state health departments and hospitals. It gave insurance companies license to pull the IV plug, and it convinced many physicians to pull back from intravenous treatment of any kind," Pat Smith states.

But the most notable part of the latest CDC study was not the association between Rocephin and gallbladder complications, a problem well documented in the past. Rather, there was something new: The CDC now insisted that the New Jersey patients didn't actually have Lyme disease. In contrast to what had been reported at the Wall Township meeting by David Dennis just months before, the CDC now said that just a small fraction of the New Jersey patients met the definition for Lyme disease. Less than 5 percent of the patients had an erythema migrans rash, the CDC reported, and a mere 13 percent had a "major late manifestation"—one of the objective signs on the short list, like grossly swollen knees or meningitis, required by scientists like Steere before late-stage Lyme disease could be diagnosed.

"It wasn't just a matter of misdiagnosis," Gubler said. "The misdiagnosis was creating another public health problem—removal of gallbladders—and that is what the diagnosing physicians and the patients who wanted to have Lyme disease didn't fully understand."

A whole community of patients said to have Lyme disease in October was disenfranchised by February, and the rude dismissal was national news.

According to Gubler, the CDC's reversal had to do only with methodology. In the first study, a survey, patients had self-reported their symptoms. "You just couldn't rely on patient self-reports." So the second effort had tapped hospital records, and those documents—considered more reliable than patient memory, Gubler claimed—indicated that the patients' descriptions of their own illnesses had been wrong. Incredibly, the same team that rejected medical records in favor of patient reports in Missouri was, virtually simultaneously, rejecting patient reports in favor of medical records in New Jersey. In each case, the decision served to lower the number of patients who could be diagnosed with Lyme disease.

Not surprisingly, an avalanche of criticism poured down on the CDC's "technique." Brian Fallon, the Columbia psychiatrist, complained that in the clinical setting, diagnosing by CDC criteria would result in "gross undertreatment and unnecessary morbidity from what is, after all, a treatable disease."

Acting on behalf of the Governor's Council, Ken Fordyce requested a meeting with CDC officials in Atlanta. His notes on the encounter in March 1993 are scribbled on a pad from the Courtyard Marriott, where he stayed.

The two officials assigned to handle the meeting told Fordyce that the "hot button" was overdiagnosis. They feared that in giving the Lyme diagnosis, other "unknown entities" would be missed. Anyway, Lyme disease needed a positive Western blot for diagnosis, they insisted, but many of the Jersey patients had equivocal or negative tests.

Fordyce countered that the researchers hadn't gone beyond the hospital charts for diagnostic records and those records were incomplete. Most of the evidence—everything from blood tests to neuropsychiatric evaluations to MRIs—had been filed in the treating physicians' private office files, not at the hospital. But the CDC had never bothered to ask.

Besides, he added, many children had recovered as a result of the treatment. The report had painted a picture of irresponsible physician behavior, yet families were warned of adverse reactions. Many of the children received weekly sonograms to look for gallbladder complications. And whenever problems arose, the antibiotic therapy was stopped. He handed the scientists letters from six families of patients who had gallbladders removed during the study period, and these contradicted the CDC report, often point for point.

"I am the parent of one of the fourteen young patients who lost gallbladders to the use of Rocephin in the treatment of Lyme disease," one letter read. "I am sorry that the CDC found such a paucity of laboratory results or documented clinical evidence to support the diagnosis of Lyme disease. However . . . my daughter Meghan's lab results are not to be found at Jersey Shore Medical Center. Meghan was diagnosed in Hamburg in the office of Dr. Joseph Salerno with the lab test having been done at the Newton Memorial Hospital." Perhaps if the CDC had contacted her family or her family physician, the writer said, the mistake could have been avoided. Her daughter's positive lab test was attached.

Other letters, often pages long, were much the same.

"Perhaps we should have looked further into this," one of the CDC officials commented.

But if Ken Fordyce had hoped for a retraction of the study—or an apology to the patients—he had come to the wrong place. In the aftermath of the gallbladder study, David Dennis would face an angry response in New Jersey, Fordyce told the CDC.

"In that case, maybe we shouldn't do further work in New Jersey," the CDC officer said.

Anyway, their work in New Jersey was done. Dorothy Pietrucha, the unnamed physician under fire in the gallbladder study, was never officially charged with anything. But slowly it became uncomfortable for her to do her job. Although it didn't happen immediately or all at once, eventually Pietrucha would tell the rising tide of children clamoring at her Jersey Shore office to seek a different port—and they did, many defaulting to Charles Ray Jones in Connecticut.

The most dramatic change brought by the study, not just in New Jersey but nationwide, was the added difficulty patients faced in obtaining the Lyme diagnosis. These patients just didn't have Lyme disease, the CDC had announced in *JAMA*; now people without the rash would need to get sicker, more symptomatic, advance deeper into the territory of the major late manifestations Allen Steere had designated, before diagnosis would be considered and treatment dispensed.

Right after the gallbladder study, in the style of a one-two punch, *JAMA* ran another article, this one entitled "The Overdiagnosis of Lyme Disease," by Allen Steere. Published to over-the-top publicity in April 1993, the second article asserted that only a fraction of patients diagnosed with Lyme had ever had the disease. Steere had reached his conclusions after studying 788 patients referred to his clinic as Lyme disease sufferers over the course of some four and a half years. He determined that 23 percent of them had active Lyme disease. Another 20 percent had once had Lyme disease but now did not; instead, these patients had another syndrome triggered by Lyme—most often, chronic fatigue or fibromyalgia. The remaining 57 percent, Steere asserted, had never had Lyme disease at all, explaining why antibiotic therapy had failed to make them well.

The patient community was alarmed. From their perspective, Lyme disease was drastically underdiagnosed and undertreated; and a diagnosis missed too long could potentially ruin one's life. How many of them had been turned away, again and again and yet again, by local practitioners, until what had been early, easily treatable disease became disseminated, late-stage infection, responsive to antibiotics, if at all, only with medication delivered at high doses, and over several months? How many now suffered permanent debility, fighting insurance companies frantically for an extra month or two of antibiotics to prevent progression of symptoms that worsened over time?

As expected, responses poured in. In a letter published in *JAMA*, Joe Burrascano complained that Steere ignored guidelines that Lyme be diagnosed clinically, based on signs and symptoms, not blood tests. Instead, Steere seemed to render diagnoses based largely on serology—but only with tests run at *his* lab. By hinging diagnosis on his tests, exclusively, while discounting tests by others, said Burrascano, Steere was engaged in a cycle of circular thinking, in which serology defined the disease as opposed to the other way around. "My experience is that the predominant problem with these patients is underdiagnosis and undertreatment," Burrascano said.

Yet Steere's study, trumpeted in the media nationwide, had a chilling effect on family doctors and pediatricians, who took it as a cue to withhold diagnosis and treatment unless evidence of infection was overwhelming or absolute. That meant patients without the rash were, in most physicians' offices, required to progress to late-stage disease, when objective inflammation and positive blood work could provide unambiguous proof. One result was that fewer patients lacking true infection were saddled with the Lyme label and, thus, fewer received antibiotics without cause. Still, with *B. burgdorferi*'s habitat pushing outwards and wooded suburbs more populated than ever, more people got Lyme disease; and with doctors more reluctant to render the diagnosis, more real Lyme disease patients—especially those without the rash—slipped through the cracks. These patients were forced to retrace Polly Murray's footsteps in their quest for a diagnosis, as if she had never paved the way for them at all.

Though the *JAMA* articles had stirred hard feelings, there was one project everyone could sign on to: the quest for a standardized test. For all Steere's insistence that Lyme was overdiagnosed and Burrascano's insistence that it was underdiagnosed, the truth is that without an accurate test Lyme was simply often misdiagnosed. A better test, or at least a standardized one, was what patients said they needed, and the scientists agreed. Not surprisingly, the idea of a "better test" was relative. To the patients, "a better test" was one that would enfranchise more of them to diagnosis. To scientists like Steere, a "better test" was one that could stanch the tidal wave of "Lyme pretenders"—the patients from New Jersey, Missouri, and points beyond clamoring for diagnosis at the gate.

To resolve the matter once and for all, the CDC and the Association of State and Territorial Public Health Laboratory Directors (ASTPHLD) cohosted the Second National Conference on Lyme Disease Testing, in Dearborn, Michigan, in October 1994. The goal was to select a new blood test standard to aid in the diagnosis of Lyme disease. But with the endorsement of new, even narrower criteria at the meeting, the scientists (who did the voting) got just what they had hoped for, leaving more patients than before outside the diagnostic gate.

The new Dearborn standard for serodiagnosis of Lyme disease was the same one Jason would pass with flying colors and Mark and I would fail in the year 2000, six years hence. It included the ELISA to screen potential patients for possible Lyme disease, and the Western blot to confirm that positive ELISA results were actually right. The so-called Dearborn Criteria replaced the potpourri of blood-test patterns previously considered positive for Lyme disease with just two Western blot patterns, one for early disease and one for late.

Serodiagnosis of early Lyme required the presence of antibodies associated with early infection, known as IgM (for immunoglobulin M). Early patients were required to generate IgM antibodies that could be picked up by the ELISA, a test that some studies showed missed 20 to 30 percent of patients or even more. Only those patients who passed the ELISA screening test could go on to take a Western blot. Based on a study by microbiologist Russell Johnson of the University of Minnesota, the Dearborn panel decided that three IgM antibodies especially common in early Lyme disease mattered most. Patients who generated two of the three IgM bands within a month of the tick bite were considered positive for Lyme.

Far more controversial was the test standard adopted amidst a firestorm of protest for the diagnosis of later Lyme disease. Here, too, patients first had to pass an ELISA, though this time by generating immunoglobulin G (IgG) antibodies, associated with advanced infectious disease. Those who passed the ELISA were sent on to step two, the confirmatory Western blot. Instead of the three bands counted in early Lyme, the Dearborn panel chose a second blot pattern for late disease, this one derived from a study Steere himself had conducted in collaboration with Frank Dressler of Germany in 1993.

To determine the *one true antibody pattern* and encode it in a test, Steere and Dressler performed immunoblots on several dozen classic Lyme disease patients known to have a strong antibody response. In the end, they decided that patients with bands indicating at least five of the ten most common IgG antibodies had *true Lyme disease*.

On the surface, the recommendations seemed to bring order to chaos. But to the patient community it was one more slap in the face. For one thing, the Steere team had used just a single strain of *B. burgdorferi* to derive the standard, and that strain came from Europe! Was this really the best match for diagnosing hundreds of U.S. strains, including some eliciting alternate antibodies not on Steere's list?

For another thing, the committee had compressed the time frame over which antibodies were expected to appear. In 1986, a comprehensive study conducted by Steere had documented antibodies to as many as eleven spirochetal proteins appearing in a sequential pattern over months or years. Yet now the Dearborn committee was asking to see five bands appear at once as early as just two months after the onset of the disease—a bar that even classic patients (like Jason) might not meet.

But the most divisive part of Steere's new "Lyme standard"—and a source of feuding ever since—was the decision to remove two highly specific *B. burgdorferi* proteins, outer surface protein A (OspA) and outer surface protein B (OspB), from the test. These were both so specific to the Lyme spirochete that they could come from nothing but exposure to *B. burgdorferi* and were even candidates for making Lyme vaccines. According to the Dearborn committee, the reason for the cut was merely statistical. In the classic patients Steere had worked with, OspA and OspB were not among the ten most common bands. It's not that these bands didn't result from Lyme disease; they certainly did, and no one denied it. It's just that, statistically, Steere said, tests weren't *more* accurate when OspA and OspB were counted in because the other, more prevalent bands, showed up as well.

Yet the omission of the two markers on Western blot testing worked against some of the sickest patients, those infected longest before being diagnosed: OspA was barely expressed right after a tick bite, but its levels increased in the human body with time. Those in the latest stages of Lyme disease were far more likely to express antibodies to OspA and OspB, even as other borrelial proteins dropped away. Without Osps A or B to serve as markers, many of the sickest patients no longer met any diagnostic standard. By excluding these patients from diagnosis, they were excluded from treatment as well.

Ken Liegner, with his practice of late-stage patients, was particularly disturbed. In December of 1994, with the consequences of Dearborn hitting home, he wrote a letter to Marc Golightly, director of the diagnostic lab at Stony Brook: "This is not just some sort of game to play with people's lives," Liegner said. "I am savvy enough to understand how ridiculous these interpretations are, but most clinicians would not have a clue."

To make his point, Liegner enclosed what he considered the two most egregious cases he'd seen since the standard had changed. The first patient, a former valedictorian, was now having trouble maintaining B's and C's—and "it is not psychological," Liegner wrote in his note. Her Western blot—called in as a negative by Stony Brook—would have been fully diagnostic if the lab had counted the presence of OspA. The second patient reacted to six *B. burgdorferi* proteins, including the hijacked OspA and OspB, and would have been fully diagnostic if either band had been allowed. Instead Stony Brook's lab report read, "These results are not specific for the diagnosis of Lyme disease." The patients needed treatment but as far as their insurers were concerned, they were out of luck.

"Credible laboratorians like yourself must speak up against the irrational and arbitrary criteria the CDC is using," Liegner wrote, imploring Golightly for help. It was absurd to rely on a European isolate as a reference strain when it couldn't possibly reflect the disease in the United

States. Perhaps Golightly could at least *alert* patients negative on Dearborn but actually diagnostic according to Lyme patterns seen in the United States. Otherwise, patients would get burned.

Liegner received some satisfaction. "Golightly agreed to report all bands on the blot, not just the CDC-specific bands, for my patients," Liegner explains, adding that Stony Brook accommodates him to this day. Liegner understood that the lab director did not want to go to war with him over Dearborn. "That's how the Nazis came to power," Liegner says he told Golightly at the time. But he also thanked him for his help.

In the end, I came to see the Dearborn criteria as an acceptable bar for surveillance purposes only. Although recognized by many of those I spoke with as a gross underestimate of the true incidence of Lyme disease, cases positive by Dearborn are certainly diagnostically pure. They constitute the top of the Lyme pyramid, classic in every way. As such, they offer a credible leading-edge indicator for epidemiologists tracking the disease as it expands its terrain.

But in its second role, as a blood test for detecting real-world patients, it is deeply flawed. In the strip malls, village centers, and medical suites along the winding country roads where our pediatricians, family physicians, and internists welcome their trusting suburban clientele, Dearborn is embraced as unassailable. Originally earmarked as definite only for surveillance, it is now being used, more than ever, to diagnose and treat. In the absence of a rash, doctors usually accept the decree of Dearborn above everything else.

As my family trucked to pediatricians, neurologists, rheumatologists, and infectious disease specialists not just in our local area but throughout the great teaching hospitals of New York City, from 1994 through 2000, the notion of Lyme disease was soundly rejected by doctors, again and again. I lay the blame squarely on the back of Dearborn and its widespread misuse. Improper reliance on the Western blot pattern—calculated, statistically, in 1993 based on a narrow set of patients, using a strain of *Borrelia* from Germany—is the single greatest reason why physicians miss the Lyme diagnosis in patients without a rash, and why they put off treatment until long after some patients can be easily cured.

⁙

For years after the ascendancy of Dearborn, the machinery set in place to stanch the tide of Lyme diagnoses churned on, unmindful of changes already wrought. As the decade passed, Leonard Sigal's conception took on a fashionable new name—Pseudo-Lyme disease—and headlined at medical conferences as an epidemic far more threatening than Lyme disease itself. As if on autopilot, the great campaign to rein in Lyme diagnoses powered on, but those who fueled it never seemed to look inward or glance back. If they had, they might have had some questions: Had they balanced their message of overdiagnosis with appropriate warnings of underdiagnosis? Had their alarm rung so loud it deafened colleagues to the cries of legitimate Lyme disease patients? Was the fixation on *B. burgdorferi* so implacable that other infections in the tick were routinely ignored? Had they enabled an epidemic right in our own backyards?

In 1996, *Yale Medicine* published an article with diagnostic and treatment instructions that made Dearborn seem broad. The article, apparently disregarding recommendations in the most conservative of the peer-reviewed literature, instructed doctors to forget about diagnosing Lyme disease early, in the rash stage, and to wait until major late manifestations of the disease appeared before considering treatment at all. The magazine's directives were so extreme they made Allen Steere, by then at Tufts, look like an antibiotic cowboy on the loose.

"If you suspect the tick was attached for at least 36 hours, observe the site of the bite for development of the characteristic skin rash, erythema migrans, usually a circular red patch, or expanding 'bull's-eye,' " the article said, perpetuating the myth that most Lyme rashes actually assumed the specific shape. But "not all rashes at the site of the bite are due to Lyme disease. Allergic reactions to tick saliva are common." Therefore, "antibiotic treatment is not necessary, is costly, and may cause side effects." While Steere advised that physicians diagnose the EM rash as Lyme disease, and treat it with antibiotic early, the article in *Yale Medicine* was telling doctors to watch and wait. And there was more: Should the patient develop symptoms of later-stage Lyme disease—defined narrowly by *Yale Medicine* as "arthritic swelling of a joint, most often the knee, or facial nerve palsy"—the physician was to "have a test done. If the test result is positive," *Yale Medicine* went on, "have a more precise test done. Only if this test proves positive should a course of antibiotic therapy begin. Expect some symptoms to linger for up to three months. No further antibiotic treatment is necessary."

In other words, contrary to the most conservative of the mainstream directives, *Yale Medicine* instructed physicians to let patients advance to late disease before they even considered testing—despite the fact that some 20 percent of patients allowed to advance so far into symptomatology might never get well. Then, unless that late-stage patient passed the series of blood tests endorsed at Dearborn, treatment was *still* to be with-held. Finally, while Steere instructed that persistently sick Lyme disease patients be given a second course of antibiotic treatment just to be sure, *Yale Medicine* said no.

Tom Grier, the longtime president of the Lyme Disease Coalition of Minnesota, was fit to be tied in 1996, when the article arrived at the Minnesota Department of Health in St. Paul. Investigating further, he learned it had been dispatched to every state department of health receiving a CDC grant for development of diagnostic and treatment guidelines. Those health departments, in turn, sent the reprint to physicians throughout the United States.

Once Minnesota health officials became aware of the *Yale Medicine* language, the reprint was pulled. The advice from *Yale Medicine* was in direct conflict with Minnesota guidelines for the diagnosis and treatment of Lyme disease. But in states without an advocate as vigilant as Grier, the *Yale Medicine* article took flight. While patients falling short of the CDC surveillance definition had always struggled for a diagnosis, the widespread distribution of the *Yale Medicine* article meant that many patients actually *meeting* the CDC case definition—patients like Jason— would be left behind, as well.

In 1999, Pat Smith, by then president of the Lyme Disease Association of New Jersey (a group that would later morph into the national association), and Duane Gubler of the CDC, were still going back and forth over the original school district study of 1992. On February 11 of that year, Pat Smith pressed Gubler one more time to get the original school study into print:

I am writing to you as someone who is in the trenches in the war against Lyme disease—you may remember the yet-to-be published school district survey you sent the CDC to NJ to complete. As I have pointed out many times since then to you, that survey contains a wealth of data that could be productively used by many investigating the impact of Lyme. Yet it remains unpublished.

As President of the Lyme Disease Association of New Jersey, Inc., I must work with people every day who are afflicted with this dreadful disease. Many times I am reminded of the question you chose to ask on that survey: "Is your life consumed by Lyme disease?" The answer now as then is the same—a resounding YES. Thousands of individuals are sick, their children are sick, there is a national epidemic which is taking away lives, yet the CDC seems to continue to participate in the same charade now as six years ago when we first met. What will it take to enlighten you to what is happening? Just what is it you are waiting for to act? When will you finally agree to spread the word that Lyme is serious, and that chronic Lyme needs long-term treatment? Please let me know, because I would like to be able to tell my daughters and the hundreds of thousands who are sick before their lives end that someone in government recognized their plight and tried to save them or at least spare some of their suffering.

A couple of weeks later, Duane Gubler wrote back: "Do not feel that because the results of the study were not able to be published that your efforts and ours were not well worth it," he wrote. The CDC programs emerging, in part, from that early, unpublished study included physician- and nurse-training programs, a new diagnostic standard for laboratory tests, and even the impetus for LYMErix, a new vaccine. By sounding the alarm through her school study, Pat Smith had played a role in all of the above.

As Patricia Smith pondered the outcome—the doctors drummed out of New Jersey, the restrictive diagnostic standard approved at Dearborn, the new vaccine, with rumors of adverse reactions already pouring in—she was filled with incredulity and a sense of the unreal. Was she really responsible for all of *that*? A promise-turned-menace (or menace-turned-marvel, depending upon where you stood), the CDC's vanquished school study was one more signpost along the tortuous road through Lyme.

30

The Long Road Home

Framingham, Massachusetts, 2002

Like Jason and others before him, the Statlenders determined that they had no choice but to cross the line—to leave the respectable but ineffective ministrations of the mainstream for the edgy counterculture of Lyme. It was that or ride the train they were on to the end of the line. It had been so many years, and so many wasted efforts—and this could be one more of them. But what did they have to lose?

The plan was to get the children tested for tick-borne disease first, this time through the controversial Lyme lab, IGeneX, in Palo Alto, California. "We don't put much stock in that lab," one mainstream expert told them, complaining that its broader criteria and lower thresholds led to overdiagnosis. But others explained that IGeneX tested for more strains of *Borrelia* and reported more bands, including fourteen separate regions of the spirochete's protein coat and the markers indicating OspA and OspB. For those who thought Lyme was underdiagnosed and that patients like the Statlender children were being missed, IGeneX was viewed as the best place to go.

When the results came back, they were enlightening. Eric and Amy each had what IGeneX considered "equivocal" results on the Western blot—some evidence but not enough to rule Lyme in or out. Each had tested positive for *B. burgdorferi* DNA. Seth's Western blot was florid, lighting up bright and meeting the CDC's stringent serological standard for late-stage Lyme disease in full. He also tested positive for a coinfection, *Babesia*.

"Given the limitations of lab testing in general for Lyme disease, and the likelihood that whatever was ailing our kids was stemming from the same etiology, Russ and I felt that their combined findings painted a picture," says Sheila Statlender. "Finally we had more pieces of the puzzle, and based on that, we moved on."

Given the implicating results, they decided to take the children to see Charles Ray Jones one at a time, starting with Eric, whose illness was relatively more recent and somewhat less entrenched. After examining Eric and evaluating his test results and his risk of exposure, Jones made the clinical diagnosis of Lyme disease and started him on antibiotics—Ceftin and Zithromax—that very day.

"Within two and a half weeks, Eric's auditory processing problem cleared significantly. It seemed like a miracle," Sheila says. "His interactions with friends and teachers improved, and he followed most conversations without confusion or delay." He was still fatigued and still in pain, but slowly, over months, he began to get well.

Next to visit Jones was Amy, whose combined symptoms had become so severe and debilitating that she rarely left the house. Previously an avid reader and top student, she now had so much trouble concentrating she couldn't pick up a book. She was so exhausted and shaky that she couldn't walk down the block, and so sensitive to touch, light, and sound that she needed the refuge of a darkened, quiet room. She, too, was put on antibiotics the day she walked into Jones's office—though at an especially low dose in deference to her sensitive gastrointestinal tract. Despite that abundance of caution, the medicine, Zithromax, just made her sicker. "Only this time, we realized it was a Herxheimer," Statlender says, so they kept on.

Finally, there was Seth. Of the three, the onset of his illness could be traced more easily back to that initial, acute onset six long and awful years before. He suffered pain and exhaustion, along with recurrent high fevers, swollen glands, and migraine headaches. He had trouble concentrating. Many of his symptoms were moving targets: At various points, for example, he developed restless legs, making sleep difficult, or vomited multiple times daily. His blood pressure plummeted, causing blackouts. Like Amy, he was extremely sound- and light-sensitive, and so intolerant of heat that he slept, throughout the winter, with his air conditioner on. He, too, was prescribed antibiotics as well as anti-malarials by mouth.

Even if related, the illnesses and treatment that followed sent each of the three along different paths. While Eric was getting stronger, Amy and Seth seemed to drift in the ebbs and flows of the disease—they'd get better, then they'd get worse, and then better again. The part of Seth's illness that clearly seemed due to *Babesia*—the night sweats and insomnia— eventually relented. But the part that appeared to be Lyme—the fatigue, fevers, tremor, and focusing problems—did not. Jones cycled Amy and Seth through various oral antibiotics, but none seemed to help much. They would have Herxheimers, causing the temporary flare of symptoms. But they failed to get the pickup at the end.

"Six months after we started, they weren't clearly getting better," says Sheila of the older two. "We were plagued with guilt. We hadn't found a tick or a rash on either of them, nor had we ever thought to check. We had never taken any precautions whatsoever, in terms of Lyme disease prevention." Jones recommended that they up the ante by switching to intravenous delivery of antibiotics. They consulted a second specialist, who concurred. Moving forward with some degree of apprehension, they worried that it could be too late for their older children—that treatment had been delayed too long.

31

⬥⬥⬥

Reporting Our Pediatrician

Chappaqua, New York, 2001

L ooking around, talking to folks, I could see there were many like us in Westchester County, in the neighboring counties and states, and across the United States—people diagnosed years after having been infected by a tick bite and allowed to become desperately ill. Given my personal experience, I suspected that large numbers of bona fide Lyme disease cases still hadn't received a proper diagnosis. Especially chilling was an observation I tried to put out of my mind as we ourselves sought help: Even after they were treated, so many of the late-stage patients I met never seemed to get well.

One day, seeking explanations, I picked up the phone and placed a call to Ned Hayes, at the time chief of epidemiology at the Bacterial Zoonoses Branch of the Division of Vector-Borne Infectious Diseases at the CDC. I explained my concern about the reluctance of the physicians of northern Westchester County to diagnose tick-borne disease. "You should send someone out here to educate these doctors," I said.

But Hayes told me, point-blank, that I was wrong. "Westchester doctors are extremely well trained and educated on the topic of Lyme disease," he informed me from his office in Fort Collins, Colorado. There would be no need for the CDC to enlighten the doctors of Westchester, he said, or to change anything at all.

Yet one didn't need to be a rocket scientist (or even an epidemiologist) to suspect he'd made a mistake. Simply by living in Chappaqua, I often met people the doctors may have missed. Waiting in line at Rite Aid, I stood right behind a young woman who'd moved to town a year before, from Italy, transferred with her husband for a promotion on his job. While he spent the day working in Manhattan, she gardened avidly in her lush Chappaqua yard. Only now she had heart palpitations, a tingling in her fingers, and a noticeable numbness in her face. I could hear her query the pharmacist as she waited to receive her physician's medication of choice for this problem: an antidepressant.

"The doctor says these symptoms are from stress," she explained to the pharmacist. "Can that be?"

I couldn't help but intervene. "Have you considered Lyme?"

"Oh yes, but my doctor says these aren't Lyme symptoms," the woman replied. He had refused to discuss the possibility, she told me, or to run a Lyme disease test.

There was another neighbor, a bright and charming woman around age sixty who had once been a beauty. But now she was so bent and arthritic she had to walk with a cane. One day I summoned the nerve to question her symptoms. "There's no diagnosis," she informed me.

"What about Lyme?" I asked her.

"I had that a decade ago," she said, "but I had a month of antibiotics. Now the doctor says it's something else—he just doesn't know what."

One cannot inhabit the northeastern suburbs without seeing the damage—in the children with headaches that never go away, the forty-year-olds with limps, the teenagers too fatigued to study or engage fully in the activities of life. Do they, in fact, have Lyme disease or some other tick-borne infection? If they haven't presented to most local primary care physicians with the bull's-eye rash, or possibly, the tick attached, even classic patients may never be evaluated for Lyme though they are at ground zero for the disease.

One afternoon in the office of a local psychiatrist known for treating the neuropsychiatric consequences of Lyme, I learned that the same pediatrician who'd misdiagnosed Jason's Lyme for years had a steady exodus of other young patients now deeply symptomatic with a host of neurological ills. "I have thirteen of his patients suffering the result of misdiagnosed Lyme disease right now," the psychiatrist said.

Disturbed that our pediatrician should be allowed to continue without at least a warning or review, I registered a complaint with the New York State Department of Health's Office of Professional Medical Conduct, the OPMC, in March 2001. I did not want to sue the physician, or to jeopardize his livelihood; indeed, as time went on I came to understand he had just been doing what he had been trained to do. On a personal level, I actually liked this friendly, affable young doctor. But I nonetheless felt bound to protect future children by registering my experience with the state agency designated to investigate such issues and, if appropriate, impose corrective action before even more patients were hurt.

My complaint was particularly solid because Jason had a Lyme pedigree. The Northern Westchester Hospital physician who had finally diagnosed him, after all, was Peter Welch, a physician whom the OPMC considered one of its top experts. (Welch had just been declared the state's witness against Joe Burrascano, by then up on charges in New York for overtreating Lyme.) With many specific signs of Lyme disease and eight positive bands on a Western blot from LabCorp, Jason met the stringent case definition established by the CDC itself. He had spent summers playing in a forest in a known Lyme hot spot. He had a large, classic Lyme rash—though not a bull's-eye—that any medical practice should have insisted upon seeing, yet Jason was told not to come in. Among the signs and symptoms of Lyme disease recorded on his medical chart were severe headache and fatigue, inflamed and pained knees, migratory joint pain, whole-body shooting pain, a transient heart irregularity detected by an electrocardiogram, and heightened sensitivity to light and sound.

The OPMC duly investigated my complaint and did not, in the end, question the veracity of my report. But there was nothing to be done. "Lyme is difficult to diagnose," an OPMC nurse told me over the phone.

"In this case it shouldn't have been," I told her. "If a case like this is missed, and dismissed as 'not Lyme,' then whom do the doctors of northern Westchester deem worthy of the diagnosis?" Wasn't something wrong with this picture?

Apparently not, according to the New York State Department of Health. "The Office of Professional Medical Conduct has completed its review of your complaint," I was told in a letter from Medical Conduct Investigator Patricia Biski, R.N. Medical records had been gathered and reviewed, she wrote, and the physician I reported interviewed by the OPMC itself. "The available evidence pertaining to your complaint does not represent misconduct, as defined by law," Biski's letter said. "We fully understand the nature of your complaint and your concern that [your son] was not diagnosed with Lyme disease for two years." (I reckoned it more like seven, but only two years had passed since the giant rash.) "While we are unable to provide you with specific details of our investigation please be advised that all aspects of your complaint were carefully considered during our medical review. Our review showed that [your doctor's] treatment did not deviate from accepted medical standards. Consequently, we have no basis upon which to proceed further at this time and our review of this matter is now closed. A permanent, confidential record of this investigation will be retained on file in our office. In the event that new complaints are received that suggest a pattern, your complaint will be reconsidered."

What had once seemed unthinkable was now put in writing for me by the health department itself: Not treating Lyme disease, even for years, even if the case was so classic it belonged in a textbook, even if patients became disabled, and even if they were children, violated no medical code in New York State. Instead, it was treating the disease aggressively, comprehensively, and beyond the narrow guidelines accepted by insurance, that brought on censure and risk. On the day I sent the complaint, seven of just eleven physicians still willing to treat late-stage, disseminated Lyme disease beyond the narrow guidelines were under investigation in New York State.

It was spring of 2001, more than a year since Dr. Welch had anointed Jason with the diagnosis of Lyme. He was still so ill—too tired to see his friends or participate in sports. After half a day of school he came home so exhausted all he could do was climb into bed. I pondered my letter from the state. Nurse Biski had said that my complaint would be kept on file, and reconsidered should new complaints, suggesting "a pattern," emerge. I didn't understand the last part: If the doctor's actions were acceptable in a single case, wouldn't a pattern of this behavior be acceptable, too?

32

✦

The Lyme Inquisition:
Doctors on the Run

Along with the effort to limit diagnosis and curtail treatment, the academics on the "right" began organizing to shut down the offenders—frontline physicians like Joe Burrascano and Charles Ray Jones—at the heart of the dispute. A 1990 letter from Allen Steere to George Kraus, health director of the town of Milford, Connecticut, shows the strategic thrust: "I think it is unfortunate that the Lyme Borreliosis Foundation and the doctors connected with them . . . have become major spokesmen for Lyme disease . . . they are the principal force leading to the overdiagnosis and overtreatment of this illness. Do you have any ideas regarding what to do about this?"

The brainstorming resulted in several strategies. One was to report physicians who veered away from Steere's guidelines and toward Burrascano's to state medical boards, where they could be investigated and sanctioned, and thus reined in.

It was all part of a new and angry litigiousness that had, by the 1990s, permeated the consciousness of the doctors and scientists who toiled in Lyme. Once just scientists and clinicians, they were now expert witnesses in court cases and defendants charged with medical malfeasance. Routinely investigated by state medical boards for exceeding the standard of care, the community doctors were forced to spend tens and even hundreds of thousands of dollars to fund their defense and then, despite their efforts, could be drummed out of Lyme or the practice of medicine itself.

Ken Fordyce, head of the Governor's Council, and Kerry Fordyce, president of the Lyme Disease Association of New Jersey during much of the 1990s, felt patients were in a bind: "Each day I would have forty or fifty calls from people who needed help, and had nowhere to turn," Kerry Fordyce says. "We had just a handful of doctors willing to treat, and I would have to call and beg them to take one more."

The whole thing was difficult because, while all treating doctors were at risk, a few of them had accepted kickbacks from the home-infusion companies selling intravenous antibiotics, raising ethical concerns. "We were in an impossible situation," Ken Fordyce says. "We couldn't allow those physicians to continue, because they were undermining everyone's credibility. As patient advocates, we had to push them out of Lyme ourselves. Yet every time one of them was forced out, that meant more patients couldn't be treated."

In New Jersey, the laser light of investigation burned not just the questionable doctors, but the honest ones, too. Dorothy Pietrucha was squeaky clean, but in the aftermath of the CDC's gallbladder study, her Lyme practice was compromised.

The husband-and-wife physician team of John Drulle and Emilia Eiras was swept up in the inquisition. These doctors not only would never dream of accepting kickbacks, they actually treated impoverished patients for free, sometimes paying for medicine themselves. The pair, brought up on charges for "the overdiagnosis and overtreatment" of Lyme disease by the State Board of Medical Examiners in 1992, had to hire an attorney to defend themselves. It might have gone badly, if not for a fluke: A nurse familiar with the Lyme controversy attended a party and overheard a State Board member discussing the plan to "get one of those Lyme doctors." He even mentioned the target: John Drulle. The nurse testified on behalf of Drulle and Eiras. Given the bias implicit in her report, the charges were dropped. The Drulles survived and continued to treat Lyme patients. But most New Jersey doctors who faced charges of overdiagnosing and overtreating Lyme disease decided to negotiate without publicity; they moved out of the state, or stopped treating Lyme disease at all.

Despite the carnage, most observers say the war between the doctors didn't go nuclear until the summer of 1993, when the U.S. Senate Committee on Labor and Human Resources, chaired by Ted Kennedy, scheduled a hearing on Lyme disease. To the horror of the patients, the sole expert witness was to be Allen Steere. Over the next week, patients bombarded Kennedy's office with thousands of faxes and calls and the upshot was inclusion, at the zero hour, of additional testimony from some chronic patients and the first Lyme warrior, Joe Burrascano himself.

And so it was that on August 5, 1993, Joseph J. Burrascano Jr., M.D., stood before the Senate committee as hundreds of Lyme patients looked on. Donning green ribbons to show solidarity with the cause, the patients there that day were poised for battle, but few had expected Burrascano's words to raise the ante so high:

> There is a core group of university-based Lyme disease researchers and physicians whose opinions carry a great deal of weight. Unfortunately many of them act unscientifically and unethically. . . . They adhere to outdated, self-serving views and attempt to personally discredit those whose opinions differ from their own. They exert strong, ethically questionable influence on medical journals, which enables them to publish and promote articles that are badly flawed. They work with government agencies to bias the agenda of consensus meetings, and have worked to exclude from these meetings and scientific seminars those with alternate opinions. They behave this way for reasons of personal or professional gain, and are involved in obvious conflicts of interest. . . . Some of them are known to have received large consulting fees from insurance companies to advise them to curtail coverage for any antibiotic therapy . . . even if the patient will suffer. This is despite the fact that additional therapy may be beneficial, and despite the fact that such practices never occur in treating other diseases.

Then Burrascano got to the heart of the matter, the targeting of the Lyme doctors:

> Following the lead of this group of physicians, a few state health departments have even begun to investigate, in a very threatening way, physicians who have more liberal views on Lyme disease diagnosis and treatment than they do. Indeed, I must confess that I feel that I am taking a large personal risk here today by publicly stating these views.

The persistent undertreatment of Lyme disease, he said, was partly inspired by politics and partly by insurers' and scientists' bottom lines; whatever the reason, the outcome—"[undertreated] patients with advanced disease [who] rarely return to normal"—the damage done was knowable in advance. "Long-term studies on patients who were untreated or undertreated demonstrated the occurrence of severe illness more than a decade later, reminiscent of the findings of the notorious Tuskegee Study, in which intentionally untreated syphilis patients were allowed to suffer permanent and in some cases fatal sequelae," he said.

Those in the audience could hardly believe their ears: Joe Burrascano had the unmitigated gall (or was it the courage, the *balls*) to accuse the academics of pulling a Tuskegee, allowing patients to progress to late-stage disease, knowing full well they needed treatment but withholding it just the same. Like the discovery of the spirochete itself, Burrascano's words were cataclysmic—once uttered, they could never be taken back. Invested before long with the indelible stamp of legend and the heightened power of myth, Joe Burrascano's 1993 Senate testimony made the fight more intensely personal than it had ever been. The doctors he maligned were not likely, now, to let things drop.

When Allen Steere spoke an hour later, his version of reality was so different it didn't seem possible he could be describing the same disease. Aware he had been demonized, Steere nonetheless addressed the committee calmly. Reserved where Burrascano was voluble, middle-aged where Burrascano was youthful, cautious where Burrascano was impulsive, Steere could still play hardball, and his points issued forth with the bite of a star pitcher's curve. In short, he held his own, describing an easily diagnosable, easily curable illness with few complications and little resemblance to the condition Burrascano called chronic Lyme. Allen Steere may have been an object of contempt to patients at the hearing, but to the rest of the world he was still the foremost authority on Lyme disease—which he did not, quite frankly, think most of these people had.

Repeating the conclusions of his "overdiagnosis" article, Steere summarized the "post-Lyme syndromes" of fibromyalgia and chronic fatigue. Such patients would not respond to more antibiotic, he said. Then Steere looked directly at the sickest of the patients to testify, a teenager named Even White, a young man so disabled he was crumpled in a wheelchair and could barely talk. "In my seventeen years of work in Lyme disease," said Steere, "I've never seen a case like *that*."

When Steere was done, Senator Howard Metzenbaum of Ohio asked him if he could diagnose *anybody* at his clinic.

"Yes," Steere said.

Why, Metzenbaum asked, did Steere seem to think the tests were so reliable while Burrascano did not?

"Because he doesn't get it," shouted a patient in the audience. The crowd jeered.

That's when Joe Burrascano pulled out a blown-up photograph of a spirochete, positively identified as *Borrelia burgdorferi* by the NIH's Rocky Mountain Labs. "It comes from a patient treated with antibiotics for thirteen months," Burrascano declared.

Joe Burrascano's fighting words had elevated him to hero status in the eyes of his minions, the chronically ill Lyme patients. But his public accusation that mainstream academics were actively engaged in conspiracy and the knowing abuse of patients to further their own agenda had been damaging, to himself most of all. His words outraged his adversaries—and turned him into a high-profile target, marked for demolition to the end of time.

Karen Forschner of the Lyme Disease Foundation got a whiff of the future a few months later, in January 1994, at an NIH meeting on chronic Lyme disease. "Toward the end of the meeting," she recalls, "Dr. John LaMontagne, a director of the National Institute of Allergy and Infectious Diseases, said to me, 'Someone should sue Joe Burrascano for his testimony.' When I asked why, he replied: 'He committed slander and someone should get him for that.' "

The first Lyme doctor to fall in the aftermath of the hearing was not Joe Burrascano but William Brown of Portland, Oregon. Brown said he'd learned how to treat Lyme disease after contracting it himself. He'd spent nine years in physical decline, shunted from diagnosis to diagnosis though the treatments didn't work and he didn't get well. After considering explanations including reactive arthritis and atypical multiple sclerosis, he finally discovered that he had Lyme disease. He was treated with two weeks of intravenous Rocephin, and temporarily improved, but thereafter relapsed. Finally, adapting techniques of the Lyme doctors in the East, he treated himself with long-term regimens of oral antibiotics, in combination, and recovered. Before long he was using the techniques to treat patients.

Brown's legal problems started when he came to the attention of a reviewer from the HMO Kaiser Permanente, which questioned his diagnosis of patients without positive blood work and his willingness to treat them long term. The reviewer turned him in to Oregon's Board of Medical Examiners for "overtreating and overdiagnosing" Lyme disease.

At the disciplinary hearing that followed, Brown was grilled for hours, the bounty of charts and literature he'd brought to defend his treatment strategy totally ignored. Of the six patients reviewed at the hearing, five had dramatically improved, but Brown was sanctioned. In fact, he was allowed to stay in practice only if he met a condition: that he sign a consent letter agreeing he would no longer treat Lyme disease. He signed it on April 1, 1994.

Across the country, in Bristol, Connecticut, a board-certified internist named Phil Watsky had been targeted as well. Watsky's nemesis was someone he had never met: Lawrence Zemel, director of pediatric rheumatology at nearby Newington Children's Hospital. Zemel had heard secondhand reports, mostly from families of children he treated, that "Watsky was prescribing months of IV antibiotics, contrary to mainstream Lyme disease therapy." Initially Zemel wrote him off. But when he learned the Lyme disease hotline 1-800-TICKBITE, located in the offices of a home-infusion company, was referring patients to Watsky, he'd had enough.

Taking action in September 1993, Zemel reported Watsky to Donna Brewer, chief of the legal office at the Connecticut Department of Health (DOH). Zemel literally proposed a sting operation to catch Watsky off guard. "Have one of your staff investigators pose as a patient, complete with vague symptoms and negative Lyme results but insisting that she has Lyme disease," he wrote in his letter. He offered to "rehearse that individual" himself.

Although health officials never did the sting, by the summer of 1995, the Connecticut DOH had arrived at Watsky's doorstep demanding the medical records of two specific patients, neither of them involved in making the complaint. The health department immediately dropped an unfounded allegation that Watsky took kickbacks from IV companies. They also dismissed charges of impropriety involving one of the patients whose records had been seized.

But the second record, involving an adult, was sent to pediatrician Henry Feder of the University of Connecticut for review. Like so many Lyme patients, the individual had tested negative on the ELISA test but positive on a Western blot. Symptoms were nonspecific—there were no swollen knees, no nerve conduction abnormalities, just the garden-variety symptoms of fatigue and pain that physicians like Sigal referred to as vague. That December, Watsky was called into the state health department, where he was grilled for two and a half hours on every aspect of the second case.

It actually appeared as if the department's attorney would rule against him based on their insistence that the CDC case definition, including the two-tier blood testing voted in at Dearborn, be followed to the letter. If the patient had been negative by ELISA, why had Watsky even ordered a Western blot? They pointed to the gallbladder study in New Jersey as evidence that Watsky had put his patient at risk.

In the end, Connecticut dropped charges for lack of evidence— Watsky had been able to prove, among other things, that he had nothing to do with the home-infusion company using his name. But Brewer sent Watsky a written warning: The state remained concerned over the health dangers of long-term antibiotic therapy. Watsky should keep this in mind because they might "reexamine" the case at any time should more information emerge. Watsky found that while the charges had vanished, the fallout had not. As a result of the investigation, two managed care plans denied him participation. Before long, Watsky had backed off from the treatment of Lyme disease.

As the nineties inched to a close, it was in Michigan where the battle waged fiercest of all. The target was an earnest young doctor named Joseph Natole, of Saginaw, who, quite by chance, had taken Lyme patients under his wing. Natole's disastrous journey started naïvely with his very first Lyme disease patient, Jane Huegel. A member of an HMO called the Blue Care Network, Huegel began suffering panic attacks, a stiff neck, swollen knees, a grinding headache, and fatigue in 1978. Yet every time she took her complaints to a doctor at the HMO she was referred "to another doctor who referred me to another doctor. One doctor told me I had headaches because I smiled too much." But her problems were never resolved. The HMO published a monthly newsletter, including profiles of new doctors arriving on staff, and in 1988, Huegel noticed a blurb about one who seemed intriguing: Joseph Natole, thirty-two, at the start of his career.

At first Huegel consulted Natole for a urinary tract infection. But by 1989, the panic attacks, stiff necks, and headaches she had been dealing with for a decade became increasingly severe. "I just felt horrid," Huegel says. So she sought the help of Natole, again. Natole did a thorough physical exam and was unable to match the strange symptoms with a particular syndrome or disease. But when Huegel mentioned how much time she spent outdoors in the woods, Natole had a thought: "Maybe you have Lyme disease," he said.

"What's that?" Huegel asked.

To confirm his hunch, Natole—who had never before seen a case of Lyme disease—ran a blood test, an ELISA. When it came back positive the next day, he ran more tests, finding that Huegel had spinal meningitis. Natole attributed this to Lyme disease and placed Huegel in the hospital for ten days of IV Rocephin. For the first time in a decade, Huegel's symptoms started to abate. Natole then sent Huegel's blood to the University of Michigan, where experts advised him that the infection was on the wane. The antibiotics had done their job, they told Natole, so Huegel should be taken off medication and sent home.

Huegel reports that five days after her release from the hospital, she relapsed and was "just as hideously sick as before."

"I don't know what to tell you to do," Natole said, when informed.

But now that she had a diagnosis, Huegel began to investigate on her own and quickly discovered the publicity booting up, thanks to the efforts of the Forschners and their new group, the Lyme Disease Foundation. "The LDF had nurses on call back then," says Huegel, who consulted with one and was told that if Natole himself called, guidance could be dispensed. That is just what happened: Huegel implored Natole to call the LDF nurses. Faced with an incurably sick patient, Natole finally did and was referred to Joe Burrascano. Guided by Burrascano, Natole placed Huegel back on antibiotics and this time, she reports, she began to get better for good.

"You know how it is," Huegel told me over lunch at an Applebee's in Saginaw. "Once you have Lyme disease you start to recognize it in others, and I did." Today, a small, rounded woman who looks like a cupid out of Botticelli, Huegel has trouble walking. It is Huegel who draws the blinds shut over our window at Applebee's so the sun doesn't irritate our eyes.

The rest of the story is Shakespearean, complete with tragic hero, high-minded intentions, and a fatal flaw. As Huegel went about her daily life in Saginaw, she began noticing others with her symptoms. She called Natole and asked if he would see them. Tentatively, he agreed. "That's how he got into the Lyme business," explains Huegel, who would found the Michigan Lyme Disease Association and serve as its president for seven years. Most of the 250 individuals Natole ultimately diagnosed and treated, says Huegel, began to get well. But right from the start, the diagnoses seemed to make the Michigan Department of Health nervous. For one thing, Natole reported fifty cases of Lyme disease right off the bat, in 1989—before reporting was even mandatory—from counties said to lack the spirochete or the tick.

He popped up on the radar screen again when state authorities investigated a home-infusion company called the Caremark Corporation, a dispenser of intravenous therapies. Caremark had been paying fees to referring physicians. As Natole's load of IV patients expanded, Caremark came to call, and offered him compensation. After reviewing the offer with his attorney, who told him it was legal, Natole signed on, insisting he would allocate a significant share of the Caremark profits to Lyme disease research. Good intentions or not, the Caremark connection would be a permanent stigma, making Natole especially vulnerable as a target for state authorities seeking to root out the overdiagnosis and overtreatment of Lyme disease.

As time passed, Michigan required that doctors report all cases of Lyme disease, and, obviously, Natole had an abundance. Yet with the state insisting there was no Lyme disease in lower Michigan, Natole's reports were red-flagged. Who was this doctor in Saginaw, and why did he have so many Lyme disease patients in an area devoid of Lyme disease, the health department wondered. Was he the *same* Dr. Natole involved with the suspect company, Caremark?

In the grindingly slow process of medical hearings, it took a year and a half for Natole to come to trial for the way he treated Lyme disease. (The Caremark issue was not part of the charges.) The testimony against him came from Allen Steere.

Critiquing Natole's doctoring case by case, Steere outlined diagnostic guidelines even more restrictive than the intentionally narrow CDC case definition intended for surveillance. Although Steere testified that patients could sometimes be seronegative, he required serological confirmation from all those whom Natole had diagnosed. When Natole diagnosed an erythema migrans rash, Steere disqualified it because Natole's description in the patient chart lacked sufficient nuance or detail. If Natole's patient had a swollen knee, Steere required positive serology. If an ELISA was positive, Steere wanted confirmation by Western blot. If the Western blot was called positive at one lab, Steere insisted the band pattern would be nondiagnostic at *his*. For confirmation of neuroborreliosis, Steere required that Natole's patients have not just objective clinical signs confirmed by ELISA in turn confirmed by Western blot, but—after all these hurdles—a lumbar puncture to test cerebrospinal fluid, even though cerebrospinal fluid rarely tested positive, even in definite cases of neurological Lyme.

The most notable part of the testimony was Steere's insistence, in every instance, that Natole's patients satisfy the Dearborn criteria. Although Steere's deposition was taken three months before passage of the new serological standard at Dearborn, and although all the cases under consideration had been diagnosed literally years before Dearborn was a gleam in Steere's eye, the rheumatologist nonetheless invoked the requirements of Dearborn (even if not by name)—including two-tier testing and the presence of specific bands—as the bar Natole's patients needed to pass to qualify for the diagnosis of Lyme disease. Natole and Steere would never have been in sync. But by invoking a serological standard of the future as a requirement for competency in the past, the Michigan Board of Medicine asked the family doctor to jump a surreal bar that required the skills of a psychic, not an M.D.

Jane Heugel was one of the patients Steere reviewed. Even though she had three positive ELISAs, and a decade's worth of headaches and panic attacks had abated after treatment with antibiotics, Steere still called the handling of her case negligent. As far as Steere was concerned, Huegel had never had Lyme disease, and shouldn't have been treated for it at all.

By February 1998, Natole's medical license had been temporarily suspended on a Lyme conviction, and he'd been indicted by federal authorities who alleged he conspired with Caremark to overbill insurance companies. He pleaded not guilty and was released on bond. That case was finally settled out of court and the records were sealed. In the end, Natole continued treating patients but, like Brown, not for Lyme.

By 1999, in the midst of the dot.com boom, as other Americans were planning parties for the new millennium, Lyme patients did a count: Pietrucha, Brown, Watsky, Natole, and dozens of others had been driven out. And Burrascano—along with ten of his practicing colleagues from the hyperendemic regions of New York State—had been under investigation for years.

It was in July of that year when Joe Burrascano was finally interviewed by New York State's OPMC and his patient files seized. By the next fall, the Lyme scene in New York State had reached a frantic, angry pitch. Patients had written to ask for an explanation as to why so many Lyme doctors were under investigation in New York State, and the OPMC had written back, citing the CDC and *The Medical Letter,* among others, as its Lyme guide: "Rarely, if ever, have . . . published guidelines indicated that anything more than two [to] three weeks of antibiotics are required to cure Lyme disease," the office said.

To the state legislature, the OPMC's apparent endorsement of a treatment formula, in writing no less, was cause for alarm. No matter what the disease, if the strategy was to identify and investigate physicians who followed a less popular treatment methodology, it was overstepping OPMC's mandate and misusing the law. So outraged were lawmakers that even as the OPMC began investigating Burrascano, the legislature scheduled hearings to investigate bias at OPMC.

On November 9, 2000, hundreds of Lyme disease patients rallied in Burrascano's defense outside the Plaza Hotel in Manhattan. They had come from across town and as far away as Oregon and California to support the doctor they insisted had returned them to health. "Today, we draw a line in the sand with our treating doctors on one side and the ivory tower establishment on the other," Pat Smith, now president of the national Lyme Disease Association, told the crowd. "Whoever dares to cross the line from this point forward and threatens our doctors' right to treat needs to understand that we will . . . in turn attack you with all the science, bodies, and medical and legal expertise it takes to eradicate you as a threat."

In the wake of this uproar, as my own family struggled with Lyme disease, Burrascano's trial commenced. Every few weeks for the next year, he faced a room of his inquisitors at the OPMC's offices on Manhattan's Lower West Side. The thing that kept Joe Burrascano's "fire stoked," sustaining him through all of it, was being "on the receiving end of a stunning amount of love." Carried on the wings of love his patients unfurled, Joe Burrascano journeyed to the dark side, where, with his lawyer, Alan Lambert, he battled for survival deep in the enemy camp.

The health department had more trouble prosecuting Burrascano than it ever thought possible, starting with its search for a witness willing to testify to "crimes" in the nine patient files culled. The problem was the evidence itself: According to sources requesting anonymity, even Burrascano's enemies felt the OPMC had failed to distinguish negligence and difference of medical opinion, mistaking the second for the first. There were many doctors in New York State who wished to dismantle Joe Burrascano—but it was difficult to convince someone to testify to negligence under oath when they felt the records didn't support it. "It was clear from the evidence I saw that it was going to be a political trial and not a medical one, and I didn't want to be part of that," said one potential witness, a professor at a New York State teaching hospital who was intensely opposed to Burrascano's treatment practices and views. The professor wanted to put Burrascano out of business, and badly, but could not honestly find incompetence in the specific records he reviewed. "I declined the honor," he said.

Going down its list of witnesses, the OPMC eventually found someone willing to sign on—Peter Welch of Northern Westchester Hospital in Mount Kisco, the doctor who'd diagnosed Jason with late-stage Lyme disease that very year. In signing up for the role of "expert," Peter Welch stepped into a quagmire that other, more prudent physicians had elected to avoid. Not only was the case based largely on differences of opinion, according to Welch's colleagues, it was difficult to get one over on attorney Lambert, a doctor himself. Lambert had managed to obtain records from patients Welch himself had seen. Since Welch was the state's witness, and, thus, a de facto paragon of doctoring, his records had been allowed in as exhibits; and it turned out that Welch had done some of the same things for which he now took Burrascano to task.

When Welch criticized Burrascano's records for failing to document a joint exam, for instance, Lambert responded with an evaluation in which Welch had failed to document a joint exam. When Welch said Burrascano had failed to evaluate blood pressure, Lambert pulled a record where Welch failed to document blood pressure; and Welch's patient had been dizzy, making the omission worse.

The first victory for Lambert—and probably the most pivotal—was convincing Administrative Law Judge Jane B. Levin to allow him to introduce evidence from the medical peer-reviewed literature. Most such tribunals relied on the expert witness as the ultimate arbiter, but with the ability to introduce outside scientific evidence the playing field was leveled in a way not usually seen.

As the weeks and months passed, the players in the hearing room scrutinized the case files exhaustively, analyzing every test, diagnosis, and decision Burrascano had made. The state's main beef, of course, was that he treated patients for Lyme disease for weeks and often for months longer than the recommendations set in stone by the Infectious Diseases Society of America and scientists like Allen Steere. Burrascano said his patients had "chronic Lyme disease," and the state held that chronic Lyme wasn't real.

The question before the panel was straightforward: Were there two standards of care for two types of patients? Or, was there just one standard of care and one type of patient—with the second type of patient (the chronic one) a bogus creation of doctors the state said were negligent and incompetent, such as Joe Burrascano?

Addressing the issue, Lambert showed that Lyme patients who failed the standard treatment could get well when more treatment was dispensed. In a 1995 paper in *European Neurology*, Pat Coyle, the Stony Brook scientist known for world-class work, reported a woman, a resident of New York City, who'd acquired Lyme disease on a camping trip through Switzerland and France. She was treated aggressively, only to recover and relapse and require treatment again. Coyle's well-documented patient had been treated on and off almost continuously for years. It was likely that such patients were more common than thought, proposed Lambert, and aggregated in Burrascano's practice—a consultancy where other Lyme doctors sent their toughest cases, the ones who didn't get well.

Take, for instance, the case of the Kentucky neurologist, age thirty-five, who'd made his way to Burrascano after his illness had plagued him for years. It had started with what seemed to be a virus, followed by neurological symptoms, including double vision and balance problems that were so severe he had to walk with a cane. The patient had undergone extensive evaluation at the Mayo Clinic, where a diagnosis of multiple sclerosis was proposed. Treated with high doses of cortisone, a steroid, the patient got sicker than ever and multiple sclerosis was ruled out. Wondering if he had Lyme disease, he consulted the world's top academic experts, including Pat Coyle of Stony Brook and Allen Steere of Tufts. Steere dismissed the idea of Lyme disease, but Coyle did not. In fact, the only tests suggestive of any disease for the Kentucky doctor were an ELISA and spinal tap, which came back borderline positive for Lyme disease. Based on these findings, Coyle recommended six weeks of IV Rocephin.

In December 1996, with the six weeks at an end but the illness still in play, the neurologist from Kentucky decided to cross the line and consult Burrascano. Burrascano doubled the dose of Rocephin and added the antibiotics Zithromax and Plaquenil to the mix. A few months later, the man reported feeling somewhat better. As months and then years passed, Burrascano tested and treated him for coinfections, continually altering the therapy step by step. By the spring of 1998, the patient reported an abatement of his symptoms; he no longer needed his cane and had returned to good health.

Yet to New York State, the neurologist from Kentucky was the perfect example of someone who never should have been treated for Lyme disease or its coinfections at all. The diagnosis Peter Welch offered for the Kentucky physician was "idiopathic disease," an illness without any explanation or any apparent treatment. Burrascano "treated him for a disease that there was insufficient evidence he had," Welch testified. And "he treated him for longer than recommendations suggest one should."

Appropriate or not, Lambert pointed out, the patient, who was, after all, a doctor himself, reported he had gotten better with the treatment.

Welch dismissed the self-report. "That's what *he* believes," Welch said.

In case after case, Welch dismissed Burrascano's approach. But with the right to introduce journal articles, Lambert prevailed. In one case, for instance, Welch criticized the way Burrascano diagnosed and treated babesiosis. Yet it turned out that Burrascano had followed the guidelines published by world *Babesia* authorities Peter Krause and Andrew Spielman to a tee.

In another instance, Burrascano diagnosed Lyme in a woman who'd been bitten by a tick, then developed the signs and symptoms of Lyme disease: joint swelling, neurological problems, and fatigue. The woman had saved the tick and had it tested. *Borrelia burgdorferi* was found. Treated, the woman got well. In this case, specifically, Welch could not support the diagnosis of Lyme disease.

The panel entrusted with deciding Joe Burrascano's fate delivered its decision on November 6, 2001, clearing him of thirty-seven charges and finding for the state in two: One patient had been inappropriately treated for *Ehrlichia* despite a positive test because he lacked the specific symptoms of fever and chills, which Welch said were required to diagnose the disease. (Many experts disagreed.) Another patient, the Kentucky neurologist, had experienced a seizure after a dose of the antibiotic Bicillin; though he had had the seizure disorder before Bicillin therapy, Burrascano should have pulled the medicine in the wake of the new seizure, said the judges; that he did not was deemed negligent, too.

To discipline Burrascano, the panel placed him on probation, requiring that his work be reviewed by a monitor for two years. It wasn't a clean sweep, but for Joe Burrascano it was an impressive victory given the dire outcome that might have been. For one thing, with a sympathetic monitor, he continued to treat his patients according to his conscience. And those judging him recognized the politics of the case. "The issues raised in this case pertained primarily to a medical debate in this field, rather than a demonstrated lack of competency," the OPMC panel of independent judges said. "We are . . . acutely aware that it was not this Committee's role to resolve this medical debate."

The panel was influenced, in part, by the inflexible stance of Peter Welch, "an arrogant witness, who appeared to be on a crusade, constantly lecturing, rather than answering, after questions were posed to him," they wrote in their final report. "Had Dr. Welch even appeared to consider viewpoints other than his own . . . it would have added to his credibility," the panel said.

Ironically, it was Peter Welch, the state's witness, who offered Jason the first act of medical kindness we'd seen in many years with the diagnosis of Lyme disease—not a difficult call given the documented history of inflamed knees, residence in Chappaqua, and eight CDC bands on his LabCorp Western blot. Not a real leap, given the huge rash. Welch had made the obvious diagnosis, but in the highly politicized milieu of New York, it had been an act of generosity, a gift.

"I'll give it to you," Peter Welch had said at the time, in conferring the diagnosis to Jason.

The phrase seemed so odd to me that I never forgot it. I knew nothing of all this, back then, and did not understand what I later came to realize: that Peter Welch had indeed given us something valuable and rare, the answer we had sought in vain for years without even knowing it, a diagnosis of late-stage, disseminated Lyme disease in New York State.

33

⬧⬧⬧

A Note from the Underground

Colorado Springs, Colorado, 2003

As the doctors had warned, the flush of energy after the photo safari began to wane, and soon Dave Martz was sicker than before. By the fall, he couldn't get out of his chair unless Dee pulled him up. He couldn't walk more than a hundred feet, or stand for more than fifteen minutes. She had to roll him over in bed and help him dress. He'd be in a wheelchair in less than six months, his doctors emphasized, so he'd better get ready to die.

Falling deeper into illness, Martz might have accepted his fate, gone on with the process of dying, if not for his son, a northern Virginia genetic engineer working on the human genome. Talking to any expert he could get his hands on, Martz's son was told that people with Lyme disease failed the blood tests all the time. Negative tests, alone, could not rule Lyme out.

Then, in December, a friend of Dave's son noticed a newspaper article published some months before in the Danbury, Connecticut, *News-Times*. Amazingly, the article described another patient, also diagnosed with ALS, who'd been treated for Lyme disease and gotten well. The man in question, Tom Coffey of Fredericks County, Pennsylvania, had been diagnosed with ALS in 2001 and given a few months to live. His steps were faltering, his speech slurred. He couldn't swallow his own saliva, let alone food, and had been scheduled for a tracheotomy and ventilation support in a few days' time.

"I couldn't cough or laugh," Coffey told the crowd at a Lyme disease symposium held at the New Milford High School in April 2003. "And I had what I can only describe as a constant pressure on my brain. I think my doctors thought I was faking it, or losing my mind."

According to the article, Coffey had questioned the ALS diagnosis, finally seeking help from a Lyme doctor, who placed him on an intensive, long-term regimen of antibiotics until he recovered his health.

"I'm just so grateful to be liberated from the hell of Lyme disease," Coffey told the group.

Martz knew he wasn't reading the *New England Journal of Medicine* here, just a local newspaper story; still, he took the quoted experts to heart. Especially compelling to him was the idea, put forth by a Dr. Steve Phillips of Ridgefield, Connecticut, that the outer proteins of the spirochetes changed, sometimes making it hard to pick the disease up on antibody tests. The implication, to Martz: To scout out Lyme, you sometimes needed to look not for traces of the spirochetal proteins detected on Western blots and ELISAs, but for *B. burgdorferi* DNA. Among the diseases that Lyme patients could be misdiagnosed with, the doctors at the conference had ticked off not just ALS, but multiple sclerosis, lupus, even rheumatoid arthritis. They also mentioned coinfections of Lyme disease, including, Martz noted, babesiosis—a ringer for malaria and treatable with the same medication, Lariam, that had coincided with the unexpected temporary improvement in his own declining health during the Kenya safari.

He knew not to get his hopes up. Amiram Katz, a neurologist associated with Yale, had emphasized the need to rule out other diseases before going with the Lyme diagnosis. "Our role is to ask first, 'What else could this be?'" he told symposium attendees. "We should wake up every morning thinking of other diseases instead of Lyme disease. We have to be careful. Misdiagnosis can run both ways and it's dangerous both ways."

Still, with a looming death sentence, Martz had little to lose. "I wasn't just a dying man scrambling for one more hope of a miracle, something that I'd seen so often in my oncology practice," he explains. Rather, in his heart, he still thought it was possible that he had Lyme disease, and that his doctors, all of them, had made a colossal mistake.

Searching around for another route to testing, Martz discovered something controversial, but, to his way of thinking, logical. It was called an antibiotic challenge test. First, he took a short course of antibiotics, the theory being that if infected with spirochetes, the treatment would kill some of them off, releasing their DNA in the blood. Then he had his urine analyzed for spirochetal DNA. The results came back unequivocally positive for Lyme disease. Antibodies to the spirochete meant merely that one had been exposed at some point in the past, but DNA in the urine, well, that implied his infection was current and active, Martz felt. After everything he'd been through, Martz found the outcome amazing. "I knew the active Lyme infection might not be causing my motor neuron disease, I knew antibiotics might not help any part of my illness," he says. But with nothing else before him except the grim business of dying, he knew he had to pursue the Lyme theory at all costs.

That Christmas, Dave and Dee made a pact: Even if by some gift of God Dave got well, they would not forget the emotional lessons learned during the months of dying, or waste their hard-earned new intimacy and human depth.

34

Second-Chance Kids

Framingham, Massachusetts, 2003

In the end, the Statlenders agreed to put their children, all three of them, on the intravenous antibiotic that Charles Ray Jones had advised them could jump-start their treatment—and slowly, with fits and starts and plenty of setbacks, they began to improve.

For Amy, the treatment didn't work until an endocrinologist diagnosed a problem with her pituitary gland that had been building for months. Her thyroid and cortisol levels were flat, he found, interfering with her metabolism. Once her endocrine function came under better regulation, however, the antibiotic seemed to kick in and her Lyme disease symptoms, including the joint and focusing problems, began to abate. It was because the spirochetes were being killed and flushed from her tissues that her Western blot finally turned fully positive, Jones felt. Soon Amy was taking classes at the Harvard Extension School and, as her balance and coordination improved, she embarked upon an exercise program. She even flew with Sheila to Mexico, accompanying Sheila's sister on a jewelry-buying trip to Mexico City and Taxco, capping the whole thing off with a dip into the healing hot springs at Ixtapan de la Sal. It was an adventure that would have been impossible only months before.

Seth got a part-time job at an outdoor supply store and, in his spare time, accompanied his father on a trip to Vermont, where they attended a workshop to learn trout fishing, a complex activity that reflected his greatly improved energy and powers of concentration. Always popular and social, he began dating and spending more time with friends. But he was reinfected with what appeared to be a brand-new case of Lyme disease on one of his fishing trips and had a serious relapse requiring that he be treated again.

The Statlenders' experience was, quite naturally, of great interest to the other Boston-area chronic fatigue parents. "As our own children were evaluated and then treated for Lyme disease, several parents from each of the two CFIDS support groups began reviewing their children's histories with new eyes," Statlender explains. Before long, several of them began stepping outside the circle of Boston's mainstream medicine, seeking Lyme tests at the same alternative labs as the Statlenders and—for those with evidence of tick-borne infection—treatment from Lyme doctors like Charles Ray Jones.

One child, for example, had lived on a street where several pets, including his own dog, had been diagnosed with Lyme disease. He had never been properly evaluated for it himself, despite years of illness. A slight droop of his left eye had been declared psychosomatic at one teaching hospital. "He ultimately tested positive for Lyme disease on a Western blot," Sheila reports. "Dr. Jones was the first after a long list of physicians to comment on his swollen finger joints." Another child had spent her summer in a Lyme-endemic, wooded area away from her family. She returned home so ill that she collapsed getting off the airplane. She had never been tested for Lyme disease. Both of these young people, like most other children represented in the two support groups, had lost years of their lives. Yet, treated for Lyme disease, they resumed friendships, returned to school, and ultimately attended college.

The story of the Boston-area CFIDS children, of course, remains complex. "Two of them, including the girl placed on the macrobiotic diet, never pursued Lyme work-ups and improved spontaneously relatively early on," says Statlender. Two others tested positive for Lyme disease but experienced such severe side effects when given antibiotics that they have required frequent breaks from treatment. "Objectively speaking, these two had been sick the longest, one of them possibly from infancy," says Statlender. "Understandably, they have gotten discouraged." They remain sick to this day.

Yet the majority of the Massachusetts CFIDS children from these two groups who pursued the Lyme evaluation tested positive on the Western blot, says Statlender. "Most of those who were able to stick with treatment have shown significant improvement, if not the return of perfect health."

PART THREE

A SEARCH FOR ANSWERS

The great tragedy of science—the slaying of a beautiful hypothesis with an ugly fact.

—Thomas H. Huxley

35

❖

Once Bitten: Accepting the Spirochete's Endless Love

Chappaqua, New York, 2002–2003

The more I learned about Lyme disease, the more disturbing it seemed. Looking out my window at the spruce forest that made us sick, I knew I had traveled far beyond Chappaqua. The forest was not just a spruce forest, not just a tick forest or a deer forest, but a daunting forest primeval of the mind—dark and glistening and full of mystery, physical but also metaphysical, biological but also metabiological, shaped not just by nature but also human manipulation of it, human interpretation of it, the imposition of our consciousness on the facts.

In the end my questions were simple: Was the infection persistent like Burrascano said or killed easily with treatment, as Steere held? Were spirochetes hiding from antibiotics in secret niches in our bodies, or had our immune systems gone haywire, attacking us long after infection was gone? Could an organism persist in us without the blatant inflammation we normally associate with infection—the grossly swollen joint, the inflamed meninges—and yet still make us sick? Finally, if infection *did* sometimes survive standard treatment with antibiotics, why all the denial? Were government officials worried about the superbugs that long-term antibiotics could spawn? So many of the big-name scientists had received funding for vaccine development—an endeavor that, by its very nature, required a circumscribed disease definition for the products to pass through the gauntlet of the FDA. Could the economic pressures of product development so early in the game, before more was known about Lyme disease, have skewed the direction of the research? Conflicts of interest were rife in the wider world of biomedicine, affecting research across the spectrum. Were the conflicts well publicized in the newspapers every day active here as well? How could so many patients be so sick while so many highly funded scientists dismissed them as neurotic and their cases as false? In this war of doctor against doctor, were egos and turf playing a role? Was this *just* an intellectual disagreement, or also an emotional one?

Only Leonard Sigal's explanation—that so many patients were somehow deluded, sick with the fear of sickness or just the burden of life and not Lyme disease or some other organic ill—struck me as too facile to believe. Because of the relapsing remitting illness I felt *inside myself* and the power of antibiotics to push it back, because I didn't think *I* was crazy, I didn't buy the theory that suburban angst was driving chronic Lyme.

Some six months after starting treatment for the coinfections of Lyme and babesiosis, I'd experienced the dramatic abatement of symptoms I had lived with for years, and I was thankful. My head stopped hurting and my vision was restored. The infernal buzzing faded. A normal, uplifting energy replaced the edgy anxiety. The grinding fatigue, so overpowering I'd slept hours each afternoon, lifted like a cover of clouds giving way to blue sky. Perhaps I was cured, I thought to myself back then.

But as time passed, I realized that my illness lingered on. Yes, my Lyme disease was treatable—I could often live life as a healthy person, and feel well. I could *pass*. But in the mode of many other chronic Lyme patients I interviewed, each time I stopped my oral antibiotic, amoxicillin, I would coast a few months and then start to sink. My fingers and arms would tingle, my eyes would blur, my knees would hurt, and numbing fatigue would set in. After each relapse I'd get retreated; each retreatment would worsen my symptoms for a day or two (the Herxheimer reaction) and then my illness would start to lift. It took no more than a month, two at the most before I felt well again, until I once more stopped treatment and spiraled down. I stayed off antibiotics for months, for as long as I could. I knew what havoc they could cause, everything from yeast infection to hard-to-treat strep. But eventually, the symptoms returned and if I wanted to function, only the antibiotics helped.

As the years passed, the notion that late-stage Lyme could be cured in a month, that retreatment was useless and the physical symptoms actually psychiatric, lost any relevance in my home. It wasn't just me but also Mark and Jason who slid back when antibiotics were pulled, riding the Lyme roller coaster: sick one month, healthy the next. Were we being reinfected right on our property in Chappaqua, and was *that* the cause of all the relapses? When you got right down to it, who really knew? Yet I was so personally fastidious when it came to exposure, and my relapses were so regular, so independent of season and so perfectly in sync with the periods when I went untreated, I didn't see how reinfection could explain my own experience with Lyme.

The murky reality was only compounded by the backstreet route to treatment. Walking through downtown Chappaqua one day, I noticed Tick Bite's shingle had disappeared. Peering inside the storefront, I found it empty. Our Lyme practitioner was gone. That week other patients started calling me. Where was she? Would they get their medical records? Who would treat them now?

Finally, I tracked her down at home. It had all been too risky, too stressful, she had a child, Tick Bite told me. I could hardly blame her, but what was she doing now? It turned out she'd gotten good-paying work at Westchester County Medical Center in Valhalla, and was no longer treating Lyme patients. In the same hospital, the well-known Lyme Disease Diagnostic Center was notorious among patients for sending them to shrinks and dismissing them in droves. "They're the only ones at the hospital not treating Lyme disease," Tick Bite now said of the Lyme clinic doctors. From cardiologists to gastroenterologists to internists, many on the hospital staff actually recognized Lyme disease beyond the narrow strictures and treated sick patients aggressively, sometimes with months of IV—but when they filled out medical charts, they didn't mention the Lyme diagnosis, avoiding a standoff with the Lyme glitterati down the hall. "A lot of people on staff can't even look those doctors in the eye anymore," Tick Bite said.

Even nurses at the Lyme clinic were quietly referring the patients elsewhere, a number of Westchester County support group leaders told me. "You'll never get treatment here," they'd tell patients who were one band shy of a "Dearborn" or lacking the rash. They'd slip them support group phone numbers on notes folded for privacy, lest anyone see.

"It's all so strange," Tick Bite said.

It truly was surreal. Hoping for a piece of suburban paradise, we instead had signed on for a tick-infested forest in Chappaqua, a community in denial. From the local medical group, which dismissed Lyme disease and barely seemed to recognize it, to the unforgiving school system, which was far more invested in Ivy admissions than helping its children in need, we were lost in the heart of darkness and couldn't seem to find our way home. Sure, we thought of relocating, just leaving, but we couldn't get it together to follow through. If only we'd had the energy and oomph to pick ourselves up and move on.

We stayed in Chappaqua out of inertia, because we were overwhelmed by the illness and too sick and exhausted to do anything else. For example, we needed to paint our house in order to sell it, but because of all our medical and private school expenses, we lacked the money to pay for it, yet were too beat up to paint it ourselves, let alone pack and look for another home. What's more, our doctors, the ones who understood Lyme, were there with us in the northern suburbs.

All I knew was that I lived at the event horizon: A science journalist with the most skeptical of mind-sets, I was disturbed to experience the same controversial disease I was investigating in my work. Yet perhaps it was my personal experience that pushed me to push the experts I interviewed, to demand more. It was politically incorrect for many academics to concede that the patients and their treating physicians could be right, even partially. But if I sat there needling them long enough, if my questions were trenchant enough and contained enough detail, enough inside knowledge gleaned from prior interviews with other scientists, they'd add nuance to what had seemed absolute—they would equivocate and many would, finally, concede that the patients could be right.

36

❖

Secrets of an Evil Genius:
The Evidence for Persistence

The first question new patients ask after finding themselves caught in the Lyme controversy is whether there's any proof that the spirochete survives standard antibiotic treatment for the disease. Part of the issue is clarified simply: Can *B. burgdorferi* persist following standard treatment, *ever*? Has persistence been shown *in anyone*? No one that I interviewed on any side of the controversy, no matter how conservative their stance, denied it had been proven in *some* patients, for sure. One of the first scientific reports involved Ken Liegner's patient, Vicki Logan, who, following aggressive treatment, had *B. burgdorferi* spirochetes cultured from her spinal fluid at CDC labs. There was the patient studied by Pat Coyle at Stony Brook and successfully entered as evidence in Joe Burrascano's defense: Bitten by a tick while camping in Europe, the woman from New York City had definite infection with *B. burgdorferi* despite her negative antibody tests; she was treated and re-treated by Stony Brook doctors for years.

In fact, live spirochetes have been recovered from treated patients almost from the start. One patient was treated with ten days of intravenous Rocephin, for instance, yet spirochetes were later grown from her spinal fluid. Scientists have recovered spirochetes from treated patients' rashes, irises, and spleens. Over the years, many such cases have been reported in medical journals, and no one suggests they are bogus or false. But since the reports involve just single patients or small groups, since they aren't part of controlled or blinded studies, and since many of the patients come from Europe, where the organism may differ, they don't prove that persistence following treatment is widespread in the United States.

Proving persistent infection in the large numbers of patients said to have chronic Lyme is hard because the standard antibody tests (ELISA and Western blot) are indirect. Like footprints in the sand, Lyme disease antibodies can be detected on the tests long after infection is gone. The tests show the spirochete was there once, but not that it is there at the time.

Proving infection persists requires that you locate the *spirochete itself*, directly, in the patients involved. That's a daunting task. Since spirochetes leave the blood to inhabit body tissue like the bladder, the heart, or the brain early in the course of infection, obtaining direct proof would mean sacrificing the patients and slicing up their organs in the lab.

It's impossible to do that experiment in humans, but scientists have taken this approach with other mammals for years. Especially illuminating is work done with dogs, where the model of borreliosis closely resembles that of humans. Spearheading the experiments was veterinary scientist Reinhard K. Straubinger, a researcher at Cornell's James A. Baker Institute for Animal Health. First Straubinger placed infected Westchester County ticks on each of nineteen beagles and allowed the ticks to feed. Some two months later, he tested the beagles and found that all but one had been infected with Lyme *Borreliae*. Straubinger treated twelve of the infected dogs with high doses of either doxycycline or amoxicillin—the treatment most commonly used in humans—and left the rest without any treatment at all. The antibiotics appeared to prevent or cure lameness in eleven of the twelve treated dogs; as they recovered, their antibody response declined as well. Meanwhile, four of the six untreated dogs developed arthritis.

Six months later, all the dogs were sacrificed. Of course, Straubinger found that the untreated dogs were still infected with spirochetes. But more interesting, he found *B. burgdorferi* DNA—suggestive of continuing infection—in five of seven *treated* dogs. Antibody levels—which had fallen during treatment—were once more on the rise six months out, presumably, said Straubinger, "in response to proliferation of the surviving pool of spirochetes."

In a follow-up of the work, Straubinger reported the first controlled study of animals treated with antibiotic after a relatively long infection period, at a time when antibody levels were high. To do his experiment, he exposed sixteen beagles to Lyme–infected ticks and allowed the infections to disseminate for four months prior to treatment. For a month, he treated twelve of the dogs with a variety of antibiotics. Then he followed all the dogs for 380 more days, finally sacrificing them and testing twenty-five tissue and blood samples from each dog for spirochete DNA. The findings: Despite a vigorous initial immune response in the dogs, DNA evidence for persistence of the organism could be found in all treated animals. Antibiotic treatment reduced the amount of detectable spirochete DNA in skin tissue by a factor of 1,000 or more, but at the end of the experiment, it was detectable at low levels in multiple tissue samples regardless of treatment used.

Elegant experiments with mice provides important insight into how the spirochete might survive. The scientist at the helm was Stephen Barthold, a veterinarian and director of the Center for Comparative Medicine (devoted to the study of diseases afflicting both humans and animals) at the Schools of Medicine and Veterinary Medicine at the University of California at Davis. Before moving to Davis, Barthold was a pioneer in unraveling the pathogenesis of *B. burgdorferi* in mice at Yale for twenty-five years.

Arriving at Yale right around the time Polly Murray wrote her fateful letter to the state of Connecticut, Barthold was on the sidelines when Allen Steere began sleuthing the mystery illness in Lyme. After the spirochete was discovered in the early eighties, Steere asked Barthold to study Lyme disease in laboratory mammals like rats and mice. Somewhat reluctantly, Barthold agreed. Little did he know that he'd just signed on to investigate the trickiest, most diabolical microbe he would encounter in the course of his career. Working with the mouse as his Rosetta stone, Barthold eventually gained insight into the unfolding of Lyme disease that few others have had.

Through his years at Yale, Barthold's observations pointed to persistence of the Lyme spirochete after antibiotic treatment, even aggressive treatment, in the mammals he studied in the lab. "You have a bacterium with a relatively small and simple genome that can do incredibly complex things. It is a fascinating organism with a lot of evolutionary intelligence, consistently capable of creating persistent infection and evading host immunity," he says. "Once infection becomes chronic, not even the strongest immune system in combination with antibiotics could be guaranteed of eliminating every last vestige of the infection."

Yet it wasn't until 2008 that Barthold followed these observations up by publishing the results of controlled experiments in mice in the journal

Antimicrobial Agents and Chemotherapy. His study consisted of two arms: One arm followed five mice that had been treated with ceftriaxone (generic of Rocephin) after only three weeks of infection, when the disease was relatively new and symptoms were at their peak. The other arm followed five mice treated with ceftriaxone after infection had progressed for four months, reaching the later, chronic form of the disease. Each of the two study arms was paralleled by a control group of mice that received only saline.

In the end, all the mice were tested and finally sacrificed so that Barthold could search for persistent infection on several fronts: attempting to grow spirochetes in culture, seeking antibodies through serology; looking for *B. burgdorferi* DNA with polymerase chain reaction (PCR); using xenodiagnosis (placing uninfected ticks on infected mammals, then testing the ticks themselves); and grafting skin from the treated mice onto uninfected mice to see whether infection would spread. In this way, Barthold was not just investigating the nature of persistence, but also evaluating the usefulness of various tests in detecting persistent infection after antibiotic treatment had run its course.

When it came to the five mice with early infection, not one had clinical signs of Lyme disease a month after treatment, and none were culture positive for *B. burgdorferi*. But tissue from two of them were still PCR-positive. And three months later, one of those mice transmitted living spirochetes to nine uninfected ticks, suggesting that at least sometimes, even aggressive early treatment may fail to cure infection.

As for the five mice with chronic infection, results suggested a window into what human patients report. Examined a month after treatment, tissue from all five animals tested positive for *B. burgdorferi* DNA. Three of the mice were able to transmit spirochetes to uninfected ticks. Three months after treatment, tissue from two of these mice still tested PCR-positive; two of the mice transmitted living spirochetes to uninfected ticks; and one mouse was able to transmit active infection to another mouse through a skin graft.

Moreover, when mice were sacrificed three months after treatment, small numbers of spirochetes were seen by Barthold in the collagenous tissue of the great vessels at the base of the heart and the tendons or ligaments of the joints. The spirochetes appeared in both treatment groups—those treated during early infection and those treated during late infection. Using immunochemistry, including markers that matched only with *B. burgdorferi* antigens, Barthold was able to prove that the structures were, in fact, Lyme spirochetes.

He also investigated whether serology, like the ELISA and Western blot tests used as the standard for human diagnosis, could detect antibodies against spirochetes following treatment. He found that as the months passed, antibody levels declined in treated mice. Yet even when antibody tests were negative, Barthold still found spirochetes in the tissues of the mice. "Results indicated that maintenance of the antibody response to *B. burgdorferi* requires active infection with a sufficient spirochete burden in tissues; antibody response declines following antibiotic treatment, despite the continued presence of low numbers of Lyme spirochetes."

Other diagnostic tests turned out to be problematic for the treated but still-infected mice as well. Barthold could get evidence of *B. burgdorferi* DNA only directly from the collagen tissue where he also found actual spirochetes. Even when he was able to find living spirochetes and pass them on to other, uninfected mice through skin grafting or tick feeding, he was unable to grow spirochetes in culture.

In short, Barthold found that after he treated acute or chronically infected mice with high doses of ceftriaxone for a month, he achieved cure by virtually every ordinary measure, from clinical signs of disease to growth in culture. Yet three months later, small numbers of spirochetes remained, hunkering down in the collagen of the heart and joints. Moreover, in the chronic mice, these spirochetes remained infectious; they could be picked up by ticks and transmitted to other mice as active infections.

Still, the treated spirochetes seemed to be altered: They appeared to be "attenuated in their ability to replicate," even in mice that couldn't mount an immune response. The finding resonates with what chronic patients report: If the surviving spirochetes of chronic Lyme disease cannot replicate, they may be impervious to antibiotics like ceftriaxone, which work by targeting bacterial cells as they divide. The persisting spirochetes could be the presumptive source of the symptoms, but may nonetheless be unable to achieve enough critical mass to cause inflammation or provoke the antibody response that experts like Leonard Sigal call the sine qua non of the disease.

"How can you say you have a disease when you have no inflammation and no evidence of antibody response—where is the illness coming from?" Leonard Sigal had asked me when I interviewed him.

A possible answer can be seen here.

The results, which confirm the dog studies done at Cornell, "offer a useful model for studying one form of antibiotic treatment failure in Lyme borreliosis," Barthold says, and indicate that "accessible indices of treatment, such as culture or PCR of skin and serologic response, cannot be relied upon for measuring treatment success.

"This study must not be overinterpreted as proof that Lyme borreliosis is refractory to effective antibiotic treatment, especially when administered during early infection," Barthold cautions. The persistent spirochetes are not immortal; if they don't regain the ability to replicate, they would eventually die off. Yet as long as they persist, they may explain the "constitutional" symptoms that chronic patients report—not the gross inflammatory signs of Lyme arthritis or meningitis, but rather what researchers term "pro-inflammatory effects." These include nuanced biochemical cascades like production of nitric oxide and activation of immune cells like neutrophils and macrophages, all of which might account for the fatigue and malaise that the patients report.

What really happens to these remaining persistent spirochetes as time goes on is, of course, unknown. Some researchers suggest that they may replicate, but very slowly, explaining why the illness goes on and on, and why long courses of treatment work for some. Some theorize that when no longer stressed by antibiotic, the dormant spirochetes become activated and resume the ability to replicate. Others have problems with putting so much emphasis on animal studies; however, since we can't autopsy humans following treatment, testing their hearts and other organs for spirochetes, studies done on people are, by comparison, crude.

"Further studies are needed to determine the eventual fate of the persisting organisms following antibiotic treatment in the context of controlled animal studies," Barthold says. In future experiments he will follow his animals for longer periods of time to see if the spirochetes ever come out of hiding, and will experiment with new, advanced antibiotics to see if they are able to better eliminate the persisting microbes when today's protocols cannot.

Other routes to treatment failure have been suggested as well. There is evidence, for instance, that the spirochete, which normally lives outside our cells, can also hide *within* them, in protected niches where antibiotics cannot go. Scientists doing test-tube studies have found that *B. burgdorferi* can hide in skin and white blood cells, surviving even when doused in Rocephin for weeks. Lyme spirochetes have been shown to persist, despite treatment, in the synovial cells of joints. At the NIH, researchers found Lyme spirochetes could strip away part of the white blood cells known as B cells; sometimes spirochetes burrowed inside the B cells, and other times they wore them as cloaks. In 2006, a group from the CDC showed that *B. burgdorferi* could invade nerve and brain cells. "The internalized spirochetes were found to be viable, providing a putative mechanism for the organism to avoid the host's immune response while potentially causing functional damage to neural cells during infection of the central nervous system," chief researcher Jill Livengood says. Skeptics point out that this kind of intracellular hiding has never been proven for *B. burgdorferi* in vivo—in the living organism—but many frontline physicians insist that treating with antibiotics like Biaxin, which can penetrate cells, may be one key to defeating Lyme.

Others point to evidence that spirochetes elude capture by encapsulating themselves in thick-walled cysts, the kind proposed by Alan MacDonald. Cysts would make it difficult for penetration by antibiotics, immune cells, or anything else. The idea floated up from the scientific ether in the early 1900s, when those studying syphilis and its spirochete, *Treponema pallidum,* under the microscope began observing a dizzying array of forms, from rods and hooks to clumps and granules to the strange cysts themselves.

For most of the twentieth century, the odd forms seen in syphilis were dismissed as artifacts—irrelevant cellular garbage floating in the glow of the microscopic field. But with the debate over Lyme disease, another spirochetal infection, some experts began asking if the strange forms, especially the cysts, played a role in disease.

One of the first to explore the issue was Dagmar Hulinska, a world-famous *Borrelia* expert from the Institute of Public Health in Prague. Hulinska studied Lyme-infected tissue under the electron microscope, and in 1995 reported "cysts" much like those in the old syphilis papers, and resembling the variants reported by Alan MacDonald several years before. By 1995, researchers were dousing spirochetes with antibiotics only to recover what clearly were spirochetal parts encased in the cysts themselves.

But could the cysts convert back to spirochetes? By 1997, the husband-and-wife team of Øystein and Sverre-Henning Brorson of Ullevål Hospital in Oslo reported just that. When they placed spirochetes in culture lacking nutrients, they became metabolically torpid and cysts formed around them. When the cysts were transferred to a culture with the proper nutrients, the thick walls dissolved and normal spirochetes emerged.

If the cysts observed in the test tube (in vitro) are being generated in us (in vivo), it could explain a lot—everything from apparently persistent infection to seronegative Lyme disease. For instance, spirochetes inside cysts wouldn't be accessible to the immune system, and so would not generate antibodies necessary to test positive on ELISA or Western blot tests. "In vivo these encysted forms may explain why *Borrelia* infection can be temporarily dormant, why a reactivation of the disease may occur when the conditions suit *B. burgdorferi,* and why infection may relapse after treatment with antibiotic," the Brorsons pointed out.

After all the decades that scientists had observed the bizarre variant forms of the spirochete, the Brorsons' experiment represented the first clear-cut proof that one such form—namely the cyst—was metabolically active and could, at least under in vitro conditions, give rise to normal, motile *Borrelia.* Their study suggested that cysts represented a state of low metabolic activity, enabling the microbes to survive in a hostile environment until conditions were conducive to their replication once more.

By 1998, the Brorsons had shown a potential relationship between cystic forms and neuroborreliosis as well. Noting how difficult it was to cultivate spirochetes from spinal fluid, they hypothesized that *Borrelia* might be present in the form of cysts. To investigate, they cultured spirochetes in cerebrospinal fluid in the lab, and found that within a day they had all converted to cysts. When the cysts were transferred to a medium normally used to grow *Borrelia,* they converted back to normal spirochetes in about two weeks. The observation could explain why spinal fluid so often tests negative for Lyme disease, and might explain the symptoms of neurological Lyme disease itself.

In a notable achievement, the Brorsons' basic findings were replicated in 2000 by a team from the University of Rhode Island. Seeking to speed up the process, the Rhode Island scientists transferred spirochetes to a culture *completely* devoid of nutrients, and reported that forty-eight hours later, about 90 percent had formed cysts. In 2004, scientists from Italy showed that spirochetes in culture converted to cysts under adverse conditions, from increased temperature to increased oxidative stress, a situation seen in nature as the result of aging, injury, or disease. When the same team inoculated healthy mice with Lyme cysts, they found that they converted to spiral forms *within the mice.* The longer the cysts had been sitting in solution in the lab, the longer they took to convert back.

In 2008, Swiss scientist Judith Miklossy took things one step further, using sophisticated methods—including atomic force microscopy (a technique with such high resolution it can visualize objects as small as of fractions of a nanometer) and immunochemistry—to study brain inflammation in three Lyme disease patients. The atomic force microscope captured atypical forms like cysts within the patients' brain cells, including neurons, while the immunochemistry proved the forms were *Borrelia burgdorferi,* spiral shaped or not. "The persistence of these more resistant spirochete forms, and their intracellular location in neurons and glial [support] cells, may explain the long latent stage and persistence of *Borrelia* infection," Miklossy wrote in the *Journal of Neuroinflammation* in 2008. In fact, like Mario Philipp, Miklossy had found that the spirochete and its lipoproteins could explain cell dysfunction and cell death in the brain. "The detection and recognition of atypical, cystic, and granular forms in infected tissues is essential for the diagnosis and the treatment as they can occur in the absence of the typical spiral *Borrelia* form," Miklossy found.

More evidence will be needed before the cyst hypothesis is elevated to fact. Seeking to confirm or refute the concept, New Jersey immunologist Steven Schutzer is testing human lesions said to contain the cysts for borrelial DNA. Meanwhile, physicians treating the sickest patients say cysts are one more factor to address when patients don't get well. The Brorsons, at least, have been convinced enough to incubate spirochetes and cysts with various medications in the lab. Studies conducted from 2004 through 2006 point to actual cyst-busters, including the antibiotics metronidazole (Flagyl) and tinidazole. (In 2007, they reported in the journal *Infection* that grapefruit seed extract worked in the test tube as well.) These drugs and supplements are hardly part of the treatment regimens listed in guidelines from the Infectious Diseases Society of America, but for many Lyme doctors, attempting to treat cyst forms with drugs like Flagyl is all in a hard day's work.

As for Steve Barthold, he insists you don't need cysts to explain why infection persists. "We have active arguments about cysts in our lab," he states. "One of our microbiologists believes in the cyst theory and I don't. The reason I don't is that I can look at the skin of a mouse or rat that has been infected for a year and then treated, and see fully elongated, healthy spirochetes in the extracellular spaces of the skin." As far as Barthold is concerned, the spirochetes survive, intact, under adverse circumstances and even after treatment with antibiotics, making the cyst an unneeded step. "The spirochetes are already there," he says. "If I can see fully formed spirochetes, how can I go about proving that a cyst is the way they survive?

"The lay public and to a large extent the medical community are very naïve about what antibiotics do," Barthold adds. "Antibiotics are not disinfectants. Instead, they reduce bacterial numbers by working against dividing bacterial populations. They can never sterilize a person of every last vestige of an infection. Effective therapy with antibiotics still needs the immune system of the host—the mouse, the dog, the person—to clean up the rest of the infection and effectively eliminate the invading organism."

With Lyme, that's not always possible. "In the late stages of infection you have organisms inhabiting extracellular spaces like the skin, which do not get well-perfused by blood. So antibiotics do not reach them. In addition, the spirochetes are not in a state where they are particularly vulnerable." In order to take up the antibiotic, they've got to divide, "yet they're quiescent." Since they're not dividing, the antibiotic doesn't impact them. Therefore, "to be effective in the chronic phase of Lyme disease you have to treat the individual for more and more time with increasingly higher levels of antibiotic for a cure."

The reason, Barthold says, is that "you are working with an organism which, at least in experimental animals, causes one hundred percent persistence in the face of totally effective host immunity. This is true for dogs, mice, monkeys, rats, hamsters. In any species we have ever studied, this bacteria is evolutionarily designed to persist in completely immune-competent hosts. We know that with mice, with dogs, and with monkeys, you can establish infection, you can treat these animals with antibiotics, and you can cure them by all indices," including culture, antibody response, or detection of DNA. "But then, if you sit back and wait, they become antibody-positive again, because you have not completely eliminated the infection.

"When a perfectly immune-competent host cannot eliminate the spirochete you are bound to have survival of the organism. All these factors, together, mean that the chances of not having an effective cure for patients in the late stages of infection are pretty high. Does that mean that all their symptoms and aches and pains are caused by Lyme disease? That I cannot answer. But I do believe there are patients who are not completely cured of infection, because it goes along with the biology of the spirochete and the biology of what antibiotics do. We have known this right from the beginning through our study of the mouse and other animal models of Lyme."

Sitting in Barthold's spacious California office, the sun shining through, I felt a sense of the unreal. Had I not recorded the interview, had I not replayed it for myself many times and transcribed every word, I might have found it hard to believe that so much evidence for the patient experience had been observed starting from those early days at Yale.

37

Mother Makes Four

Framingham, Massachusetts, 2003–2004

With her children in treatment for Lyme and its coinfections, it occurred to Sheila Statlender that she might be infected, too. Her hands and feet tingled, she suffered the radiating pain of sciatica, and though she was a devoted runner, her stamina now suffered because she ran out of air. And really, hadn't she enjoyed the same yard, hiked in the same deer preserve, and taken the same exact trips as her children? She wasn't nearly as sick as they were, but something wasn't right. Of course, she was stressed and tired, as she'd told herself for years: She had three children, and they were sick. Yet now she wondered if the symptoms could be her body's expression of Lyme disease.

It was certainly possible, Charles Ray Jones said.

Getting her blood tested proved a revelation: Her Western blot for Lyme disease was highly positive, and her Western blot for babesiosis showed evidence of exposure as well. Eric was getting better. Slowly, excruciatingly, Amy and Seth were, too. Might not Sheila benefit from treatment, much like them?

Yet treatment for Lyme disease and *Babesia* seemed to stir up her symptoms, causing flare-ups of the usual suspects like neck pain, aching joints, and tingling. Once provoked, moreover, the heightened symptoms seemed not to resolve. "Rather than seeing improvement, my symptoms became more obvious and pronounced," says Sheila. Under the care of one Lyme physician she cycled through several oral antibiotics—minocycline, penicillin, Biaxin, and Plaquenil. Each new antibiotic exacerbated the symptoms—throbbing neck, worse tingling and sciatica, increasing fatigue. Herxheimers, the doctor suggested. But with each new trial of antibiotic, she fell only further into illness, because none of the so-called herxes were going away. By the time she was done with all these "cures," her fingers were swollen, her neck was throbbing, and not just her knees but also her elbows, wrists, and other joints were inflamed. Her sacroiliac joint ached, and tendonitis migrated from one limb to the next.

With the new, more severe presentation she finally consulted another physician, who happened to have a specialty in neurology. The new doctor, located closer to her home, initially continued the oral antibiotics and then tried intramuscular injections of Bicillin, which didn't help at all. "He also explained that while a lot of my symptoms were arthritic, some of them—the sciatica, the tingling and occasional numbness in my extremities, and a slight sway when I stood with my eyes closed—were suggestive of neurological involvement," she says. "My biggest concern—the one that drove me to try intravenous treatment—was my knowledge of what Lyme disease had done to my children over time, and my fear, as an educated person who highly values her mind, that my cognitive functioning could become impaired."

The new doctor treated her with Rocephin, but she had some early side effects that made it impossible to continue. "Literally overnight, I retained fluid and put on ten pounds," she says. Then, after two and a half weeks on the medicine she found she had developed several gallstones. But her Lyme doctor had given her Actigall, which helped the stones resolve. "My primary care physician was calling me with the names of surgeons, but my Lyme doctor suggested that if I could wait it out, the stones might dissolve on their own." That's exactly what happened. Although Sheila's gallbladder was saved and the bloating abated, her Lyme symptoms progressed. Then she tried intravenous Claforan and that, too, caused her symptoms to flare. After a year of treatment for Lyme disease, Sheila Statlender was sicker, by far, than if she'd never been treated at all.

In a final try, her Lyme doctor prescribed intravenous vancomycin and for the first time, she began to experience improvement. "First the sciatica resolved, then the tingling left, then the stiffness and body aches dissipated. After a few months I felt better, much better," she reports. Four months into the treatment she felt her energy returning, her body felt more flexible, and the aches and pains in her joints continued to fade. Another turning point came with the addition of the drug tinidazole, which was said to penetrate cysts. Stopping the tinidazole she relapsed; resuming it, she continued to improve, and sustained her gains.

Like her children, Sheila was not yet out of the woods. Even as the Statlenders shed their illness there would be more relapses and plateaus along the way. Yet the disease that had once seemed implacable was now movable, changeable, possibly fixable: "Our children were able to participate in activities and friendships outside of their home; in other words, to have lives," says Sheila. "This was a magnanimous, magnificent reprieve."

38

❖

The Big Sleep:
Our Younger Son Falls Ill

Chappaqua, New York, 2003–2004

If you had asked me in 2000 whether Lyme would be pivotal in our lives three years hence, I would have said no. But with positive tests for tick-borne infections other than Lyme disease, our cases were complex. As careful as we were, we risked reinfection in the hyperendemic hamlet of Chappaqua. And most damning, we'd been diagnosed late, so that infection had smoldered inside us, disseminating unfettered for years. The best way to sum it up would be to say we kept getting better slowly, despite the relapses that set us back almost to square one.

Mark had pushed his symptoms back with simple doxycycline. Yet almost three years after his treatment had begun, he continually relapsed within weeks each time he tried to stop the daily dose. First he would urinate all through the night and his neck would resume the crackle, then he would lose his cool. He would begin to get irritated at the slightest of provocations and his brain would become so fuzzy, his memory so porous, that his boss would be prompted to ask, "Are you off that medicine again?"

I, too, required one round of antibiotic after the next. My great desire was to get off these drugs because, by this time having interviewed so many experts, I knew just how dangerous they were when used for so long: If you were exposed to other, random infections, long-term antibiotics could make them antibiotic-resistant and turn them into "super-bugs." It's not a trivial issue: According to the most thorough such study ever done, nearly 19,000 people died in the United States in 2005 after being infected with drug-resistant bacteria that spread through nursing homes and hospitals. Along these lines, some Lyme patients I met had been found to have infections in their sinus and elsewhere that were near impossible to wipe out. By killing even ordinary germs before your immune system kicked in, antibiotics could—over the long haul—weaken your natural defenses. They could kill off the good bacteria in your gut, making you nauseous and queasy. With the protective flora gone, moreover, you were prone to yeast infections—candida—which, if untreated with medicines like Diflucan, could cause symptoms every bit as devastating as Lyme disease. Over the years, reporting the Lyme beat, I'd met more patients than I could count who'd ended up suffering yeast infections following all those antibiotics. A worst case outcome was infection with *Clostridium difficile*, often called *C. difficile* or "*C. diff*," a bacterium that causes symptoms from diarrhea to life-threatening inflammation of the colon. There were people who had tried to treat their Lyme fruitlessly, for years, without realizing Lyme was no longer the germ they needed to cure. For those on intravenous antibiotic, the line delivering the drug directly to the vein could get infected; such people had been hospitalized, and one woman I knew of had died. As the CDC pointed out, the most common intravenous antibiotic, Rocephin, could cause the gallbladder to fail. In a maddening catch-22, another academic expert told me he had evidence that long-term treatment could make *B. burgdorferi* itself resistant to antimicrobial drugs. No, long-term antibiotic was no panacea—it certainly didn't seem to be an all-out cure for relapsing-remitting Lyme disease like mine, and it carried enormous risk.

The cycle of damage that could be done with long-term antibiotic was almost endless, and yet, despite the risk, nothing was worse for me than the return of my Lyme symptoms. For me this included the grinding migraine with its nausea, the buzzing in my arms, the fuzzy thinking, and a profound exhaustion that forced me to bed for hours each day—until I finally relented, going back on treatment and pulling myself back up.

By 2003, whatever component of my illness had been caused by *Babesia* appeared to be gone, because antimalarials like Mepron made no difference whatsoever in how I felt. Instead, it was only amoxicillin, at sufficient dose, that banished the headaches and extinguished the electric current that coursed through my arms and legs. The fact of the matter is

I could not function without new rounds of antibiotic, no matter what the risk: Almost nothing is as risky as losing your mind to a dense, confusing fog. Without antibiotic for two or three months my slide was so rapid, and my condition so poor, that I could not stay up long enough or think clearly enough to work as a science journalist and earn money to pay the bills. When you are caring for children, especially sick children, your thinking had better be clear. Amoxicillin saturated my blood, tinged my breath, and inflamed my gut, but it cleared my brain and banished the weird buzzing and the infernal headache. It was my salvation and vice.

Only Jason was living proof that we might emerge intact. Through his senior year of high school he played varsity basketball and nurtured close friendships. His brain was so retooled that, studying AP Physics, he devised formulas that were faster and tidier than the ones in the text. Taking the antibiotics that Dr. Jones prescribed, his bone pain lessened and his nausea subsided. The old Jason, the funky, fun, argumentative Jason, the boy we thought we'd lost, had made it back. If Jason was our loss leader in discovering the illness, our canary in the coal mine, he was also the white dove who flew back to our teetering ship, carrying the olive branch of health. When he was accepted to Brown University in spring 2003 we dared ask ourselves whether our luck had finally turned.

Perhaps it was the melody of hope, so long absent but now playing through our days, that inspired our younger son, David, to take off his shoes and socks one afternoon and roll joyously in a mountain of leaves by our driveway. Watching him dance in the leaves I knew were home to ticks, I thought he might just as well be swimming in a vat of plutonium. "Get out of that pile," I screamed frantically, but to no avail.

With the inimitable style of a newly minted teenager, he looked at me sideways and said, "You sound like a nut."

When, a few weeks later, he started falling ill, it didn't seem like Lyme disease—not any Lyme I'd experienced myself. For our family Lyme had meant swollen knees, tingling fingers, crackling necks, numbness in our arms and legs, jabbing pains, headaches, nausea, extreme sensitivity to light, and a confounding mental fog. But the new illness, when it came, carried none of these discomforts. More like the wash of a gentle breeze, it had just one symptom: somnolence, a deep and pleasant and unending sleep.

Slowly, imperceptibly, so that at first we did not notice it, David started to sleep more—at first he just went to bed earlier, but eventually, as weeks and months passed, he could barely wake up at all. Under the direction of a local pediatrician who referred us to specialists, we began investigating in a thoroughly mainstream mode. But from neurologists to psychiatrists to immunologists to endocrinologists, no one could explain the somnolence, and no one found anything wrong. Finally revisiting the Lyme issue, we sought counsel with Charles Ray Jones. But he, too, sent us away. Whatever this odd illness was, he said, it surely wasn't Lyme disease.

Another disabling mystery illness, but *not Lyme disease,* had come to call on our family. It's hard to believe, but on what we hoped would be the back end of our Lyme nightmare we found ourselves seeking the cause of another inexplicable illness that caused our second child to drop from his life just as the first had done before. We spent eight unbearable months consulting a round of experts before Ken Liegner, seeking an explanation, ran a lab test that picked up 14,700 gene copies of *Mycoplasma fermantans,* one of the controversial coinfections thought to coexist with *Borrelia burgdorferi* in the tick. Sure, the diagnosis was edgy, open to question—Liegner said so himself. But over the course of months, after consultation with half a dozen physicians, it was the first objective evidence of anything specific to emerge. Liegner sent us to Eugene Eskow, a New Jersey doctor who'd published an article on *Mycoplasma fermantans* from tick bites. Eskow said that David's single symptom, somnolence, together with the DNA evidence and a couple of other objective immune markers he was able to detect through blood tests, were classic for *Mycoplasma* infection, often associated with chronic fatigue. Along with Ken Liegner, Eskow treated David with antibiotics he'd found effective against *Mycoplasma fermantans.*

Like his brother before him David, too, began to get better, but not entirely. He improved, he fell back into sleep, he improved again.

"Maybe we have some Lyme in the mix here," Ken Liegner suggested to us.

I knew then that Lyme—or whatever it was that dogged us—would not leave without a terrible, knock-down blitzkrieg and the fight of our lives. How we wished to be done with Lyme disease! But it wasn't done with us. Just like that, David (who had just three bands on his Western blot and so could not be diagnosed officially) joined me and Mark in the fields of Lyme where we toiled, another of Lyme's mutts.

39

Houston Calling

Houston, Texas, 2004

Asking around for someone to take his case, Dave Martz was finally referred by a colleague to an old med school buddy: a Dr. William Harvey, formerly of Colorado Springs but by then practicing in Houston. As a courtesy, Harvey fit Dave in quickly, arranging for an appointment in February 2004. He even took Dave and Dee out to dinner the night they arrived in town.

Right off the bat, Harvey agreed that Dave probably had Lyme disease: It wasn't just the positive DNA test, but other signs and symptoms Harvey associated with the disease, from itchy, peeling skin to swollen joints and arthritic pain so severe it could be managed only with a hundred milligrams of OxyContin a day.

Harvey had his own take on Lyme disease, which he explained to Dave and Dee over the evening meal. In addition to being spread by ticks, he theorized, Lyme could also be transmitted human to human, through blood, sperm, breast milk, or other bodily secretions. Harvey's version of Lyme—"human borreliosis," he called it—could be transmitted much like HIV: sexually, between lovers, and from mother to child in the womb.

Harvey told the Martzes he'd hit on the radical theory a few years back, after large numbers of systemically ill patients in his Houston practice began testing positive for *B. burgdorferi*—despite the fact that no more than 2 percent of the ticks in southeast Texas carried the spirochete at all. Most of these people had been sick for years, and more often than not, their family members were sick, too. If they weren't getting the disease from tick bites, he hypothesized, perhaps they were transmitting it between themselves.

Deferring to the test results, and thus presuming that the patients had late-stage disseminated Lyme disease, Harvey began treating them with antibiotics and found that across the board, most patients improved within three to six months. After a lifetime of illness, many got well. Hoping to unravel the mystery, so at odds with mainstream thought on Lyme disease, Harvey ultimately published his theory in the journal *Medical Hypotheses,* a treasure trove of fascinating ideas that had yet to be proved. Writing in the journal, he proposed two types of Lyme disease: The first was the conventionally accepted illness spread by ticks, and the second was "a much larger . . . pool of *B. burgdorferi*–infected humans with a clinical presentation of extraordinary variability, global geographic distribution, and far greater prevalence." In any given individual, said Harvey, the infection could smolder under the radar, unfelt for years before it might suddenly explode. If not treated with antibiotics, the patient could be sick for life. By positing the possibility of a hidden pandemic of mammoth proportions and global reach, Harvey's theory appeared outrageous to mainstream scientists. But for his odd group of patients, it at least suggested a mechanism for their plight.

It also appeared to explain Dave Martz. Might not Martz have been infected after exposure to the bodily secretions of a dying ALS patient in the back wards of the tiny Las Animas Hospital some forty-eight years before? Martz might have harbored the infection for years before expressing it as ALS.

Based on such concepts, in fact, Harvey had already treated a number of ALS patients with IV Rocephin—with varying results. The first patient had come to Harvey at the very end of his rope, so sick he couldn't talk anymore. Harvey treated the man with a gram a day of Rocephin, but it did no good; if anything, the patient only got sicker. Another patient, not as far into the disease, was treated with two grams of Rocephin a day. His disease was halted in its tracks. A third patient, a doctor, had come in with early ALS; like Martz, he could still walk, talk, sit down for a meal. Harvey treated this man with four grams a day of Rocephin, and he got well.

Why was the Rocephin working? The explanation that made most sense to Harvey was that it was blasting spirochetes, but there was another theory, too: Rocephin had been found to stimulate a gene that limited the amount of a neurotransmitter called glutamate. Excess glutamate at the nerve endings had been tied to ALS, and suppression of the molecule was one theorized treatment for the disease. The theory had so much weight, in fact, that government-backed trials of the Rocephin treatment for ALS patients already were under way.

Whatever the mode of action, for the dying Martz it was worth a shot. He truly had nothing to lose. By the time he left Houston, Harvey had agreed to treat him not just for Lyme disease but also babesiosis— signaled by Martz's dramatic response to Lariam and his severe chills and sweats. Martz returned to Colorado Springs with prescriptions for Mepron and Zithromax (treatment for babesiosis); Rocephin at four grams a day (for Lyme disease); and Flagyl (to treat the cystic forms of the spirochete that might emerge in response to the Rocephin).

Traveling at Godspeed to his final reward, David Martz had a central catheter inserted in the large vein near his heart for delivery of the Rocephin. He was just weeks away from a wheelchair, but if so, he was going to get there through Lyme country. "I was determined to see this through, come hell or high water," he says.

40

·⊹·

Putting Treatment to the Test

Evidence for persistent infection, compelling to Lyme doctors who treat it and patients who say they suffer from it, hasn't convinced most infectious disease doctors that long-term treatment really works. Alan Barbour, today director of the Pacific-Southwest Regional Center of Excellence for Biodefense and Emerging Infectious Diseases at the University of California Irvine and one of the world's foremost spirochete experts, has posed the question: "What does it *mean* to persist?" Barbour does not dispute the objective findings of scientists like Straubinger and Barthold, but contends that even if some spirochetes survive, they may not be present in sufficient quantity to cause disease. While Lyme doctors treat empirically in trial-and-error mode, hoping to see improvement, researchers like Barbour demand treatments be proven in clinical trials before they'll accept that they work.

It was on October 18, 1994, that the NIH hosted a powwow for scientists to brainstorm ways of gathering the evidence for or against longer-term treatment, at last.

"This is a pressing issue. We have been forced to come to grips with it," Stony Brook neurologist Patricia Coyle began. Coyle saw hundreds of patients at Stony Brook, and found that "all regimens had treatment failures. We honestly don't know the best antibiotic, the best delivery method, or the best length of treatment." A stickler for precision, Coyle defined the controversial entity, chronic Lyme disease, for the group:

"Chronic or intermittent problems beginning at the time of clinical Lyme disease and persisting months to years despite adequate antibiotic treatment." As to the cause, the issue of persistent infection versus post-infectious response was "definitely an open question," she said.

Then, addressing Allen Steere, Coyle asked: "What percentage of these patients do *you* think have persistent infection?" She looked at him, waited a bit, and when he didn't respond, she added, "I think it's actually a significant number."

"I agree that some patients who have post–Lyme disease syndrome are persistently infected," said Steere. "I fully agree."

In the aftermath of the meeting, it seemed inevitable that long-term treatment for Lyme disease be put to the test. What was the appropriate treatment length, particularly for patients who did not respond to the recommended regimens? Did further treatment help? Which medicines worked best?

A call for proposals went out, and two came in. The first proposal came from Ben Luft's team at Stony Brook. The second came from the New England Medical Center (NEMC) and infectious disease specialist Mark Klempner, in collaboration with Steere at Tufts. The Stony Brook plan attempted, at least in spirit, to embody the philosophy of the Lyme doctors by treating for months and combining antibiotics, including ones that crossed the blood-brain barrier and penetrated cells. The complexity of the plan made it costly, the NIH said, explaining why it opted for the truncated experiment from the NEMC.

It was a sweltering day in July 1996 when Ken Fordyce of the New Jersey Governor's Council and Carl Brenner of the Lyme Disease Coalition of New York and Connecticut traveled down to Bethesda to discuss the decision with the NIH. NEMC had proposed testing long-term regimens by treating chronic Lyme patients with a single drug—Rocephin—for a single month. Rocephin was known for its poor intracellular penetration, and one month of treatment with Rocephin was *already* the standard of care. The protocol could be considered "long term" only in the sense that patients enrolled would need to have been treated before. "Everyone knew that the clinicians were treating much longer than that," says Brenner. "It was an amazingly shortsighted plan because, clearly, it would do nothing to resolve the issue. If one extra month of treatment ended up showing no benefit, the obvious criticism would have been that they should have tried treating longer term."

In the end, John LaMontagne, director of the National Institute of Allergy and Infectious Diseases and Phillip J. Baker, the new head of

Lyme Disease Programs at the NIH, took the arguments to heart, to a degree. In fact, they established an advisory committee (including two patient advocates, four scientists, and a clinician) so the Lyme community could have a role. Brenner was appointed to the committee, along with a second patient—Phyllis Mervine, the California woman who *still* lived "off the grid" high in the Coast Range. Mervine had, in the intervening years, been successfully treated for Lyme disease with a long-term regimen of the antibiotic doxycycline. She'd gone on to found the Lyme Disease Resource Center (now the California Lyme Disease Association, or CALDA), where she worked to raise consciousness out West.

When the newly appointed advisory committee convened on August 14, 1996, moving beyond the decades of bad blood was a challenge, to say the least. NIH officials had placed a few security guards around the conference room for fear, Phil Baker explained, that unruly patients would barge in and force a physical confrontation. One patient in attendance recalls a surreal close encounter during a meeting break, when he was inside a bathroom stall. Baker and some scientists from Tufts entered the bathroom and, thinking they were alone, began to talk.

"These patients aren't nearly as disruptive as I thought they would be," said Richard F. Kaplan, referring to Brenner and Mervine along with several patient-observers. Kaplan was the psychologist charged with evaluating study volunteers through a battery of neuropsychiatric tests.

"We managed to get a pretty good group. The ones here today are the responsible ones. This collection is okay," Baker replied.

The patient considered walking out and joining the discussion, but not wanting to cause embarrassment, he remained in the stall until the bathroom was clear.

Despite the rocky start, the committee did excellent work that day in accordance with its mandate, which was broad. Not only was it to review and comment on the design of the current study, it was also charged with helping to interpret results and participating in future studies on chronic Lyme.

By now, Klempner had made some changes himself, and the protocol he submitted for review included a single month of Rocephin followed by two months of doxycyline, a drug said to penetrate inside cells. In addition, he wanted to add a group of patients testing negative on standard antibody tests but still diagnosed, unequivocally, with Lyme disease because of an EM rash. Without a direct test for infection, Klempner proposed evaluating patient improvement by asking subjects to fill out questionnaires. Brenner and Mervine requested that the study team try testing for *B. burgdorferi* DNA through polymerase chain reaction.

Even with the longer treatment timeline and the additional months of doxy, Mervine was worried that the study wouldn't show much, and she expressed her doubts. The timelines and doses involved, after all, were *far* less than those the Lyme doctors said they needed to see any real results for patients so chronically sick. "But Klempner and NIH assured me that this was just the first in a series of treatment studies, and that they would look at longer trials in the future, when this was done," Mervine says. "My fears were allayed."

Yet finding patients for the study proved a daunting task. For one thing, entry requirements were steep. Not only did accepted subjects need to document prior treatment, they also had to have either a physician-documented EM rash or one of Steere's classic late major manifestations accompanied by five of the ten CDC-designated Western blot bands—in other words, they had to represent the top of the Lyme pyramid most patients couldn't ascend.

But it wasn't just the entry requirements that served as a barrier. Carl Brenner arranged a presentation for doctors and patients in Katonah, a heavily endemic Westchester town, in the spring of 1997, but few bothered to attend. For those who did, the skepticism was so thick you could cut it with a knife. "I would like to refer some of my patients," one doctor said, "but I'm not convinced that I'd be doing them a favor. They may get three months or if they wind up in the placebo group, they may get nothing. I worry that I could be jeopardizing their health."

Thanks to recruiters in the Lyme patient community like Phyllis Mervine, Klempner eventually rustled up 129 patients—78 in the seropositive group and 51 who were seronegative. Each group was split in two, with half receiving antibiotic treatment and half receiving placebo. Because the study was double-blinded, neither the physicians nor the patients knew who was assigned to which group. Klempner would determine the value of the treatment by analyzing the lab tests and the patient questionnaires.

Perhaps it was Carl Brenner's faith in the purity of science that blinded him to the rumblings of politics and forces in play behind the scenes. Before the study was even complete, an expert panel from the Infectious Diseases Society of America (IDSA) published clinical guidelines for treatment of patients with Lyme disease. When it came to chronic Lyme, the panel concluded, it just did not exist—never mind that the NIH was spending millions on a treatment study of it even as the guidelines went to press. Insiders on the IDSA committee reported shenanigans. First was the removal of a committee member, Sam Donta of Boston University, who fought for inclusion of the chronic Lyme diagnosis along with longer treatment. Second was the demotion of Ben Luft, unceremoniously removed from his role as committee chair. Luft's great transgression? He'd wanted to hear Donta out. With Donta gone and Luft demoted, the widely distributed new IDSA guidelines—disenfranchising the chronic patients still being studied—became the standard of care.

Publication of the guidelines in November 2000 coincided with the halfway point of the study. As in any drug trial, it is at this juncture that monitors examine the results and decide if the second half of the study should go on. Given all the limitations, no one, least of all the patient community, was particularly shocked when the monitor found no benefit to the treatment. The study was halted at once.

The uproar started later, in June 2001, when the findings were published to fanfare over the Internet by the *New England Journal of Medicine,* which declared them so urgent they couldn't be held for print publication in July. The Internet release was accompanied by a press release from the NIH: "Clinical Alert: Chronic Lyme Disease Symptoms Not Helped by Intensive Antibiotic Treatment," the NIH declared. Instead of announcing the failure of *this one* treatment in this limited group of patients, NIH had applied results to all treatments for all patients with chronic symptoms of Lyme disease.

Media coverage was intense. "Antibiotics don't cure chronic Lyme disease," announced *Time* magazine. The *New York Times* quote of the day was from Leonard Sigal: "Lyme disease, although a problem, is not nearly as big a problem as most people think. The bigger epidemic is Lyme anxiety." To patients who'd been hearing the same Sigal sound bite for more than a decade, it was astounding that the *Times* could trot it out as news yet again.

In one sense, the study had validated patients: Klempner showed they were very sick and in a lot of pain, as impaired as those with congestive heart failure and sicker than people with type two diabetes. But as to the major question—the utility of long-term treatment—the scientists were unequivocal: The antibiotics didn't work because the chronic patients weren't infected. In fact, bowing to patient requests, the researchers had screened the subjects' blood for *Borrelia* DNA. "Significantly, more than 700 different blood and cerebrospinal fluid samples were collected from the study volunteers. None of the samples showed evidence of persistent infection with the Lyme agent, *Borrelia burgdorferi,*" the NIH Web site said. The agency's next step would be investigating autoimmune and other noninfectious processes to determine the cause of chronic Lyme.

All in all, most patients were stunned. They hadn't been counting on Klempner to prove they were chronically infected, or even that longer treatment worked—they viewed this study as a first step only. But they never expected the scientists to apply the results of the limited trial to all treatment protocols for all Lyme disease patients. They had never expected the NIH to orchestrate such an overwhelming blitz of PR.

Carl Brenner felt betrayed. All he'd wanted was a role in the scientific process, but he'd been used as window dressing to convince patients they had some oversight, when clearly they did not. As soon as the report hit the Internet, he was deluged with e-mails and phone calls from patients frantic that their treatment might be withheld.

"How do you think it looks to Phyllis's and my constituency when the study is suddenly and prematurely concluded, rushed into print without the Committee's input . . . and then blasted out to the press with such force that it becomes front-page news on the *New York Times* . . . I'm sorry, I'm not naïve—I know a thing or two about academic politics," he wrote in an e-mail to the sympathetic committee chair on June 14, 2001.

Brenner, who'd had mixed response to antibiotics himself, wasn't even a devotee of the long-term school of thought. "I hope you understand that I am griping here about the process, not the results," his e-mail went on. "I am not at all wedded to the idea that long-term antibiotic treatment is necessarily effective for chronic Lyme disease symptoms. (Although I don't rule it out, either.) But I sure as heck would be hard-pressed to make the case that this study of only 100 patients has shut the door on that possibility. Unfortunately, the study's authors seem to be far less reserved in their conclusions. I am really trying to be objective here, but I am finding it difficult to accept that this has been a fair process."

To some in the Lyme community, the study appeared to be a straw man, designed to fail. Sam Donta expressed concerns in a letter published in the *New England Journal of Medicine*. Citing the experience of doctors who typically treat chronic Lyme, he noted that stable improvement in patients was generally observed only with protocols lasting far longer than three months, and with antibiotics better able to penetrate the cell. Others complained that the dose of doxy used was too low to penetrate the central nervous system, and that the study hadn't looked at drugs for treating cysts. Brian Fallon protested that Klempner's patients had a hodgepodge of later symptoms—some neurological, others arthritic—making the small group too heterogeneous to define.

Yet the biggest problem may have stemmed from the two things the patients had in common. The first of these was that all had previously failed antibiotic therapy for Lyme disease—making them far more likely to fail again.

The second, interrelated commonality was that some 75 percent of the patients had been admitted to the study based on a physician-diagnosed rash, the classic sign of *early* Lyme. These rash patients had been treated at time of diagnosis, says Phil Baker, a treatment strategy that mainstream studies show should cure 95 percent. "All of the patients enrolled in the study had to have been treated with a standard course of antibiotics that should have cured their initial infection. Evidence of such treatment had to be documented in their medical records. If they weren't treated appropriately for their initial infection, they would not have been enrolled in the study. Why? Because they could still have an unresolved active infection, rather than chronic Lyme disease," Phil Baker explains. Yet these patients had *failed* that treatment—because here they were in Klempner's study, after all, still sick.

Lyme rash patients who failed early treatment were, in no uncertain terms, outliers, with failure due to unusual strains of infection, immune problems, or some other unexplained cause. Whatever their issues, they were a world apart from the vast majority of chronic Lyme disease patients, who were typically diagnosed late and never received early treatment—though it would likely have cured most of them, had it only been prescribed. Using this tiny minority to explain the experience of the overwhelming majority was an unfounded intellectual leap.

For Phyllis Mervine, the final disappointment came in the fall of 2001, when she lobbied for concessions from NIH—especially a softening of the "Internet Alert" declaring that *all long-term treatment* had now been proven ineffective for *all patients* with chronic Lyme disease. Toward that end, she requested another meeting of the advisory committee in which the issues could be aired. After a heated exchange of e-mails, a meeting was scheduled for November, but by then 9/11 and the anthrax attacks had turned everything on its head and the meeting was canceled. It was in April 2002 that Carl Brenner and Phyllis Mervine received letters informing them that the Lyme Disease Advisory Committee—by now renamed a "Panel," and so governed by different rules—had been disbanded for good.

As far as the NIH was concerned, Klempner's two study arms had done the job. "In view of the number of publications that emerged from his work and the large amount of new information they provided—his are the most informative clinical studies that have ever been conducted on chronic

Lyme disease. [They] demonstrated for the first time that these patients experience significant pain and certainly require appropriate treatment. Since extended antibiotic therapy is not beneficial, *alternative approaches* must be explored. If one truly wishes to help these patients, that would be an excellent way to establish common ground where all those who have been engaged in this controversy can work together toward a common objective," said Phil Baker, who oversaw the work at NIH from beginning to end.

Insurance companies took heed. Again and again, as patients sought coverage, the Klempner study was invoked as the reason for denying claims.

But even Baker agreed that the Klempner study "may not have provided all the answers," and it wasn't the final word, not even at NIH. Other studies had been commissioned in the mandate to answer the chronic Lyme question, and in the years that followed, these were published as well.

The next to roll off the press was a study by Stony Brook neurologist Lauren Krupp. To be accepted into the Krupp study, a Lyme patient had to be suffering from severe fatigue six months after his or her antibiotic therapy had come to an end. Fifty-five patients signed on. For twenty-seven days running, half the patients received IV Rocephin and the other half placebo.

Unlike Klempner, Krupp found a significant difference between the treated group and the placebo group. Six months after the study's end, 64 percent of treated patients and 18.5 percent of placebo patients showed improvement for fatigue. Krupp did not find a corresponding benefit for cognitive function, but then again, the patients had been selected on the basis of exhaustion. Since the patients didn't have severe cognitive deficits in the first place, said Krupp, "that may have contributed to the lack of a treatment effect" there.

Why did Krupp's results differ from Klempner's? One reason, says Brian Fallon, could be her decision to focus on a homogeneous set of patients notable for a single, consistent presentation. It is entirely possible that antibiotics may aid fatigue but not memory, he says—or that the patients were not particularly cognitively impaired in the first place, so that small improvements would be difficult to detect. In the end, despite the positive results, Krupp's paper contained a disclaimer mentioning adverse reactions to antibiotic and so recommending no more than a single, short-term course of treatment for the persistent symptoms of Lyme disease, including fatigue.

A third NIH treatment study, published in the October 2007 issue of *Neurology,* came from Fallon and his team at Columbia Presbyterian

Hospital in New York, where the Lyme and Tick Borne Diseases Research Center had just been launched. Like Krupp and Klempner, Fallon admitted only the most classic and well-documented of Lyme disease patients, even requiring that each and every subject have a currently positive Western blot. As with the two previous studies, Fallon's well-documented Lyme patients had to have been treated before; adhering to an especially rigorous standard, they had to have been treated with at least three weeks of intravenous antibiotic to sign on.

Among the three studies, Fallon's was unique. All participating patients had the classic neurocognitive signs of Lyme disease, including impaired short-term memory and verbal fluency. And, as dictated by study protocol, all received a significantly longer-term regimen of ten weeks of IV antibiotic (or the placebo equivalent of that amount). Instead of measuring improvement largely through subjective patient questionnaires, moreover, Fallon conducted objective neuropsychological tests of memory and other aspects of cognition (such as verbal fluency and psycho-motor functioning), and performed state-of-the-art brain imaging, including MRI for brain structure and Positron Emission Tomography, or PET, for brain function. (PET scans measure blood flow and energy metabolism in the brain.)

Would the treatment lead to solid changes? Could improvements in memory be validated by changes in brain imaging? When the study was unblinded, the team was able to plot the trajectory of three separate groups: patients treated with Rocephin, patients treated with placebo, and healthy patients who weren't treated at all. Looking at fatigue, physical dysfunction, and pain, Fallon found the Rocephin-treated patients who started out with greater symptom severity showed greater improvement than the patients receiving placebo. These same patients given Rocephin three months later showed continued improvement in pain and physical functioning. In this regard, Fallon had confirmed the findings of Krupp.

On objective tests of memory and overall cognition, however, the news was not as good. Healthy controls and patients on placebo improved slightly over time, the result of "practice" by taking the test more than once. But for treated patients, the graph careened: Two weeks after therapy's end, the line soared sharply upward to indicate significant improvement in cognition. Three months later, the line plummeted to once more coincide with that of placebo controls. Fallon noted that the initial improvement was in multiple aspects of cognition, not just memory as initially expected. As in Oliver Sacks's classic book *Awakenings*, which described patients who rose to consciousness only to fall back down the tunnel of darkness, the treated Lyme patients briefly recovered their former powers of cognition, only to relapse. The recovery and loss of cognition was paralleled by alterations in blood flow and energy metabolism on PET. Like Krupp of Stony Brook, Brian Fallon of Columbia found that additional antibiotic treatment pushed back the symptoms of chronic Lyme, even if imperfectly and just in part.

Commenting on the reversal, Fallon says it's *possible* that Rocephin was treating memory loss by killing *Borrelia,* but he actually leans another way. In this group of patients, he thinks, the Rocephin may have been impacting neurotransmitters and deftly protecting the brain. Rocephin stimulates the production of the brain's glutamate transporters, he explains, harking back to the ALS study so notable to David Martz. The more glutamate is removed from the extracellular space by these transporters the less glutamate is awash in the brain. Since too much glutamate can be toxic, drugs that suppress it—like Rocephin—may treat the cognitive deficits of Lyme. "Basically the relapse was too rapid for infection to thoroughly explain it," says Fallon, "so I'd look for another cause." To Fallon, the psychiatrist, the rapid relapse was similar to what might happen if you pulled someone's Xanax—and faster than the return of an infectious disease like Lyme.

Many disagree, mentioning clinical observation and theories of persistence to reframe the debate. Joe Burrascano says that relapse after just ten weeks of treatment is fairly standard in his chronic patients across the range of antibiotics, even those with no known impact on the brain. Others contend that Rocephin induces cysts, which may convert back to spirochetes in weeks. Still others point to intracellular hiding: "Take away extracellular antibiotics like Rocephin too early, or maybe at any time, and the spirochetes come out of hiding, allowing the disease to return," says Pennsylvania physician Harold Smith.

Of course, since Rocephin repairs the brain even without infection, it's impossible to know, in the end, which mechanism is at the root. Either way, Rocephin might make the symptoms go away. After millions of dollars and years of research, the NIH treatment trials were a wash. In telling us how to treat, they resembled nothing so much as a Rorschach test: Every individual faced with the data saw only vindication for his or her own point of view.

Writing an editorial on the Fallon study in the same issue of *Neurology,* the well-known neurologist John Halperin suggests that Lyme patients may have no more cognitive loss than anyone else. "Interestingly, in studies of the general population, symptoms such as those described by these patients are reported by up to one-third of individuals, with severe cognitive symptoms in two percent," he says in an article entitled "Prolonged Lyme Disease Treatment: Enough is Enough."

ILADS president Daniel Cameron sees it another way. There were just 37 patients in the Fallon study and 221 patients in the three studies overall, he said, "far too few to conclude 'enough is enough' right now." Writing in the journal *Epidemiologic Perspectives & Innovations,* he said the results were "not generalizable to the overall Lyme disease population" because patients selected to participate had been sick for too long, and had failed the same treatments, often many such treatments, before. Indeed, Cameron's own study with the oral antibiotic amoxicillin has tied treatment success to timeliness of the diagnosis—with the length of delay predicting whether a patient might respond at all. Yet the three NIH studies reported treatment delays from months to years—and enrolled patients refractory to treatment from the start. In the Klempner trial patients were sick an average of 4.7 years before entering, and in the Fallon study, 9. Because these patients had failed the very same treatment before, often many times before, this made it all too likely that they would fail them again.

As for the chronic patients—the sickest of them—the studies did nothing to light the way. Those kept afloat on an ocean of antibiotics kept on taking them. Those who failed to respond often found other, alternative treatments: hyperbaric oxygen, Rife machines said to kill bacteria by bathing them with electromagnetic waves, or herbal extracts like Samento and Cumanda. Some were treated for heavy metals and others for exposure to mold. Some patients reported these therapies helped, but others ventured further, finding their answers online. One Web site promoted a Lyme treatment of vitamin C and salt. Another sold a pill called the *Sputnik,* advertised by its manufacturer as an "alternative parasite zapper" that switched itself on "in the electrolyte environment of the stomach," emitting "electric pulses, of a definite shape, range, and frequency." The sickest patients sometimes felt so desperate they spent tens of thousands of dollars on dangerous "miracle cures": A doctor from Atlanta gave five Lyme patients commercial-grade weed killer; a doctor from Topeka, Kansas, stands accused of murder, charged with injecting his Lyme patients with Bismacine, containing the potentially poisonous metallic element bismuth. One of those patients died. It was all in response to the pain and frustration, the lack of answers, the mess and insanity of Lyme.

Papers were duly published, opinions freely swirled. Yet none of the studies accounted for the mix of coinfections or the alternate species of

Borrelia. None reflected the zeitgeist confronting the Lyme doctors, who strive to bring such patients back through a *brew* of treatments aimed at all sorts of infection and physiological imbalance—much of it not even Lyme disease—prescribed in sequence, empirically, over the course of months to years. If Lyme vox populi is a mélange of tick infection and immune dysfunction, environmental insults and damage already done, then the ivory tower studies and the patients on the ground will always inhabit two worlds. Were such studies ever to elucidate the disease of five Western blot bands and swollen knees, they would still shed little light on the vast epidemic of "Lyme."

Because the NIH studies were so limited, and especially because the hunt for infection was indirect, they spawned only more rancor and spin. The impasse had been foreseen by some people right from the start. "I felt uncomfortable at the thought that human treatment studies would rely largely on indirect evidence to make conclusions about infection," reflects Carl Brenner. "There were so many ways for such leaps to be misleading. Patients could be persistently infected without responding to the treatment, or conversely, they could be uninfected but respond to antibiotics due to anti-inflammatory or other effects. You couldn't infer infectious status based on treatment response."

The danger of making unjustified leaps had been worrisome to Brenner and his fellow patient Barbara Goldklang. In the early 1990s they'd both been members of the research-oriented nonprofit Lyme Coalition of New York and Connecticut. Back then, the group had urged the NIH to fund studies in rhesus monkeys, where disease is close to our own. Just like humans, rhesus monkeys get the erythema migrans rash; their antibody patterns and ours are almost the same. But unlike humans, rhesus monkeys can be sacrificed in the lab. After the study is done, their tissues can be necropsied, and instead of inferring infectious status indirectly (as, say, Klempner had), researchers could go right in and (like Straubinger and Barthold) see if the spirochetes were there or not. As luck would have it, microbiologist and primatologist Mario Philipp of the Primate Research Center at Tulane was proposing just such a study as the final Klempner protocol was being developed. To Brenner's and Goldklang's delight, the NIH agreed to fund the work.

In 1996, while serving on the advisory committee for the Klempner study, Brenner saw a perfect chance to make one of the rhesus monkey studies serve as confirmation for the human trial already under way. Due in part to Brenner's urging, the NIH agreed to make the rhesus monkey treatment regimen exactly the same as the treatment regimen used by Klempner on his human patients—except that instead of relying exclusively on tests like Western blots for antibodies and PCR for DNA, they would also sacrifice the monkeys and look for the spirochetes themselves. Thus, Philipp would be performing a sort of fact-check of Klempner's work. "From the beginning I pushed the advisory committee for a statement that the Klempner study would not be released before the Philipp study—that they should be published concurrently." Because it could look more deeply and examine what was happening inside, "Philipp's work would be the gold standard," Brenner says.

Even though the advisory committee embraced the recommendation for simultaneous publication in writing, it was not to be. The Klempner study was ended early and spit out at the speed of light, while the Philipp study was held up for one reason after another (including Hurricane Katrina) for years.

Some thirteen years after the study's commission, results have yet to see the light of day. Yet word from a number of academic insiders is that the work replicates in monkeys the mouse studies done by Barthold at Davis and the dog studies done by Straubinger at Cornell, posing a challenge to the NIH conclusions that have determined patient care for years. Indeed, if small numbers of living, infectious spirochetes remain behind, invulnerable to antibiotics, we will have to investigate their role in the disease. Increasingly, evidence suggests that low-level infection in some patients can cause the kind of "pro-inflammation" that may be at the root of the pain and fatigue that chronic patients report.

Barthold thinks such findings could well explain patient complaints, but argues for caution nonetheless. These kinds of results must be "scrutinized, criticized, and reproduced by others," he says. And "the presence of bacteria that remain after antibiotic treatment is not unusual. More than 90 percent of people exposed to tuberculosis carry the bacteria without disease. Herpes virus, cytomegalovirus, papilloma viruses, all can cause devastating disease, even cancer, yet we walk around with them in our bodies every day."

Yet *Borrelia* isn't a virus—it's a bacterium, and as such produces products even in a torporous state, says Eugene Davidson, professor of biochemistry and molecular biology at Georgetown University Medical Center and department chair from 1988 through 2003. "It exports things that make people feel ill."

Davidson has found that the spirochetes can "go cryptic. That means the organism is silent, it is hidden, and you can't see it," says Davidson, who's worked with *Borrelia burgdorferi* in species from mice to rhesus monkeys since the early 1990s. "At a certain stage in the disease it appears to be gone, and you do not know that the host is infected, yet you can get a recrudescence through a trigger that no one yet understands."

If, as Barthold says, we all carry a *range* of cryptic organisms, then why might *Borrelia,* in particular, make us feel so sick? "Just because one organism doesn't make us sick doesn't mean a second one can't," Davidson explains. "*E. coli* can usually live comfortably in the gut, yet there are strains of *E. coli* that export highly toxic materials and cause great physical distress. There are organisms that produce materials capable of making us sick, even in tiny quantities, because there's such a strong response on the part of the host. Even an organism that's relatively quiescent is able to produce inflammatory materials, provoking cytokine responses that cause reactions in the host. Low levels of metabolic activity in the organism could fall below the detectable limits of our technology, but they are still eliciting inflammatory cytokines, and as a result of that, the host doesn't feel well. These cryptic *Borrelia* may be so quiescent they are almost like spores; yet even if they replicate slowly, they are using resources, even while hidden from view."

If the animal work tells us anything, it is that the human treatment studies have been overinterpreted, oversold, and misused. Using twentieth-century technology and antibiotics, these studies were able to provide some answers about specific treatments for specific patients. But due to their flagrant limitations, including the inability to autopsy participating patients, they could *never* have done what some scientists claim: shed the laser light of Truth on the deeper questions, the haunting and *still-open* questions of Lyme.

Here's an observation from the peanut gallery: Scientists like Allen Steere and Mark Klempner continue to search for the elusive "autoimmune trigger" of chronic Lyme disease year in and decade out. They *believe* it exists, but have never found the proof. For Lyme's old guard, it is a search for the Holy Grail. Would they ever consider the remaining spirochetes, the ones now documented in a roster of convincing animal studies from their colleagues and peers, as the trigger instead? At least these spirochetes have been found. They provide a direct explanation for what patients report. At least now we know they are *real*. If we could eliminate those spirochetes with twenty-first-century antibiotics or treat their immune effects with targeted immune-modulating drugs, might not that ease some of the misery called chronic Lyme?

41

※

Busted Flat in Chappaqua

Chappaqua, New York, 2004

To paraphrase Tolstoy, every happy family is the same, but each Lyme family is unhappy in its own special way. We had moved to paradise, only to find it toxic. We had children, only to mire them in disease. Our life was so exhausting and expensive, with so much regret, it drained us to the bone. I think of 2004 as the year I threw up my hands and relinquished unto the spruce forest my last naïve hope.

At first things seemed to be looking up. More than three years after starting treatment, Jason was completing his freshman year at Brown University, and he was nearly well. His mind was clear enough to handle math and physics and philosophy. He played basketball. He went to parties. He had friends. After flirting with the abyss, in what seemed like a miracle Jason had returned to us. Dr. Jones wanted Jason to continue on antibiotics to clean up the last few remnants of Lyme disease—the now-tolerable stomachaches, bone pain, and fatigue that lingered on. But Jason was a college kid and following a schedule of pills was the last thing on his list. Despite the flickering symptoms, Jason rejected more treatment. He preferred to think of himself as healthy; and for the most part, he was.

Yet spending some weekends at home in Chappaqua, Jason was, naturally, exposed to the tick forest surrounding us and so, to Lyme disease. We'd done our best to clear our property, creating a lawn out front where once we'd had just forest, filling our flower bed with wood chips, and spraying all of it with pesticide to kill the ticks. We had even expanded the driveway, carving, under a canopy of trees, a macadam circle large enough for shooting hoops. Jason and his friends spent many an afternoon playing basketball in the circumference of our driveway, yet every so often someone would overshoot. One day I saw Jason dive into the brambles to retrieve a basketball barefoot. "Get out of the woods," I'd shouted down the driveway the same way I'd implored his brother to get out of the leaves, to no avail. And the truth is that wasn't his only exposure. It was impossible to live in Chappaqua without risk of Lyme disease. And it wasn't just Chappaqua that held risks. He'd brazenly gone on a camping trip with friends that year to an island rife with ticks and deer. Even the campus green at Brown University, surrounded by city streets near downtown Providence, had Lyme ticks: One friend sitting on the green had pulled a tick from her leg only to find, a short time later, an erythema migrans in that very spot. She later tested positive for Lyme disease.

None of us really knew how Jason had been reinfected, least of all Jason. He did not want to think about Lyme disease anymore. He did not want to restrict his movements, avoid the environment, or even take precautions. "Just leave me alone on this issue," he warned me. The dirge had lasted too long; he'd had enough.

But despite such sentiments, by late spring 2004, Jason began to sink. First three round bull's-eye rashes, as perfectly matched as triplets and each the shape of a rosebud, appeared along his shoulder blade and neck. I captured them with a Polaroid. They must have been secondary to a primary rash, one we'd never seen, the doctor said. After that Jason's bone pain, stomachaches, and fatigue returned in force. His Western blot, highly positive in 2000, had turned negative over the years until, by 2003, he had not a single positive band. By late spring 2004, his blot was once more positive, with so many bands it again exceeded the exacting requirements of the CDC. No one, not even the doctor, could be sure that Jason hadn't just relapsed. But to me, this appeared to be a reinfection, caused by another tick bite. For the second time in a row, Jason had a textbook-classic case—a *new* case—of Lyme disease, one that had gone untreated for months.

By now age twenty, Jason was no longer a pediatric patient—it was as good a time as any to leave the care of Dr. Jones and take him to Joe Burrascano, who treated adults. Burrascano prescribed oral antibiotics, but Jason wanted none of it. He was a young man sick of being sick— sick of thinking about Lyme disease, sick of swallowing pills. With the infection still new, moreover, he wasn't that ill, not yet. Even the return of his Lyme disease and warnings it would get worse were insufficient incentive for Jason to comply with treatment. Back at Brown, to my horror, Jason continued to avoid treatment, and he continued his descent. Joe Burrascano was furious. "Follow the treatment," he told Jason at one of his appointments, "or please just don't come back." For a very long time, Jason didn't.

Jason's reinfection was the end of the road for us. Now we had two sick boys: The older one, Jason, up in Providence, was falling back into illness. The younger one, David, still in Chappaqua, suffered from God knows what. He was too exhausted to roll in the leaves anymore, too sick to leave his room or his bed, too fatigued to go to school.

Mark and I trucked uneasily on: Mark appeared to function with a low dose of daily doxycycline, going to work and playing tennis, but whenever he ran out and tried to go cold turkey for a while, the symptoms came back in force, and he would resume the drugs. I, too, cycled up and down: Taking amoxicillin, I was asymptomatic. Stopping the antibiotic, I crashed. With our medical bills mounting and new infections complicating illness from the past, we knew we had to leave Chappaqua. It was time to get out of Dodge.

42

⟡

Resurrection

Colorado Springs, Colorado, 2004

Back home in Colorado Springs, Dave Martz asked a local physician, a friend, to oversee directives from Dr. Harvey of Houston. Martz took his *Babesia* treatment at home and received Rocephin for Lyme disease in the doctor's office daily, waiting to see what might emerge.

Changes were dramatic. His stamina improved, and by the end of the first month, his pain and arthritis were totally gone. Where once he could endure no more than an hour of conversation, now he engaged with company for five hours at a shot. He could get in the car; he could go to the mailbox and collect the mail. At the end of two months, he could cross his legs—something that had become impossible. At the end of three months, he could stand up from a chair, walk and move around, and do deep knee bends, all without help.

His overseeing doctor, an infectious disease specialist, was speechless. "I cannot explain this," he said. But after he sent Martz's blood to the Lyme lab at Stony Brook only to have it come back negative, he was reluctant to continue the antibiotic in an open-ended way. Martz's situation was virtually unheard of, and this kind of treatment for Lyme disease was *way* outside the mainstream. This wasn't the Northeast—it was Colorado, it just wasn't done. Treatment like this, the doctor explained, put his reputation and practice at risk.

Martz understood, so he approached his close friends in oncology— where the clinic was used for intravenous infusions of chemotherapy on a daily basis, and he wouldn't stand out. They agreed to let him infuse his Rocephin with the cancer patients, and the treatment went on. "If I hadn't been a respected physician, it never could have happened," Martz says.

Extended treatment paid off. By the end of the year, Martz's legs had straightened, and the fasciculation was gone. In fact, Steven Smith, the neurologist who'd given Martz his death sentence, pronounced the ALS now gone. "By December, I was normal," Martz says.

Thinking back over his case, Martz hypothesizes that he was infected with versions of *Borrelia* and *Babesia* years ago, as he cared for a dying man in a dusty Las Animas ward. The infections, he theorizes, triggered the ALS. "If they hadn't been treated, the ALS would have gone its course."

Ultimately, the case was important enough to merit a write-up in the journal *Acta Neurologica Scandinavica*. Doctors had debated Rocephin as a treatment for ALS for years, commented coauthors William Harvey and David Martz. Then, in 2001, it was learned that the antibiotic might work by limiting the expression of the neurotransmitter glutamate—the same mechanism Brian Fallon suggested for his Lyme patients whose memories had soared but then plunged. Harvey and Martz had an alternate theory: "Chronic neurologic infection with a spirochetal agent such as *B. burgdorferi*," they wrote, might be triggering the ALS. It was possible, they added, that coinfection with *Borrelia* and *Babesia* in particular had heightened Martz's risk—and that he got better while similar patients did not because of the especially high dose of Rocephin and treatment for both infections at once.

43

⬥⬥⬥

Lyme Disease and Immunity:
The Search for the
Golden Fleece

Why does Lyme disease cause some people to get so ill they can barely function while others, similarly infected, don't get sick at all? Why do antibiotics cure many Lyme patients, while in others illness persists? The answer lies, at least in part, in the immune system: As with eye color, emotional temperament, and height, many immune traits are inherited and programmed by our genes. When it comes to our immune systems, we are all unique. By interacting with an infection, each person's immune system can change the nature of the disease. Conversely, a disease can activate, suppress, or otherwise damage an immune system that was previously working well.

For years, most of those arguing over chronic Lyme disease have taken one of two sides: Some insisted the illness was due largely to persistent infection; others said that infection was gone, and that an immune system gone haywire was to blame instead. For years, these protagonists have asked the same, impossible question: *Is it thee or me?*—the microbe or the immune system?—as if we are dealing with two mutually exclusive possibilities, as if infection and immune disturbance can't be in play at once.

An advocate of the immune-only theory is Mark Klempner, who led the first chronic Lyme study for the NIH. Klempner found that a significant number of his Lyme subjects had a gene commonly found in those with multiple sclerosis. The gene, known as DQB0602, was almost eight times more common in Klempner's persistently sick Lyme patients than in the public at large. This did not, of course, mean that chronic Lyme disease and multiple sclerosis were the same; but it suggested to Klempner that Lyme, like multiple sclerosis, could be an autoimmune disease in which the body attacked itself. (For his unusual group of patients, including the significant number who failed early treatment for the rash, it could make sense.)

Klempner and Steere suggested the controversial theory of "molecular mimicry" to explain how they thought it worked. A human protein (in this case the one produced by the special gene) and a spirochetal protein were, coincidentally, so similar in structure that the body mistook them for each other. After infection, the theory went, antibodies generated against the spirochete ended up attacking the human look-alike protein, the so-called mimic, embedded in the patient's cells. Since supply of the mimic was endless, the attack could go on forever, perpetuating symptoms of the disease even when infection was gone.

Steere took the concept much further, finding that a third of the Lyme patients had the gene for a molecule similar to the antibody for the spirochetal protein OspA. He theorized that patients with the gene would be at higher risk for a particularly severe, inflammatory version of Lyme disease, especially Lyme arthritis. In experiment after experiment, he searched for the mimic in Lyme arthritis, but has never found it to this day, leading him to theorize that another, still-unknown immune mechanism may be in play.

Proving molecular mimicry "would obviously lead to an entirely new approach to therapy," with a focus on drugs suppressing the dysfunction in the immune system, Klempner said. Though molecular mimicry remains to be proven or disproven for any disease, some doctors say that by addressing the issue now, a subgroup of chronic Lyme patients can finally get well. They point not only to Steere's work but also to that of Norman Latov, professor of neurology and neuroscience, and director of the Peripheral Neuropathy Clinical and Research Center at the Weill Medical College of Cornell University in New York. Looking for cross-reactions that could account for some neurological symptoms, Latov zeroed in on OspA, too. While Steere theorized that OspA might lead to more severe joint disease, Latov discovered that the protein cross-reacted with neuronal tissue, a finding he published in the *Journal of Neuroimmunology* in 2005. The process damaged the myelin sheath protecting the nerves, much as was seen in MS. But while MS largely damaged the *central* myelin sheath, in Lyme disease, myelin in the peripheries—the arms and legs—were also damaged. Using techniques of immunochemistry, Latov found evidence that antibodies against OspA could react with central myelin (in the brain and spinal cord) and myelin lining nerves at the peripheries as well.

To deal with the disease process, some doctors have begun implementing treatment with intravenous immunoglobulins, or IVIG, an amalgam of antibodies donated by tens of thousands of healthy individuals, combined into a single pool. This treatment is considered the first-choice therapy for patients with chronic inflammatory demyelinating polyneuropathy (CIDP), which is similar to the neuropathy seen in patients following Lyme disease. With similar disease processes, physicians felt similar treatment would help.

"Something in IVIG appears to block the OspA antibodies from reacting with the mimic, and it doesn't have the disadvantage associated with steroids or chemotherapeutic agents of activating low-level infection," says Orange, Connecticut, neurologist Amiram Katz, a clinical faculty at Yale School of Medicine, who finds that the treatment can help. To qualify for the pricey therapy (about $10,000 to $20,000 a month) patients undergo a skin biopsy right in Katz's office. The samples are sent off for analysis to see if a shortage of nerve fibers might signal autoimmune damage and account for the tingling and pain. If damage can be documented through biopsy along with nerve conduction studies, insurance will pick up the bill. And Katz says that in qualified patients, improvement in the neuropathy may be seen within two months. "This is not an infection anymore. The damage has been done and we are correcting it. The patients are feeling better, their tingling and nerve pain are diminished. In addition, they usually report having more energy and clarity of thinking," Katz says. (It's worthy of note that even as scientists collect evidence and clinicians tap their theories to help patients heal, the Infectious Diseases Society of America has included IVIG on the list of therapies to be avoided in chronic Lyme.)

While this kind of autoimmunity may turn out to explain a few incurable patients, most frontline scientists believe that something far more common, but also more nuanced, explains the persistent symptoms in most. The complexity starts with the changeability of the spirochete itself. In most bacterial diseases, small numbers of microbes remaining after treatment are routinely mopped up by the immune system, but Lyme spirochetes can persist even in the face of a robust immune response, evading the immune system with ease. One trick used by *B. burgdorferi* to accomplish this feat is changing its protein coat constantly, thus eluding the antibodies that destroy most other germs.

As the infected individual generates antibodies against one set of Lyme proteins, the spirochete cloaks its outer surface with an entirely new set of proteins, making it unrecognizable to the immune cells targeting it. In the process, Lyme turns into a moving target that can evade the mammalian immune system for months and years.

This observation was validated in 1997, when University of Texas microbiologist Steven Norris discovered the engine of change in *B. burgdorferi* genes. Like a kaleidoscope that is constantly changing the image on its screen, the special segment of DNA discovered by Norris constantly churns out novel gene sequences; these new genes in turn direct the production of new proteins. As the proteins randomly change, the spirochete's coat morphs, making the immune molecules that might once have killed it impotent in its wake. Experiments with mice demonstrate "promiscuous recombination" of the genes, producing a vast array of proteins at rapid pace. The system is so extensive, Norris said in the journal *Cell,* it can "potentially produce millions of antigenic variants in the mammalian host."

In 2006, Norris reported that the entire mechanism wasn't merely random, but could also respond to cues in the environment, aiding the spirochete's survival from locale to locale. What's more, the process could be dialed up or down by changing the temperature and acid content of the surrounding tissue and cells. The news is good. "Many steps in the pathway between a gene and its functional product may be exploited to maintain control of this process," Norris says. In other words, in the future, suppressing the mechanism of protein change could be one effective way of giving the immune system a boost and helping to keep Lyme under control.

In short, Norris understood what most of the top-bench scientists explained to me: Lyme disease was an infectious disease *and* an immune dysfunction. In the later, chronic stages of the disease, cure would mean dealing with both aspects at once.

Hoping to explore the realm where infection and immunity meet, Steve Barthold worked parallel to Allen Steere back in the early days at Yale, studying mice. To get to the bottom of things, Barthold infected a group of mice with *B. burgdorferi* spirochetes and waited until they developed an immune response. Then he transferred their blood (containing antibodies but not spirochetes) to mice that had never been exposed to the disease. When he later exposed the healthy mice to *Borrelia burgdorferi,* they appeared immune. It was clear that antibodies from the blood of the first group had literally served to "vaccinate" the second group. Because the blood contained all the antibodies needed to protect the mouse, offering a thick coat of immunity, Barthold called it the Golden Fleece.

What fascinated Barthold was his observation that even after infected mice made a Golden Fleece of immunity and seemed to recover, he always found living spirochetes in their tissues later on. If the mice weren't sacrificed, moreover, disease would come back periodically, as in human patients. The implication: The Golden Fleece could work to suppress the inflammatory signs of Lyme disease, even if some spirochetes remained.

To understand all this better, Barthold set out to learn what aspect of the immune system could eliminate inflammation (and thus, most measurable signs of disease) but not the actual spirochete. One way to find out was to compare normal mice with the ultimate "control" mice—those lacking any immune system—referred to by scientists as "severe combined immunodeficient" mice, or SCID mice, for short.

As expected, when Barthold injected SCID mice with *Borrelia,* he found that they stayed sick; it made sense because without immune systems they were incapable of making antibodies (a Golden Fleece) of their own. Yet when Barthold injected the Golden Fleece made by normal mice into infected SCID mice, the SCID mice, too, were cured of signs of the disease.

As the years went by, Steve Barthold's quest was to unravel the mystery of the Golden Fleece: If he could figure out how it worked, he would gain extraordinary insight into the disease and might even find a cure. Inside the mammal—the mouse, the hamster, the human—*B. burgdorferi* was changing its protein coat continually, donning a new, unrecognizable "costume" as soon as antibodies against the old one were made. Because the spirochete was so changeable, it was virtually impossible to isolate it from an animal at any given moment and assume that the organism captured was the same as spirochetes operating earlier or later in the course of disease.

Barthold could conceive of just one way to track the natural history of the disease in the body: through the rich and complex fabric of the Golden Fleece itself. Because the Golden Fleece could ultimately rid mice of all signs of the disease, he reasoned, it probably contained antibodies against every iteration of the spirochete from beginning to end. Like time-lapse photography where the period of exposure is prolonged, the Golden Fleece would amount to an amalgam of the accumulated history of Lyme disease. Each part of the spirochete expressed in the mouse, and each matched piece of the Golden Fleece represented another layer of Lyme.

Hoping to deconstruct the disease as thoroughly as possible, Barthold decided to start with a single, easily measurable sign, Lyme arthritis. What spirochetal proteins caused it? And was there a fraction of the Golden Fleece which, if injected into SCID mice, could cure only Lyme arthritis but not the rest of the disease? Eventually, using sophisticated molecular techniques, Barthold found a mouse-made antibody in the Golden Fleece that appeared capable of resolving Lyme arthritis but not any other aspect of Lyme disease. It matched, like lock and key, a spirochetal protein that Barthold named "arthritis-related protein," or ARP. "No one knows the function of ARP for the spirochete," he says. But whenever an antibody to ARP is injected into a Lyme-riddled SCID mouse, severe Lyme arthritis resolves; if ARP levels surged high enough, he later learned, Lyme carditis would resolve, too.

As technology has become more powerful, Barthold has wielded the Golden Fleece to deconstruct Lyme disease, one antibody, one spirochetal protein, and one tissue at a time. In 2006, he reported that an antibody to another Lyme protein—decorin-binding protein A (DbpA), so-called because it attaches to a molecule called decorin—could also eliminate the symptoms of Lyme carditis and Lyme arthritis in the mouse. What is especially fascinating is just how precise the impact is: The treatment eliminated the heart inflammation, and thus, outward signs of the disease, but it got rid of spirochetes only selectively. Indeed, after treatment with antibody to DbpA, spirochetes were eliminated from the heart base and synovium but not vascular walls, tendons, or ligaments. At Barthold's lab, the hunt is still on for other immune components of the mouse cure—and by extension, our own.

It was Steve Barthold's work that served as inspiration for Janis Weis, an immunologist at the University of Utah, who wondered why Lyme varied not just from tissue to tissue but also from individual to individual, even when the initial load of infection was the same. When she started out in 1992, she was well aware of the burning debate in Lyme: *Thee or me?* Was chronic disease associated with chronic persistent infection, or was it caused by the immune response of the host? There were two paths, and many scientists traveled just one. But Weis reasoned that the deepest understanding of the disease would mean traveling both paths, at once.

At first, she set out to learn what *Borrelia* did to the acting armies of the immune system, the white blood cells called lymphocytes. Generally revved into action only after exposure to foreign organisms, lymphocytes include the T cells that engulf and destroy microbes, and the B cells that produce specifically targeted antibodies against them.

Culturing mouse tissue in the lab and exposing it to *Borrelia,* Weis learned that B and T cells damaged the spirochetes. But it was a more generalized inflammation—provoked before these immune cells *ever appeared*—that damaged the *mouse*. "The initial response was so powerful," she says, "we knew it had to play a role in the disease."

Weis soon realized that some mice got far sicker than others, even when exposure to infection was exactly the same. Were some mice (and some people) just less susceptible to inflammation? To find out, she crossed severely and mildly arthritic mice over generations so that all kinds of intermediate combinations emerged. In the end it took years of interbreeding to create 400 mouse lines, each one at a different point on the spectrum, from those prone to severe inflammation to those incapable of any inflammation at all. When Weis infected the 400 mouse lines with *Borrelia,* she found a full spectrum of disease severity, correlating with the genetic background of the mouse. Depending upon where mice fell on the spectrum, even a small number of spirochetes could provoke and sustain their genetically predetermined variety of disease. No matter where on the spectrum an individual fell, when *all* the spirochetes were eliminated the signs of disease went away.

The work suggests, at first, that controlling inflammation could help reduce symptoms. But while runaway inflammation is bad, the converse turns out to be worse. Mice without an inflammatory response don't appear sick at first, but nor are they able to control infection. In the end, says Weis, such mice develop runaway infection and are sickest of all.

To help explain her observations, Weis began hunting for the cell receptors that *Borrelia* proteins would need to latch on to to provoke the inflammatory response. The receptor she found turned out to be a molecule called Toll-like receptor 2, so named because it functions almost like a toll. If *Borrelia* "pays the toll" by latching on to the receptor, then inflammation starts up.

Mice without the receptor developed little inflammation, but they also had no way to stanch infection. The spirochetal load in such mice eventually became immense: The mice were so overwhelmed with *Borrelia* that they, too, eventually developed inflammation, probably through another pathway, and ultimately became more disabled than mice with the most pro-inflammatory genes. Of course, where you fall on the spectrum may never make a difference unless you have Lyme disease. "This same system exists in humans, and probably explains why different people have such different disease outcomes," Janis Weis says.

The mouse findings in Lyme arthritis have been extended to the brain through monkey research at Tulane. Working with untreated rhesus monkeys (in experiments separate and apart from the study done to check the Klempner results), microbiologist Mario Philipp says his findings shed light on human neuroborreliosis—Lyme in the central nervous system and brain, the most devastating consequence of late-stage disease. Philipp ultimately found that the process described by Janis Weis—early damage caused directly by the spirochete—was what damaged the monkeys' tissue most. Based on his knowledge of just how destructive that inflammation could be, he theorized that spirochetes in the brain were driving a form of cell death called "apoptosis," in a similar but slower version of the mechanism already proven in Alzheimer's and AIDS dementia. His hypothesis: Infection inflamed the brain (just as it did the joints), and this in turn caused the death of brain cells, a degenerative process that might continue as long as the spirochete or its proteins lingered on.

He had good reason to suspect this was the case. It was well known that in the normal brain, the neurons responsible for sending messages and executing cognition were supported by a scaffolding of larger, structural cells called astrocytes. In neurodegenerative diseases like Alzheimer's and AIDS dementia, large-scale death of the neurons led to an increase in the number of astrocytes, a process known as astrogliosis. When Philipp sacrificed some infected monkeys, he indeed found proliferation of the astrocytes and cell death in the frontal lobes of their brains.

When he cultured the astrocytes in a dish with proteins from the spirochete, he found that some of those astrocytes reproduced at an abnormally high rate, proof of astrogliosis. Others died, a sign of apoptosis, or cell death. Philipp's next step is searching for death not of the astrocytes, which are just support cells, but of the neurons themselves. "We are predicting that we will find it," he says, "and are setting up experiments along those lines."

Today Philipp says his model of neuroborreliosis is similar to Weis's model of Lyme arthritis, involving an initial inflammatory response provoked and sustained by living *Borrelia*, often at very low levels—the kind of levels Barthold has found in his treated yet persistently infected mice and Straubinger has found in his dogs. "There is no need to imagine an autoimmune engine for this disease," says Philipp. "The spirochete is the direct cause. When people remain sick, the cause is either the spirochete or the remnants of its lipoproteins, never fully cleared."

The monkey research has validated the complexity of Lyme disease in other ways as well. Indeed, in sync with *Borrelia burgdorferi*'s continually changing protein coat, researchers have found that one set of spirochetal genes operate in the monkey's heart and another set in the central nervous system. Different genes operate in monkeys with normal immune systems than in those that are immune-suppressed. Each gene codes for different proteins, and, by extension, different forms of disease.

Such findings belie one-size-fits-all treatment guidelines and a cookie-cutter view of the disease. Lyme in the mouse and the monkey (and by extension, in us) is so complex it can produce a different disease in each organ of the body and every person it infects.

"Mammals are not clones, so each individual may respond to an infectious agent in a different way," Georgetown's Eugene Davidson says. "Add to this other infections, the variety of strains, and the ability of bacteria to mutate, and you can begin to understand the variability of the patient response. The cryptic nature of the organism makes it all the more complex."

What does it mean *to persist*? Alan Barbour has asked.

For each and every Lyme patient, the meaning of persistence is unique.

44

How I Cured My Own
Lyme Disease

Stamford, Connecticut, 2004

Casting about for a new place to live, we found a nearby city—a straight shot up the Interstate from Jason in Providence, close to the Harvey School, where David would be enrolled. David's health had been fragile the year before, but our fingers were crossed that after the summer, in the nurturing and close-knit Harvey family, he might reenter the world. We moved to our new home, a twelfth-floor apartment in a high-rise in downtown Stamford, Connecticut, in June 2004.

It was from that high vantage, inside a white brick tower atop a platform of concrete, no longer exposed to ticks, that I finally got well. With Tick Bite out of the picture, I'd long since taken a more assertive role in my treatment. In the course of writing my book, after all, I had clocked hundreds of hours interviewing scientists of every Lyme persuasion and the most skilled of the Lyme doctors. I'd read thousands of pages in medical journals. I'd spoken to hundreds of patients, some of them doctors or scientists, who'd successfully rid themselves of seemingly intractable Lyme. Tapping the concept of Paul Lavoie, who viewed Lyme as layered, an onion to be peeled, cognizant of the coinfections, I sought to peel my illness empirically, one step at a time.

After my nurse practitioner prescribed Mepron and Zithromax, for instance, my night sweats and migraines evaporated. I understood that those drugs in tandem targeted *Babesia,* and logically concluded that the worst of these headaches came from babesiosis, which now was gone. Treated with amoxicillin, my thinking cleared up and my exhaustion relented. Stopping amoxicillin, the fatigue roared back, so I restarted amoxicillin. I spoke to Tom Grier, the activist from Minnesota who was trained as a scientist and worked in pharmaceuticals. Grier told me he'd been sick for years until he ordered roxithromycin from Europe. In this one instance, I too ordered an antibiotic—roxithromycin—from Europe, and found it resolved my swallowing problem and put an end to the choking, but that was it, so after six weeks, I dumped roxithromycin and went on to something else.

Could Lyme form cysts? Just in case it did, I was treated with Flagyl. Could the spirochetes hide in cells? Whether or not they did, Biaxin combined with Plaquenil penetrated the body's cells and also worked for Lyme disease; for whatever reason, that drug cocktail alone relieved the infernal buzzing and tingling all over my body, detaching me finally from the neurological power grid of Lyme. By 2004, I felt I had peeled away many layers—but an infection or some kind of illness, *whatever it was* (and who really knew if it was Lyme disease now) seemed perpetually to lurk beneath. No matter what I did, when I stopped medicine altogether, a grinding fatigue and malaise always eventually returned.

I was describing the situation to Joe Burrascano during an interview when he stopped to tell me how he'd cured his *own* Lyme disease in 1998. He'd been on the antibiotic Ceftin for twenty-six months when, with all his symptoms finally gone, he decided to stop treatment cold. Slowly his Lyme disease returned, but instead of resuming treatment at the first sign of relapse, he'd let himself fall far back into illness before starting the Ceftin again. He repeated this cycle once, then again. "After the third cycle, which produced the strongest herx I had in years, the symptoms never came back," Burrascano said.

With my situation much like his—asymptomatic on treatment but relapsing when off—Burrascano conjectured that a few rounds of Ceftin might work for me as well. "Remember to let yourself fall to the bottom," he admonished. "Don't be afraid."

Be brave, I told myself silently after stopping the first round of Ceftin. *Courage,* I thought as the headaches and nausea, the brain fog and confusion, the fatigue and joint pain returned with a vengeance, as the buzzing intensified and I choked on my food and my fist reformed the claw. Back at square one, in bed, I restarted the Ceftin and treated three months to the abatement of symptoms—then let myself crash . . . down, down, down to the bottom of the Lyme pit, again.

Three times, Burrascano said.

With so many chronic patients who never got well no matter what the treatment, I feared I might fall down the deep dark well of Lyme, never to reemerge. Yet Burrascano had explained the premise, encouraging me to go on. Antibiotics like Ceftin killed spirochetes only when they were metabolizing nutrients. But the intensity of the attack also made spirochetes rush for cover, causing them to stop metabolizing or, he theorized, convert to hard-shelled cysts. A course of treatment therefore might kill some spirochetes but cause others to hide out, temporarily leaving the patient without any symptoms but still harboring the germ. Only when treatment stopped and the adversity was gone would the spirochetes return to normal, multiplying in number and causing the symptoms again. When symptoms were bad, then the infection was on the move, and antibiotic could kill spirochetes. So that's when you stealth-bombed them with Ceftin, dousing more spirochetes with each such onslaught until, you hoped and prayed, you killed them all. It was a grave mistake to keep the dose low, Burrascano had warned, because that would selectively kill the weaker, more reachable germs, leaving a stronger, deeper infection behind.

For two cycles running I was treated with high-dose Ceftin, then fell back down the Lyme hole. But after my third round of Ceftin, in December 2004, my Lyme symptoms left forever. There were no more relapses. I tossed my antibiotics. Like Joe Burrascano, I was well.

I knew my so-called cure proved nothing and could help no one but me. Just another patient story among the thousands already told, it existed outside science and beyond the pale of evidence in the vaguest nether reaches of Lyme. Standing on my terrace high above Stamford I glimpsed the red neon Target sign, *my* kind of bull's-eye. I could see the crisscross of roads with traffic, the people walking to movies or dinner at nearby cafés. Past the bustle of the city I saw the woods that held the deer that carried the ticks that transmitted the spirochetes. I now lived on concrete, but forest ringed the city like a crown of thorns. "We haven't moved far enough," I told Mark. We were out of the literal woods and I myself was well. But my boys were still sick and Lyme still held us captive. *After you take Lyme out of the girl,* I wondered ruefully, *could you ever take the girl out of Lyme?*

45

⬦

Pay It Forward

Colorado Springs, Colorado, 2005

For Dave Martz, purging his nightmare year and just moving on was unthinkable. If he'd learned anything from his father, the minister, it was the need to give back. So in February 2005, seemingly rid of ALS and recovered from Lyme disease (though at 85 percent of his former stamina) he decided to open the Rocky Mountain Chronic Disease Specialists, a practice aimed at treating folks like himself, with Lyme-like versions of ALS. Such patients had all been diagnosed with atypical versions of motor neuron disease. In general, they were younger than the average ALS patient (who was late middle age), with rheumatic problems, major pain, sensory neuropathy, and cognitive dysfunction. Many experts held that such patients really always had severe forms of Lyme disease and that the ALS label was a mistake—but not Martz. Instead, he theorized that these were usually cases in which true ALS had been triggered by Lyme.

The literature now was rife with reports of such anomalies: Lyme-triggered Parkinson's had been reported, as had Lyme-associated Alzheimer's. And there was the older work on Lyme-like ALS from the neurologist John Halperin at Stony Brook. A third of the Halperin patients had responded positively to antibiotics, as had Martz himself.

"I took my inspiration from *Field of Dreams*: Build it and they will come," Martz states. And indeed people did come, more than Martz could handle alone. Soon he was hiring staff, including a physician assistant.

William Harvey himself came out from Houston to work in the new practice three days a week. A neurologist was hired part-time. The crew trained with the likes of Joe Burrascano and Charles Ray Jones.

The patients themselves, Martz adds, were highly credible. They'd been dismissed by other physicians but not by Martz. "Many were extremely successful in their own fields, some of them very wealthy, before they ever got to me." In fact, the patients who found Martz often arrived from across the country or around the world—to get there, to even *know* about Martz in his little corner of Colorado, meant they had to have resources, intellectual or financial, or be blessed with sophisticated friends.

Before long Martz was learning more about this patient group from the clinical perspective than had ever been known. For one thing, they had to be treated very early in the game—usually before they lost the ability to walk—or as Halperin found with the sickest such patients, the treatment might do nothing but make them worse and rush them toward death. For another, these people had to start treatment slowly, at doses lower than for ordinary Lyme patients. True, Martz himself had recovered on large doses of Rocephin, but he'd been the exception. Such doses could give patients herxes so violent they might not get through them; in contrast, as long as the patient came in early enough in the course of illness, the smaller dose might work. "Slow and steady wins the race," Martz states.

One young man who sought Martz out was referred by his physical therapist in Illinois. He was so ill he was wheelchair-bound. He could walk three or four steps at most, and had trouble speaking and swallowing. Meeting the patient for the first time over lunch, Martz was troubled by the degree of his debility, yet because the man could still walk, even if haltingly, Martz agreed to take him on. So he treated him with Rocephin and evoked "a wonderful response from that level of disease." He improved so much that eventually he was able to walk some 200 steps on his own and took a vacation in Disneyland. Sadly, he died suddenly from something unrelated to either ALS or Lyme disease—blood clots in his legs.

Another patient, a woman, came from Albuquerque. Wheelchair-bound, she could not even get on the exam table without several people pitching in to lift her up. In addition to clear motor neuron disease, she had arthritic symptoms, severe pain, and cognitive problems. Martz put her on a regimen of antibiotic and had her take a hotel room in Colorado Springs for a couple of weeks so he could monitor her closely. "Two weeks after she arrived I saw someone ambulating through the parking lot with a walker. It was her!" Martz says. Today the woman from Albuquerque can walk without a walker or even a cane. "She's up and around, continuing her life," says Martz.

This kind of success occurs with just a percentage of the Lyme-like ALS patients who have sought Martz out. Of the 130 such patients that Martz has treated, he's helped 30 achieve subjective improvement; half a dozen have had a striking return to relative health. Yet only a few, including the woman from Albuquerque, have resumed anything like normal function. In fact, none of the patients achieved the spectacular response of Martz himself. "They all came in sicker than I was when I started the therapy," Martz states. That, he says, is the key. As a doctor with connections and exquisite access to the cutting edge, he was able to get ahead of the curve to get well.

As for Martz himself, health is sustained only if the treatment goes on. He's tried to cut the IV cord periodically, but without his Rocephin, Mepron, and Zithromax, has found himself rapidly sinking into the symptomatology of Lyme, babeosis, and ALS. As soon as the infusions stop, stamina plummets and the whisper of fasciculation returns. "My disease is still there," says Martz. "It's suppressed, but not cured."

46

A Family Affair

Framingham, Massachusetts, 2005

If the fall from health had been slow torture for the Statlenders, the climb back up was excruciating. For three years running they had been treated with the range of antibiotics proffered by their doctors, taking the roller-coaster tour through the hairpin turns and double-down dips of Lyme. They were healthier and stronger now than they had been in years, but progress had been erratic, and they still had so far to go.

For one thing, Eric's case had not proved as simple as they had hoped in those first, flush months, when his pain and auditory processing deficit had given way swiftly to the treatment. He had, since that period, plateaued, and his illness, though not as disabling as Seth's and Amy's, proved stubborn. There was profound fatigue, light sensitivity, insomnia, headaches, and flare-ups of full-blown disease. There were days when he could not get out of bed or get to school, not even the little Montessori program which, gentle as it was, ultimately proved too much for him.

Though needle-phobic, Eric finally followed the lead of Seth and Amy, embarking upon intravenous antibiotic treatment, too. And from that point forward, says Sheila, he steadily began to improve—as long as he didn't push things, he could live his life, home school, have friends. Even as he got better, Eric, like his siblings, was finally testing floridly positive on a Western blot, meeting CDC criteria for late-stage Lyme.

Almost thirteen, he announced that he wanted a bar mitzvah. He longed to read his Torah portion in front of his friends and family in the synagogue he'd attended since he was small, and he wanted to party later on. Sheila and Russell agreed, although not without some trepidation.

"I could not believe we were planning a bar mitzvah when our children were so sick," Sheila recalls. "But Eric wanted it very much."

On IV Rocephin for a few months, he was healthy enough that June to go through with the ceremony—but it was perhaps even more remarkable that Seth and Amy, who'd been sick for so long, got through the hectic day. "They were both so pale and thin," Sheila recalls, and Amy's arm was bruised from the recent placement of an intravenous port. Seth, newly infected some months before on a fishing trip, had suffered a severe relapse requiring a second round of IV antibiotic. "His Lyme Western blot lit up again like a Christmas tree," Sheila recalls.

Sheila was amazed that Seth had the energy to run the bar mitzvah's poker tournament, a task of focus and energy that had recently seemed beyond him.

It was a harbinger of more good things to come. Not only was he working ever more hours at the outdoor supply store, he was also focused enough to read extensively for the first time in years. Following his passion, he consumed all he could about ecology, natural habitats, and the arcane rules of fly fishing—how to choose and attach the flies, how to cast the line, and which kinds of bait would work best at which Massachusetts riverbeds for the maximum payoff in pike, salmon, and trout. When customers came for fishing supplies, they consulted Seth not just on fly rods and tackle but also on which shallow flats and tidal rivers were home to the best striped bass and bluefish in the state.

When Seth won two large poker tournaments, each one carrying a significant monetary prize, it represented a show of strategic thinking that would have been difficult for him not so long before. Sheila had to admit that, compared to the deck she thought he'd been dealt, things were looking up.

47

⋯⋄⋯

Red-Flagged at Blue Cross: The Role of Managed Care

Wherever I went, Lyme patients asked me how this could have *happened* to them—what in the world explained the rejection, the intransigence of the medical establishment, and the weirdness of their plight? Some believed in conspiracy: Lyme was a secret government experiment gone awry and now part of a cover-up; Lyme was a bioweapon, a mutant microbe that had escaped from Plum Island; Lyme was the sinister effort of a One World Government to enslave us by infecting our yards and dulling our minds. If any conspiracy existed, I never found proof of it. Instead, I found a money trail, and it was hardly hidden.

Why did it not surprise me that the 800-pound gorilla was managed care? It only makes sense. The greatest economic force working against Lyme patients is the astronomical cost of long-term treatment. The CDC's unpublished school study said it all: Treating a case of late-stage disseminated Lyme disease could cost $100,000. And as in our family, where one Lyme patient existed, a sibling or parent who'd dabbled in the same ecosystem and was likewise infected might not be far behind.

In the early days of the epidemic, before anyone grasped the scope of the problem, insurance companies could be flexible about treatment for Lyme disease, covering many weeks or months of intravenous Rocephin, and paying for a hospital stay to boot. But as the number of Lyme cases increased, cost became enormous, and the insurers rebelled. By August 1992, Prudential, Metropolitan Life, and Blue Cross Blue Shield of New

Jersey, among others, had imposed an intravenous antibiotic limit of twenty-eight days.

The policy was endorsed by Steere, whose treatment guidelines appeared in *Transactions of the American Academy of Insurance Medicine* in 1993. In a paper written for insurance company medical directors, Steere urged use of the CDC surveillance definition for diagnosis and stated that "all stages of the infection" could generally be successfully treated in ten to thirty days.

By 1995, the landscape of Lyme was littered with letters from the desperate and destitute begging their insurers for one more month of medication. The fallout from the denials became unmistakable, as thousands of patients who had responded to therapy fell back into illness and others could not get treatment at all.

Lest anyone think that insurers were simply following the trail of science—or what they thought was science—evidence shows that by the middle of the 1990s, Lyme disease had been "red-flagged" at the highest levels of insurance and managed care companies as a draining expense. As the true cost became clear, these companies established cost-containment policies for Lyme disease. While denials could sometimes be appealed, the appeal process was long, arduous, and often unsuccessful. By the time a patient was approved, if that ever occurred, the illness might have progressed to a far more debilitating stage, to the brain.

Much of what we know about the machinations of managed care comes to us from a lawsuit involving Ken Liegner's patient, Vicki Logan, and others who were refused antibiotic therapy by their New York insurer, Empire Blue Cross Blue Shield. The suit was settled out of court, in Logan's case, netting the means to pay Liegner's sizable unpaid bill, though not approval for treatment with IV. More important, it managed to obtain a deposition, under oath, from the architect of the plan, Empire's former chief medical executive and vice president, Dr. Richard Sanchez. Back in the early 1990s, Sanchez had belonged to a group called "the California Posse," known for revamping managed care out West. Hired by Empire to do the same in New York, he arrived in 1995 to find the company in dire straits. "They were losing money on every member they enrolled," said Sanchez, whose road map to profit was outlined in a report commissioned from the big-four accounting firm Deloitte & Touche. The problem at Empire, said the accountants, was rooted in corporate culture: Empire reviewers were just "not aggressive enough" to confront treating doctors and turn down their requests.

Deloitte & Touche had some solutions. One was an incentive plan that paid company employees and physician reviewers as well as treating doctors *more* when they restricted treatment and turned down claims. From the family pediatrician to the insurance company nurse, success in restricting payouts would mean financial reward. As an adjunct to this, Deloitte & Touche recommended focusing on the small number of diagnoses accounting for the greatest outlay: diabetes, heart disease, cancer, asthma, neonatal care, and Lyme disease.

Before Sanchez arrived, the company's standard for the Lyme diagnosis had been vague and its willingness to treat somewhat open-ended. But under the new mandate Sanchez endeavored to tighten things up. One costly treatment, in particular, caught his attention: the intravenous antibiotic Rocephin. In the wake of the accounting report, Sanchez required patients who wanted Rocephin to meet three conditions: documentation of an erythema migrans rash or some other explicit evidence of a tick bite; seropositivity on an ELISA screening test followed by confirmation with Western blot, à la Dearborn; and finally, all other possible explanations for the illness had to be investigated and ruled out.

The requirements set a higher bar, by far, than the surveillance standard established by the CDC. Requiring the same individual to have *both* a physician-diagnosed rash and a positive Western blot meant that large numbers of textbook-classic patients would be ruled out. After all, any physician who diagnosed a rash also treated it, unless that physician was negligent. Yet rash patients who failed treatment and went on to late-stage disease generally tested negative because antibiotics given so early blunted the immune response, a peculiarity proven at Stony Brook a few years before. Thus, a patient who met both requirements was rare. The rare patient who qualified would *first* receive six weeks of oral antibiotic. Only then, if still sick, would the patient receive the IV. Since the disease was progressive and could cause permanent damage, including brain damage, the stakes in the Lymelands were now higher than ever.

Was Sanchez aware of the Stony Brook findings when he instituted the policy? asked the lawyer conducting the deposition, a Westchester resident named Ira Maurer and a Lyme patient himself.

Yes, indeed, Sanchez testified. They'd "tightened up the definition and diagnosis . . . fully understanding that there would be people who thought they had Lyme disease or had been treated for Lyme disease or who were seronegative who were not going to meet the criteria."

But did Sanchez grasp the risk involved? "Doctor, what's your understanding as to how fast Lyme bacteria can spread from the location of the tick bite to the brain?" Maurer pressed.

"It can be as short as a week and as long as six weeks," Sanchez replied under oath. "My understanding of the subject currently is that aggressive intravenous administration very early on in any suspected dissemination of the disease is the appropriate choice."

Yet the patient with central nervous system Lyme disease early in the course of infection was out of luck. Although Sanchez said he understood the oral regimens could pass the blood-brain barrier only "poorly," with "intravenous agents much more successful," the patient in need of Rocephin would be turned down for six critical weeks. "It was our policy not to approve," Sanchez explained.

"Are you aware of any particular scientific or medical justification for the policy?" Maurer had asked.

"No," Sanchez said. "We clearly knew that some patients would not fit the classic policy or definition . . . We expected those patients to rise up through the appellate system and therefore not fall through the cracks."

Yet patient after patient, Maurer's clients included, had spent months or years appealing to Empire and other insurers as their central nervous system disease progressed. Many had never recovered as a result. Wasn't part of the calculus for profit the assumption that not every deserving patient would appeal?

"Any time you put up a hurdle, certain people will fight to get over it and others will accept it and not appeal," Sanchez agreed. That was "common knowledge," he explained.

The Sanchez reign at Empire was not a happy one. Despite the potential for personal profit, the company's longtime physicians lacked the "stomach, heart, or will" to deny so many claims, Sanchez said. They just could not operate under the new rules and sleep at night. Helping to make decisions about Lyme treatment in their stead were a stream of consultants, the same doctors who authored the papers on "Lyme hysteria" and "pseudo Lyme." Leonard Sigal, for instance, consulted for Prudential, Aetna, Blue Cross Blue Shield, Anthem, and Metropolitan Life, passing diagnostic and treatment decrees. His fee was $560 an hour in 1996, though he worked for a day rate as well. Sigal was not alone: Other top academics consulted, too. The consultancy fees would "pay for a lot of college tuition, actually," Sigal had quipped under oath, when testifying against a patient's diagnosis of Lyme.

In the end, at Empire and insurance companies everywhere, nurses and doctors who accepted the new order stayed on, and those disturbed by the rules or more sympathetic to the patients did not. It was only the patients who had no choice. The world of managed care had reconfigured medicine around them, forging a harsher, less sympathetic realm. But unless they were independently wealthy and could pay out-of-pocket, Lyme patients had nowhere else to turn.

By 1999, when the State of Connecticut held a legislative hearing on the insurance problem, denial of claims for Lyme treatment had reached a pitch. Letters of appeal to insurance companies, on file in the Connecticut State House, are heartbreaking—many patients mortgaged their houses and went into debt to pay for the antibiotics they said ultimately made them well. Others, denied coverage, became permanently impaired. As the decade came to an end it was virtually impossible to find a doctor within a managed-care network willing to treat Lyme disease for more than a month.

Testifying before the New York legislature in Albany in November 2001, LDA's Pat Smith said that the environment of managed care had cast a pall over Lyme. If doctors treated patients who fell outside the CDC surveillance criteria, insurers threatened to drop them. Most doctors, fearing reprisals or economic hardship, referred patients to the few who were still willing to take them on.

Throughout Lyme country, the power of insurers was intimidating and all too real. Dr. Alan Muney, chief medical officer for Oxford Health Plans, also testified at the Albany hearing. Oxford monitored Lyme treatment as a matter of course, he explained, taking its guidance from the treatment study published by Mark Klempner in the *New England Journal of Medicine* that July. If there was a "quality problem," including inappropriate treatment or overtreatment, Oxford might require the physician to undergo continuing medical education, Muney said. But when the doctor refused to change, he was dropped from the network and reported to the disciplinary board of his state.

"How do you explain the body of evidence you've selected, which says that they keep getting cured when, unfortunately, the cure doesn't last?" demanded Assemblyman Joel Miller of Poughkeepsie, a dentist, disturbed by Muney's stance.

"We could pay for injecting hot ascorbic acid into festering wounds if you like," Muney retorted. "But there is no evidence to say that that's the appropriate treatment. If everyone wants insurance companies to cover that, the premium will go up as a result."

It was the same year that Kenneth Liegner opened his mailbox to find a letter marked "personal and confidential" from the New York State Department of Health. "I knew right away what it was," says Liegner, recalling a chart that had been ominously requested by authorities the year before. Picking up the phone, he called the family in question to see if they had filed a complaint. No, they had not, said the patient's mother. But Liegner might be interested to learn that their family physician, who had administered long-acting benthazine penicillin on Liegner's advice, was under investigation as well.

If neither the family nor their primary care doctor had filed the complaint, then who had? Reviewing the patient's chart, Liegner noted something odd. In 1998, when he'd recommended the long-acting benzathine penicillin to the patient, he had promptly received a communication from Prudential/Aetna Pharmacy Benefit Managers demanding justification for the medication. "I supplied this in a letter of medical necessity citing references from the medical literature," Liegner recalls. He prescribed the same medicine to the patient in 2000, and again was contacted by the plan requesting that he explain his choice. "Unless I am missing something, it would appear that the only possible source of any complaint against me was the insurance company," Liegner says.

With his encyclopedic patient records and penchant for scouting diagnoses far outside the Lyme box, Liegner could brave the challenge.

It wasn't Ken Liegner, but his patient, Vicki Logan, who'd reached the end of the line. Her situation was desperate, and if he didn't intervene, she would die.

Ever since Liegner brought Vicki Logan around with 109 days of continuous IV antibiotic in 1993, he'd been on the case, collecting evidence for B. burgdorferi infection from her serum, cerebrospinal fluid, and other bodily tissues, and treating her aggressively with intravenous antibiotics when her status declined.

For many years, all that evidence had served Liegner and Logan alike. For Liegner, it was validating and a documentation of his theories. For Logan, it was the entrée to additional courses of treatment with intravenous antibiotics, which pushed her symptoms back. A partner in all of this prior to the arrival of Richard Sanchez was Logan's insurer, Empire Blue Cross Blue Shield, whose doctors and nurses were willing to authorize further courses of treatment, providing Ken Liegner could supply them with evidence that the infection was still alive.

Right from the start, Ken Liegner communicated to Empire his radical stance: "I believe Vicki requires open-ended intravenous cefotaxime for the foreseeable future," he wrote to Mary Berlin, a company case manager, in July 1993. "I know this seems to be an incredible situation but all I can tell you is these are the facts of her case. In my opinion antibiotic treatment is no solution to Lyme disease but it is the best we

have available at the present time for averting otherwise relentless neurological deterioration which has the potential to lead to death."

Sherwood P. Miller, assistant medical director of Medical Policy and
Research at Empire Blue Cross Blue Shield, would not approve open-
ended infusion therapy for Vicki Logan, as Liegner requested. "If she relapses and requires more antibiotic treatment by IV, another authorization
should be requested," Miller said. Still, as the months and years passed,
the two doctors reached an understanding.

In July 1994, for instance, Liegner informed Miller that Logan had
"deteriorated markedly since intravenous antibiotic therapy was discon-
tinued" several months earlier. "Now that she has been without treatment
for some 6+ months she has begun to develop severe polyarthralgias [pain
that travels from one joint to the next]. She has never previously manifested this symptom; to me it is a clear clinical indicator of progressing
disease. . . . I ask you at Blue Cross/Blue Shield to reconsider your position regarding intravenous antibiotic therapy in this unfortunate and severely affected woman's case."

Miller, who was not without compassion, approved three months of
treatment in response.

And so it went. Liegner documented the disease, one way or another,
year in and year out, and the insurer, in turn, approved treatment when
the decline seemed severe. Always, Liegner argued for an open-ended approach that might circumvent the relapses. Always, Miller and his colleagues parsed the therapy out a few weeks or months at a time.

But by the summer of 1995, Sherwood P. Miller and his faction at
Empire were no more. The California posse had arrived, and things had
changed. Logan's case did not meet "managed care guidelines," Empire
now said, refusing Liegner's requests. As the months passed and the letters flew back and forth, Vicki Logan deteriorated. So Ken Liegner admitted her to Northern Westchester Hospital, treating her aggressively,
come what may. Between November 1996 and April 1997, for six
months, he kept her in the hospital, and slowly brought her back. As before, she improved dramatically with treatment, but when Empire refused to reimburse the hospital, leaving a $175,000 debt, Northern
Westchester was forced to absorb it.

It was in the fall of 1997, in the wake of another frightening dive,
that Empire approved Logan for three months of treatment one last
time. Again her improvement was impressive, but with the cessation of
treatment, the slide was just as swift. Would Empire consider extending
it? "This particular patient requires prolonged, perhaps open-ended

intravenous antibiotic therapy. On-again off-again treatment, which has been all that has been possible in her case, has allowed her to progressively deteriorate, her illness unchecked," Liegner wrote.

The treatment was "experimental," Empire wrote back, insisting it needed absolute evidence of active infection with a specific disease before it would authorize more intravenous antibiotic. For a year Logan went untreated as Liegner conducted test after test, trying to find the proof. As the months passed, Logan became desperately sick, developing a life-threatening case of aspiration pneumonia, a problem Liegner attributed to infection of the cranial nerves. She'd experienced the same problem before, Liegner wrote to Empire in October 1998, "and it was felt mandatory to resume intravenous antibiotic treatment aimed at Lyme disease even though we did not then have proof of active infection with the Lyme organism. With such treatment she made dramatic recovery. Had we waited to institute therapy until we had unequivocal proof of active Lyme infection . . . she very likely would have died." Given Logan's status as a CDC-proven case of chronic Lyme, with multiple past tests showing persisting infection despite intensive treatment, Liegner implored Empire to relent. Yet even when Logan tested positive for *B. burgdorferi* DNA on a new test, and when scientists at the University of Pennsylvania found Lyme antigens in her spinal fluid, Empire refused.

"At your request she has received over 23 months of intravenous antibiotic since 1991," Empire's senior medical director, Franklin L. Brosgol, M.D., wrote to Liegner in July 2000. "The duration of her treatment far exceeds the course of treatment recognized by medical authorities as sufficient to eradicate the *B. burgdorferi* causing Lyme disease." In essence, in order to consider more treatment, Empire needed proof of active infection not through the presence of antibodies or even DNA (despite studies showing it was synonymous with living infection) but in the form of motile, living spirochetes—a feat accomplished in spinal fluid perhaps 10 percent of the time at best, even in the most classic and incontrovertible cases of patients with central nervous system Lyme. Empire would be happy to pay the Mayo Clinic to search Logan's fluids for the bugs.

It was early in 2002 that Ken Liegner began to get all his "ducks in a row" with the intent of preparing "the mother of all letters of medical necessity" for Empire Blue Cross Blue Shield in the Logan case. He had collected new specimens of blood and cerebrospinal fluid, sending them out to multiple labs and hoping he might find some evidence of active infection with which to jump-start the treatment again.

But the relationship between Logan and Empire abruptly came to an end. A family member forgot to mail the premium, and she was unceremoniously dumped from the plan. Without another insurer, she'd become a client of Medicaid. Vicki Logan was now insured by New York State.

In the wake of all this, Liegner admitted Logan to his hospital, Northern Westchester, one last time with the intent of treating her with intravenous antibiotic for months on end, as before. But without a guarantee that Medicaid would cover and with the old debt still unpaid, the hospital called for a review. It was the Ethics Committee itself that held the treatment wasn't "a wise use of scarce resources." Liegner was ordered to discharge Vicki Logan to a nursing home.

That May, Liegner arranged to meet with the Office of Medicaid Management at the New York State Department of Health on Logan's behalf. He was already under investigation by the department for overtreating Lyme disease, in danger of going to trial and even losing his license. But now that Logan was insured by the state he was determined to take them on, nonetheless. Logan was dying, he said. Why couldn't they give her the benefit of the doubt, *even now?* His frustration was fueled by more than Logan alone. She was not unique. It was Liegner who saw the sickest of the Lyme patients, their lives winnowing away while treatment was withheld; it was Liegner himself who needed the help. Chronic Lyme cases were piling up all around him—and the agents of their triage, their plight, were insurers. "Care is too expensive, so the best approach is to 'let 'em rot,'" he said. New York State wanted nothing more than to hang Ken Liegner from the rafters, something he understood. Yet his distress was so visceral he really didn't care if his intervention now might sink him later on.

The moment Ken Liegner entered the conference room at the DOH headquarters, the atmosphere was charged. "This is a dying woman," Liegner told the officials. "She's on a trajectory to death without intervention. She has documented chronic Lyme disease that improves with treatment." He asked for three to six months of IV antibiotic to start but added that "open-ended treatment would be best."

Thomas R. Fanning, director of the Division of Policy and Program Guidance, Office of Medicaid Management, pointed out that the treatment was experimental. Perhaps Kenneth Liegner didn't grasp the concept of medical necessity, Fanning added. A nursing home, like an HMO, like Medicaid itself, was legally bound to pay for necessary care, no matter what the cost. But "nine out of ten external reviewers would look at the facts in the Logan case and vote for denial of the treatment," Fanning said.

"If you say you'll pay for the treatment, I can treat her," responded Liegner. "My patients need help. One is a Vietnam veteran who had an erythema migrans rash and is now in a nursing home. He calls me every week." Suddenly, despite his best intentions to stay calm at the meeting, Liegner's face reddened and his outrage was clear. "These people are lepers, financial liabilities that no one will go near. You have the means to help them." Now he was yelling at the health department officials: "I will not allow this patient to die for lack of treatment. I will not allow it!" he boomed.

Fanning's face, too, was red, but his voice was measured and soft. "She's in a nursing home, with a treating physician. You are not the player." Vicki Logan wasn't Liegner's patient anymore, but his former patient, Fanning was pointing out. One alternative, Fanning suggested, would be transferring Logan back to Liegner's hospital, Northern Westchester, for care—only when the hospital requested payment could Medicaid even consider it.

But that was an impossible dilemma, Liegner explained, "because the hospital has already thrown her out. If I transfer her back they'll sanction me and remove my privileges, and then they'll send her packing without any treatment anyway."

But that was *Liegner's* problem, warned another official at the meeting, Foster Gesten, M.D., medical director for the Office of Managed Care in New York. Since only Liegner believed in the treatment, it was Liegner, and Liegner alone, who was ethically bound to see to it, Liegner who would be held accountable if the treatment was never dispensed and if, as a result, Logan died, Gesten said, whether Liegner was officially Logan's doctor or not. "You could be charged with negligence," Gesten told Liegner, looking him right in the eye.

"I'm already under investigation for *treating* these patients," Liegner said.

Gesten shrugged.

In the weeks after the meeting in Albany, Ken Liegner secured privileges to treat at Treetops Nursing Home, becoming Vicki Logan's physician of record once more. In that capacity, he treated her with three weeks of intravenous Claforan before Treetops, awaiting approval from New York State Medicaid, asked Liegner to hold off.

In July 2003, as Liegner appealed to Medicaid, Logan suffered three grand mal seizures and was moved to Hudson Valley Hospital Center in

Cortlandt Manor, New York. She died there of a myocardial infarction on July 17, 2003. It was Logan herself, in death, who stood poised to settle the debate about her own chronic Lyme disease. Did she have it, as Liegner said, or not, as her insurers insisted was the case? Following in the footsteps of Lyme's worst nightmares, Logan had arranged in life to be sectioned during autopsy and made into slides, her brain and other body organs dispatched to centers of research, where the hunt for spirochetes could commence. Yet even in death Vicki Logan was rejected, with the Hudson Valley Hospital pathologist unequivocally refusing to perform the autopsy and make the slides.

"She could still be infectious," the pathologist said. Hospital administrators backed the pathologist in his decision: Given the chronic Lyme, they agreed, the procedure wasn't safe.

Incredulous that Hudson Valley Hospital would refuse to perform an autopsy, Liegner placed a call to psychiatrist Brian Fallon at Columbia. Fallon arranged for the neuropathologist at the Columbia Presbyterian Medical Center in New York City to perform the autopsy, and Logan journeyed deeper into the Lymelands, again. When Columbia pathologist Jenny Libien peered inside Logan's brain, she found "lymphocytes and plasma cells throughout, indicating a chronic and ongoing process." Inflammation of the blood vessels was profound, and lesions were noted through the white-and-gray matter of the brain. Evidence for cell death in the white matter of the frontal lobes was widespread. With damage and inflammation so extensive Libien couldn't find spirochetes, but she did find Logan's brain consistent with autopsies of other chronic neuroborreliosis patients of the past. "To the pathologist, this picture is beautiful and horrible," Libien said. "The next time someone tells you it's all in your head, picture this."

Libien sent forty-two slides of Vicki Logan's brain to the National Institutes of Health, where pathologist Paul Duray had a look. "We've never seen anything like it at NIH before," said Duray. Given the grotesque level of damage and all that swelling, finding intact *Borrelia* in Logan's brain may have been impossible, akin to finding "a two-foot-tall volcano somewhere in the continental United States. But just because we didn't find it, doesn't mean it wasn't there."(Logan's brain is under study to this day.)

"Vicki Logan was killed by a system that rejected her," Ken Liegner says. Off the grid and beyond anyone's road map, she lived and died in New York.

48

✥

The Vaccine Connection:
Lyme Gets a Business Model

Insurance medicine was an ugly fact of life in Lyme, but just as damaging and far more insidious was the effort of another giant industry, pharmaceuticals, to extract *its* share of profit by producing a Lyme vaccine. By studying big pharma's decade-long effort to bring a Lyme vaccine to market, it's possible to see the circumscribed Dearborn test standard and denial of chronic Lyme in a new, more disturbing light.

The seed was planted in 1980, when Congress passed the Bayh-Dole Act giving universities and their faculty members permission to stake patent claims on discoveries they made through research funded by federal agencies such as the National Institutes of Health. Instead of leaving the ownership of intellectual property with government, the scientists now had a chance to be stakeholders and entrepreneurs themselves. The new law accelerated the rate of academic breakthroughs like gene splicing, gave rise to three-way partnerships between government, universities, and start-up firms, and spawned the modern biotech industry almost overnight. By the early 1990s, university scientists were scrambling to patent genes, proteins, and organisms, hoping to launch products and profit from the discoveries they made.

In Lyme disease, the main product of interest was a vaccine aimed at restoring ease in the great outdoors. Toward that end, big pharma made millions of dollars in Lyme vaccine grant money available to scientists; when Lyme researchers applied for government funding, a vaccine was often in the crosshairs of their view. It logically followed that many of the top researchers would apply for vaccine-related patents and launch vaccine-related start-up companies while others would become big pharma consultants, garnering sizable grants for conducting vaccine studies at their university labs. As the years went on, it only made sense that the big decisions regarding Lyme disease—the paradigmatic issues like the literal disease definition and the exact serological pattern needed for diagnosis—would take the patents and future viability of the products into account. As in the rest of biomedicine, the scientists making those decisions were, by and large, stakeholders. Their partnership with industry was business as usual in the scientific culture of the day.

In many other diseases, the interests of the patients and commercialization of the products had somehow managed to converge. There was a confluence of interest and one hand seemed to wash the other. Yet Lyme was a special case: Moving a product past the obstacles to FDA approval required great exactitude, while the equivocal status of many Lyme patients and the many strains of the Lyme organism could thwart that goal. To prove a vaccine effective, investigators had to be able to tell the difference between people who suffered infection and those who had reacted badly to the vaccine itself. The more flexible the definition of the disease—and thus, the more uncertainty associated with diagnosis—the more difficult this became. Lyme diagnosis often *was* uncertain—"shades of gray," Leonard Sigal had said—yet writing that reality into the development of a new vaccine could derail its approval.

On top of that, *B. burgdorferi*'s talent for altering its outer coat made it a poor candidate for vaccination in any usual sense. Most modern vaccines work by a simple method. A surface protein from the germ is multiplied through molecular technology and injected into the body. Our immune cells generate antibodies against the protein. Should the actual microbe later attack, the preexisting antibodies would latch on to the surface and wipe the infection out.

But the quick-change artist *B. burgdorferi,* which morphed continuously from tissue to tissue and over time, was far too nimble for such tricks. By the time the body made antibodies against any one protein, the spirochete would morph into something else. In fact, as scientists searched for vaccine candidates, only one *B. burgdorferi* protein appeared to protect mice against Lyme infection—outer surface protein (Osp) A. To Steve Barthold, then of Yale and an inventor of the OspA vaccine, this made perfect sense. It might be impossible to immunize a mammal against Lyme disease, but you *could* immunize a tick, where most spirochetes live in the midgut and don an unchanging coat made virtually exclusively of OspA. When a tick bit a mammal "vaccinated" with OspA it would ingest a surge of blood laced with the OspA antibody. The antibody would rush to the tick's midgut, killing most of the spirochetes on the spot before they could flow back and infect the human host. Because some strains of the spirochete lacked OspA, the vaccine wasn't foolproof; because it took days for a total kill inside the tick itself, there was a small window of opportunity for infection to spread, reducing the efficacy overall. Even so, industry executives thought that the OspA vaccine was a clever invention, representing a creative solution to the confounding complexities of Lyme.

It didn't take long for two competing pharmaceutical giants— SmithKline Beecham and Pasteur Merieux Connaught—to launch two potential products. The Connaught effort, with the clinical trial headed by Leonard Sigal, was killed by the company in the wake of lawsuits over side effects. But the SmithKline vaccine, with Steere leading the study, promised to make it through the pipeline at FDA.

It was in 1998 that Steere announced the success of his large-scale clinical trial for the vaccine called LYMErix in the *New England Journal of Medicine*. There was just one fly in the ointment, and it was a whopper: Steere was elsewhere proposing that OspA, the active ingredient of his vaccine, was the specific trigger for chronic Lyme.

Steere's chronic Lyme theory was based on the same molecular mimicry concept suggested by Klempner. In an act of scientific integrity, Steere even published evidence for the controversial theory in the prestigious journal *Science* the week after the release of the vaccine results— much to the ire of the manufacturer, by then called GlaxoSmithKline. Steere and Tufts immunologist Brigitte T. Huber had found a striking resemblance between a portion of the OspA molecule and the human protein LFA-1. Antibodies against OspA, Steere theorized, might mistakenly attack LFA-1 in human cells—and would continue attacking even after the infection was gone. Steere had traced the suspect human protein to the common arthritis-linked gene, HLA-DR4, which was found in a third of the population, making risk of the reaction high.

The theory provoked skepticism. Barthold, Weis, and Philipp, researchers with intimate knowledge of infection and immunity, describe some cross-reactivity with almost every microbe. Just because one molecule resembles another doesn't mean it fuels disease. Not even Steere, who felt he'd done his due diligence in alerting the world to the theory, could prove it was correct. (He's currently searching for an alternate autoimmune "trigger" to explain chronic Lyme.) *Could* the OspA vaccine drive a few unlucky recipients to autoimmune disease? Steere hadn't seen it in the vaccine trial, but found it "an issue of concern. If OspA vaccination induces joint symptoms, it must be a rare phenomenon," Steere said. But when a contingent of LYMErix vaccinees popped up to say they'd been damaged by Glaxo's vaccine through the mechanism of Steere's theory, the stage was set for a debacle worthy of Lyme.

At first the FDA approved LYMErix anyway, sending it off to market in December 1998 and declaring a leap into the unknown. "Those who did the trial," said Vanderbilt professor David Karzon, a member of FDA's LYMErix panel, "have unearthed some very interesting sinister possibilities that may or may not be real."

Yet by January 2001, amidst a hailstorm of LYMErix lawsuits, the FDA had reconvened on LYMErix at the Bethesda Holiday Inn. Among the presenters were a small army of vaccinees who said they'd been badly hurt. There was Emily Biegel, who addressed the panel for her husband, John, vaccinated in April and May of 1999. "Some of you may have seen him come in with a walker," she said. "An active outdoorsman before vaccination, John has since been through four hospitalizations, atrophy, insulin dependence, compression fractures, tremors, and twenty-five plasmapheresis treatments. He is positive for HLA-DR4."

Jenny Marra, a New Jersey hospice nurse positive for HLA-DR4, had been living with severe joint and muscle pain since vaccination in 1999. Glaxo, she complained, did not include a warning about the potential risk. "Had I known this I personally would not have taken the vaccine," she said.

Karen Burke, the mother of two toddlers from the Pocono Mountains of Pennsylvania, said that her husband, the vigorous owner of a construction business, got his second dose of LYMErix in July of 1999. By October, he couldn't roll over in bed. "My standing joke with him is, honey, at least when our kids are big enough to go to Disney World you'll be well enough to sit in a wheelchair, and we'll get to the front of the line. It's not funny, but you have to have some fun in your life," Burke said.

Stony Brook's Ben Luft, a panel member, described the "twilight zone" of the "disconnect" between patient testimony and Glaxo's denial of the adverse events.

Even Steere's scientific collaborator, Brigitte Huber, entered the fray after Karen Forschner of the Lyme Disease Foundation discovered that Huber had filed a World Trade Patent for a second OspA vaccine based on research funded by the NIH. The Huber patent, based on elaborate animal experiments, offered a genetically modified OspA molecule said to cause less of an autoimmune reaction than the OspA used to make LYMErix. Huber had literally assigned "binding scores" to the two OspA molecules, citing evidence that scores above a certain cutoff caused autoimmune disease. LYMErix tested above the cutoff, but the new molecule fell below. The patent "details the autoimmune mechanism as reality, not theory," Forschner said.

Despite all this, FDA officials ultimately kept LYMErix on the market in what it called "data-gathering mode," aimed at determining whether it caused irreversible autoimmune disease or other adverse events. The warning labels and package inserts reflected no special danger and remained unchanged.

With the vaccine still available at any suburban doc-in-the-box, the numbers of the vaccinated naturally soared. As more people were vaccinated, problems that were rare or avoidable in a screened population increasingly began to emerge. Not only were reports of more "autoimmune" cases coming out of the woodwork, but there was another problem as well: The vaccine appeared to awaken old, presumably "cured" cases of Lyme disease, Boston University's Sam Donta said. After he treated these patients with antibiotics, most got well—just as he would expect in bona fide cases of the disease.

But the confusion didn't stop there. As LYMErix recipients got tested for Lyme disease in the course of their ordinary lives, laboratorians around the country found their Western blots on fire, with almost every band lit. Discounting the OspA band on the Western blot had proved an insufficient precaution; even with that step taken virtually all vacinees tested positive for Lyme disease, whether they had the infection or not.

Paul Fawcett, director of the immunology laboratories at the Alfred I. duPont Hospital for Children in Wilmington, Delaware, and a noted expert on Lyme disease serology, observed the ability of the OspA vaccine to provoke a wide range of Borrelia-specific bands on Western blots well before the product reached market, as patients involved in clinical trials appeared for routine Lyme disease tests. Fascinated by the phenomenon, he coordinated a study of twenty adult volunteers, all employees of the hospital, who received three vaccine doses each and submitted blood for analysis. As it turned out, the elaborate banding patterns showed up in all but one subject in Fawcett's experimental group. In fact, the banding was so robust that thirty days after the second dose of vaccine, the only two commercial Western blots then approved by the FDA were "rendered virtually useless for diagnostic purposes," Fawcett says. "Many people were so reactive that they often showed fifteen to twenty bands," far more than the minimum requirement of five. What's more, Fawcett found that the odd patterns were sometimes accompanied by adverse events. Two of the twenty patients in his study developed severe arthritic pain, and the strange symptom—not generally seen in Lyme disease itself—of swelling hands, despite the fact that they had no exposure whatsoever to the spirochete.

What could be going on? Describing himself as a "fan of data," Fawcett reviewed his findings and concluded that the only explanation was a "hyperactivation" of the immune system after exposure to the vaccine. It was this activation, he felt, that accounted for adverse events.

The bizarre banding pattern was recorded as well by Philip J. Molloy, medical director of Imugen, the Massachusetts diagnostic laboratory identified by many in the mainstream as the sine qua non for diagnosing vector-borne disease, and David Persing, chief medical officer of Cepheid and one of the most respected microbiologists on the Lyme scene today. Their investigation, published in *Clinical Infectious Diseases,* concluded that the problem was not the vaccine, but the Western blot itself. Like everyone else, Molloy and Persing found that vaccination led to a complex pattern of multiple bands, including CDC diagnostic bands, on Western blots, making it difficult to determine which bands came from the vaccine and which ones from infection. "It was possible to tell whether or not they had been vaccinated," says Persing, "but not whether they had Lyme." Molloy suggested that the phenomenon was the result of instability of OspA—its degradation into smaller fragments and buildup into larger particles, resulting in Western blot tests with a diversity of bands that seemed to confirm the disease but actually meant nothing at all. One interesting implication of the finding, he theorized, was that even for those not vaccinated the banding pattern chosen at Dearborn represented nothing more than "an immune response to OspA, which is being 'counted' several times, while other bands presumed to be present are not really there at all." That would make the Western blot pattern chosen at Dearborn "irrelevant" for garden variety diagnosis, says Molloy.

As for GlaxoSmithKline, it never denied the existence of the dirty blots. "We would need more time for our scientists to study the papers and reports in depth," Glaxo communications director Carmel Hogan said at the time.

Whatever the explanation turns out to be, one wonders how researchers ever managed to differentiate between vaccine adverse reactions and Lyme disease itself. With such mixed-up results, how could they prove that the vaccine worked or that it was a vaccine at all? Researchers had tried their best to come up with a circumscribed serological definition for Lyme disease during the vaccine trials, but the utter messiness of Lyme, including all that was still unknown, may have tripped them up.

Hearing all the problems, patients couldn't help but wonder whether conflicts of interest, including potential for profit, had played a role in so much sloppiness and such a frenzied rush to market on their behalf. Thinking back over the years, they asked themselves whether the increasingly restrictive disease definition had been motivated by the vaccine. The thing that bothered Lyme patients most was the removal of the OspA and OspB markers from the diagnostic pattern chosen for the Western blot in Dearborn, Michigan, in 1994, just as the vaccine trials were getting under way. *Why* had the markers, so specific for Lyme they were vaccine candidates, *really* been purged from the Western blot? Was it to make sure vaccinees wouldn't test positive on Lyme tests? Was it a misguided effort to avoid all the confusion that the OspA molecule was causing now?

The Dearborn panel voting on the Western blot pattern had particular potential for bias. Indeed, the nine voting consultants hired by the CDC included a scientist holding the patent for OspA; the inventor of the canine Lyme vaccine, Lymevac; and Allen Steere, who was both an author of the study used to generate the hotly contested Dearborn standard as well as the lead investigator for clinical trials of the vaccine. It wasn't widely known, but the FDA had accepted Steere's so-called Dearborn criteria as the serological standard for the LYMErix trials months before the vote in Michigan ever took place.

The circumscribed view of the disease was extended, as well, to the influential *Clinical Treatment Guidelines* published by the Infectious Diseases Society of America (IDSA) in 2000. As the mainstream standard of care, the guidelines were embraced by insurers to cut antibiotic treatment for Lyme patients across the board. It's notable that eleven of the twelve IDSA panel members had economic interests related to the Lyme vaccines under development since 1993. These eleven scientists received Lyme vaccine research grants, had the potential to profit from patents and development of associated diagnostic kits, or participated in clinical trials. At least four members of the 2000 panel ran Lyme vaccine trials for manufacturers in aggregate involving some 14,000 patients, all for a fee. Of course the money would not line the pockets of the researchers directly, but it would add to the importance and viability of their labs.

Beyond individuals, many institutions had a financial interest in the success of LYMErix. U.S. government agencies, including the CDC, the National Institutes of Health, and the Department of Defense owned partial rights to revenue from more than a third of the fifty-six U.S. patents identified as especially significant for Lyme disease vaccines and tests. Companies with Lyme vaccine claims included the multinational life science giants Aventis and AstraZeneca as well as Abbott Laboratories, American Home Products, and Schering-Plough, to name a few. Yale, which held rights to the OspA patent, would have seen a windfall had the vaccine been a hit. The web of vested interest was intricate and vast.

In fact, you could see Lyme (like any other disease) through the lens of the business plans it generated. Reading through business proposals on file at the NIH, it's clear that OspA was supposed to be just a first step, one of many vaccines and test kits produced in lockstep, in an incremental plan. The next potential vaccine candidate was OspB, also removed as a diagnostic marker in the Dearborn vote. Projected revenues for the products add up to hundreds of millions of dollars annually in the United States and Europe, and there's no question but that the derailment of the OspA vaccine, LYMErix, would throw everything off track.

Why purge both OspA and OspB from the Western blot? One possible influence could be the vaccine: "There was the feeling that OspA would lose its diagnostic value with widespread use of LYMErix," points out Phillip J. Baker, executive director of the American Lyme Disease Foundation and former director of the Lyme program at NIH. If OspA was taken out, OspB, which resides on the same strip of DNA as OspA, would have to go, too.

Why limit the disease definition and dismiss chronic Lyme? One influence could be the vaccine. Vaccine development required a clinically testable disease definition to pass clinical trials and garner FDA approval. The manufacturer had to find a population free of Lyme disease, vaccinate it, and then prove the vaccine had worked by retesting the population. With an endemic population that might harbor lingering or under-the-radar infection even after treatment, without a restrictive case definition that ignored Lyme's "shades of gray," that would be impossible.

The point was made clearly by Raymond Dattwyler, the immunologist from Stony Brook, at an FDA meeting on the vaccine in Silver Spring, Maryland, in June 1994—just months before the circumscribed serological standard removing OspA was pushed through in Dearborn.

Dattwyler pointed out that the nonrheumatologic manifestations of fatigue, fever, headache, or stiff neck—the very symptoms Dattwyler himself said were often most common in his Long Island patients—"would be difficult to categorize from the point of view of a study population when one talks about vaccine trials." Later on, another meeting participant, Stanley M. Lemon, M.D., dean of the School of Medicine at the University of Texas Medical Branch at Galveston, summarized the consensus as follows: "I get the sense from the committee, again, that we don't believe that the CDC case definition can be applied, as it is, in a vaccine efficacy trial. . . . We believe that there probably should be a greater attention paid to supporting laboratory evidence of infection and stricter clinical definitions for each of the syndromes to be considered."

In short, Lyme's inconvenient complexity—its annoying fuzziness—had to be replaced by a mythical simplicity for the products to fly. With the dirty Western blots apparently unnoticed (or swept under the rug), and with the circumscribed disease definition in place, it became possible to "validate" LYMErix and get approval from the FDA.

To what extent did vaccine development *really* influence the various players? Was there a concerted conspiracy here? Deliberate collusion or fraud? I've never found any proof. Instead, money set the course. The factors that helped the various products and projects stay aloft included the restrictive Dearborn criteria (with the removal of OspA) and denial of any Lyme disease outside the definition imposed.

In the face of so many suspicions and all the uproar, LDA president Pat Smith asked her congressman, Chris Smith, to arrange a special meeting with the FDA in 2002. The day she arrived at headquarters, a dozen FDA top brass sat around a wood table the length of a large conference room, notepads in hand, awaiting their meeting with the powerful Congressman Smith.

"Where's Congressman Smith?" they asked Pat Smith when she arrived with her team.

"Oh, he had to cancel," Pat Smith explained, but she'd brought someone else: the ultimate vaccine whistle-blower, Donald H. Marks, M.D., Ph.D., former lab director for Pasteur Merieux Connaught.

In the early days of the OspA vaccine, Connaught's product, ImuLyme, had been racing neck and neck with LYMErix to reach the market first. Accusations of adverse reactions early in its history brought a rain of lawsuits, and Connaught pulled the plug. Yet the two vaccines had been nearly identical, and it was fair to say that Marks knew more about OspA's capabilities than almost anyone in the world.

Presenting his case to FDA officials, Marks said that all the issues in LYMErix had been noted in ImuLyme, too: the occasional autoimmune reaction, indicating Steere could be on to something; the relapse into old disease; and the hyperactivation of the immune system, including swollen hands and the dirty Western blots with every band lit.

"The dirty banding makes it impossible for physicians to differentiate between LYMErix vaccination, new infection with *Borrelia burgdorferi,* or reactivation of infection," Marks told the FDA officers. "The net result is that cases of Lyme disease will go undiagnosed and untreated. Adverse reactions to LYMErix will be misdiagnosed as Lyme disease and people will be unnecessarily treated with antibiotics." Physicians unaware of the potential problems could not appropriately treat the patients who were sick.

Marks reviewed twenty-two cases in which "the adverse event was not anecdotal but a medical certainty." Of four neurological adverse events, all were caused by LYMErix (as opposed to Lyme disease), with presentations from peripheral nervous system disease to memory loss to an immune-related complex of joint pain and fatigue. Rheumatologic reactions included joint pain and arthritis itself. "You'll never find statistical significance for the worst adverse events," he told the FDA, "because they are so rare." In these instances, you must weigh the risk of the disease against the risk, even if extremely low, that an individual could be damaged by the vaccine. Perhaps it was worth taking such risk for smallpox, but *Lyme disease?*

On February 25, 2002, a month after the meeting, the LDA received written answers to questions it had submitted to the FDA. In thirteen pages of response, the FDA repeated, again and again, that it saw no compelling evidence to suggest that LYMErix was unsafe. What of the Tufts patent for a safer OspA vaccine? "Theoretical concerns may spur scientists to develop what they believe are theoretically safer products," the FDA replied.

The next day, on February 26, GlaxoSmithKline quietly pulled LYMErix from the market, citing "poor sales."

As for the vaccinees suing Glaxo, their class-action suit was settled in July 2003. The settlement was so small—about $1 million—that there was only enough to compensate the lawyers. The patients would not get a dime. "The case was never about lining plaintiffs' pockets with millions of dollars, it was about public safety," said Stephen A. Sheller, the attorney who brought the suit. In fact, as part of the settlement, Glaxo agreed to add better warnings should LYMErix ever be reintroduced in the United

States. Don't laugh: While LYMErix is gone from the home turf for now, Glaxo has quietly been developing "LYMErix Europe," a product that includes the same controversial OspA molecule used here. And why not? Glaxo and the FDA maintain, to this day, that LYMErix is perfectly safe.

Following the exit of ImuLyme and then LYMErix from the U.S. landscape, other vaccines that have been waiting in the wings may eventually appear. At Baxter Healthcare Corporation, a pharmaceutical company in Deerfield, Illinois, an effort is under way to create a modified OspA-based vaccine. The new vaccine is being produced with the help of a machine called the National Synchrotron Light Source at the Brookhaven National Laboratory on Long Island. The Synchrotron bombards actual OspA with X-rays, leading to a three-dimensional computer model of the protein. The computer-model is then used to synthesize a new molecule, never before seen in nature, that can immunize against the disease without inducing the autoimmunity or the hyperinflammation attributed to natural OspA. Recently, John Dunn of Brookhaven has also patented genetically engineered proteins that combine pieces of OspA and OspC, each present on the surface of the spirochete at different points, promising a vaccine with a one-two punch.

Another possibility comes from Eugene Davidson, the Georgetown molecular biologist. Working with Alan Frey, a cell biologist at New York University, Davidson used ultrasound to break up Lyme spirochetes. The result was a mixture of every protein found in a range of *Borrelia burgdorferi* strains, encapsulated in tiny vesicles one thousandth the size of a living bacterium. The vesicles, sterilized by Davidson and completely noninfectious, nonetheless contained every spirochetal protein that might play a role in disease—sort of the mirror image of Barthold's "Golden Fleece," which contained every antibody created by those proteins. When tiny doses of Davidson's vaccine were injected into mice and, later, rhesus monkeys, the result was complete immunity against disease—just as Barthold found when he injected mice with the Golden Fleece made of all the antibodies.

And Stephen K. Wikel, an entomologist at the University of Texas, is working on a vaccine made from tick saliva. A vaccine that deters the *Ixodes* tick itself could be far more useful than a mere Lyme vaccine, since ticks carry several diseases, not just the one. Indeed, while developing vaccines that target each possible tick-borne disease would be daunting, targeting all those infections through their vector—the tick—is within reach. Wikel's goal: developing a vaccine that specifically targets the molecules responsible for helping the tick feed and transmit disease.

At least the effort goes on. No matter what vaccine ultimately emerges, if it can actually prevent Lyme disease without risk, it isn't likely that patients will protest conflicts of interest or profit for the scientists behind its success.

49

❖

Over and Out, Colorado

Colorado Springs, Colorado 2007

It's August 1, 2007, when I fly in to Denver, rent a car, and drive in the early-morning hours to the crisp, clean corporate park that houses Dave Martz's practice—the Rocky Mountain Chronic Disease Specialists in Colorado Springs. The office is new and bright, uplifted by Martz's many photos of animals in the African bush, but the day itself is sad. As seems to be happening more and more lately, another Lyme doctor—Martz himself—is pulling up stakes and shutting his doors. I arrive amidst fruit baskets and chocolates sent by grateful patients, boxes stuffed with papers and medical records and supplies. A beautiful young blond woman named Christine stops by, just to thank Martz. She'd been sick for eighteen years, ever since a tick bite in Texas at the age of seven. Her parents read about Lyme disease in *Good Housekeeping* magazine, and brought Christine out to New Jersey, where a neurologist treated her with IV Rocephin, but to little avail. Back home in Colorado her leg pain and exhaustion became almost unbearable. Labeled a malingerer and attention-seeker, she was homebound until 2005, when Martz opened his doors. Treating Christine with much smaller doses of oral antibiotic over a long period of time, he's been able to get results where others could not. Today, says Christine, her pain is gone and her life has been restored.

Yet Martz will soon be gone. He's had three heart attacks over the past two years, he explains, and his doctor has read him the riot act: Either he retires now or the work will do him in. Dee has joined the chorus. He's getting sucked back in, she says, with the clinic a 24/7 drain on his time.

Like Burrascano and other departing Lyme doctors, Martz is bound for research. Among the questions he'd like to answer: Is the disease he now calls "Chronic Lyme-Like Illness," or CLLI, a definable and provable entity? Can it be effectively treated with extended antibiotics? Is it possible that *some* patients have the motor neuron disease of ALS triggered or imitated by this infection? If so, are there clinical or laboratory red flags? What if any antibiotic regimens (drug, dose, and duration) might be effective or work best?

Martz isn't the only one following the trail. In 2006, he was called to attend the exclusive Gordon Conference on Lyme disease, an honor generally extended only to Lyme's leading mainstream lights. The usual names at a Gordon Conference on Lyme disease include Allen Steere of Harvard, John Halperin of North Shore University Hospital, Gary Wormser of New York Medical College, Eugene Shapiro of Yale. Yet the experience of the minister's son, extraordinary yet credible, was more than compelling to the small group of experts who, for part of an afternoon, respectfully discussed Martz's wild ride through ALS and Lyme.

50

The Falmouth Reunion

Falmouth, Massachusetts, 2007

After flying home from Colorado, I take off with Mark for the Cape Cod town of Falmouth (famous for its island ferries, its lighthouse, and its ticks) to catch up with Sheila and Russ. "I can't believe you actually agreed to come here," Russ says in greeting, knowing we have fled our suburban tick forest for an urban high-rise in Stamford, and that I traced my *Babesia* to Woods Hole, just miles from the Falmouth street where we now stand.

"I have no intention of stepping off the concrete here either," I swiftly assure him. Russ, who grew up on Cape Cod and has family roots in Falmouth, takes Mark on a tour while Sheila and I stay back to talk. The empty dining hall in the Statlender's elegant hotel, the Inn on the Square, provides a cool, quiet place for discussing the recent past. Every so often Sheila's cell phone rings and the news is always good: First it's Seth calling from his skydiving lesson in Orange, Massachusetts; then Eric from an amusement park in Ohio, where he's gone on a trip with a friend; then Amy who's traveling through Europe, where she's studying language and taking in the sights.

"For the first time in a decade, we can all pass for normal," says Sheila, who looks tan, athletic, and healthy, and has been bicycling around the Cape. Actually, for the Statlenders it's been a stupendous year. In March they went to Israel. "A miracle," Sheila says. "Not perfect, healthwise, but this was a feat not possible for several years." Visiting King Herod's Palace and the sacred burial ground at Bet Shearim, Amy strode out in front of them. "It was hard to keep up with her. Double, triple miracle," Sheila says. Seth went on an archaeological dig in the caves outside Jerusalem, searching the layers for evidence of civilization past. Touring the country, he was interested to learn that Israelis don't go to college until after serving in the army and traveling. It was refreshing to see different pathways in life.

"We spent years in our own, personal holocaust," comments Sheila. "It was symbolic to visit a new country and feel we could have a fresh start, too."

Still, it's hard to recover from the toll of chronic illness, even for those on the mend. None of them have yet been symptom-free long enough to stop their treatment. True, Amy spent seven weeks touring Europe—but continued her medication while abroad. Eric, on IV Rocephin for many months, stopped the treatment after feeling better, only to relapse. Now he's being treated with an oral antibiotic, and pushing his symptoms back again.

"I have to look at the glass that is half full," Sheila reflects. "We still have ups and downs, and there's serious concern that we still live in a highly endemic area, rife with the possibility of reinfection despite taking precautions. The kids had major portions of their relatively young lives dominated by a terrible illness. It breaks my heart sometimes, but then I think, this is the life that is ours."

51

❖

Getting Dr. Jones

Over the years the Statlenders have become what you may need to be in Lyme, these days, to truly make it back once infection has gone untreated for years: landsmen, insiders, trusted members of the club. With the Lyme doctors under fire, fewer of them each day are willing to widely provide the kind of aggressive, multidrug, or intravenous treatment that may be required to bring some persistently or co-infected patients back to health. With complaints to state medical boards threatening their licenses, the doctors are careful about who gets the full monty instead of treatment-lite.

One woman I met, a longtime leader of a support group in her community, suffered a devastating Lyme relapse that involved cognitive confusion, overpowering fatigue, and severe whole-body neurological pain. One of the leading Lyme doctors, a man she knew for years, treated her with soaring doses of amoxicillin for Lyme along with Mepron and Zithromax for suspected babesiosis. A few months later the woman had recovered her cognitive faculties and was ready to run laps. She was writing newsletters and running meetings, and offered to cook me meals while I finished my book.

I was so impressed I referred a second woman to the doctor: The second woman had nearly identical test results and disease signs and symptoms and was infected in the same hyperendemic area of the Northeast. Yet the doctor treated her with only very low-dose Zithromax—a single tiny pink pill a day. The woman continued to slide so badly that eventually she was wracked with pain and could no longer leave her bed, until one day months later, her husband called to ream me out for the reference. *What was I thinking? What could they do now?*

What could I say? I knew how it went. The two women were similar, except in one respect. The first was known, trusted, a longtime insider. The second was a Janey-come-lately to the Lyme scene. Aggressive treatments were risky, and adverse reactions could be profound. The doctor was already under investigation in the state where he practiced. The first woman would never have turned on him. He *knew* that. But the second? He couldn't be sure. A decade earlier this doctor would probably have treated *both* women aggressively—but with the Lyme war now so heated, he didn't want to take the chance.

With the cost to physicians so high, only one doctor has consistently treated the youngest of patients, the most vulnerable, despite the risk to himself: the defiant pediatrician Charles Ray Jones. Long past the age of retirement, with a grandchild to tend and trips to take, Jones has continued to treat by his conscience, all the while enduring attack from academic honchos at the University of Connecticut and Yale, who brand him a quack and a fraud.

Discussing the onslaught with me from his office in New Haven one day in 2002, Jones was sanguine. "I haven't done anything wrong," he said. "When the health department gets complaints against me, they toss them in the trash.

"I don't know everything," he said, "but when I have reason to know I am right in medicine or anything else, I will follow what I know." Glancing out the window of his ground-level suite, he gestured toward his nemesis, Yale University Medical Center, in plain sight down the road. "I am established enough to withstand the slings and arrows from across the way," he said that day. "Besides, I can sleep at night. I just hope for *their* sakes they are sincere in their stated belief that Lyme disease can always be treated short term." And then he was silent, as if issuing a prayer for their souls.

Perhaps Jones didn't pray hard enough. At eighty, he's hardly immortal, yet in all the intervening years since our talk that distant day, he has been unable to find a young physician to help in his practice, someone he can nurture and train to take over once he is gone. And by 2006, the complaints that once landed in the trash were being sent to prosecutors: Charges of professional misconduct revolving around the treatment of Lyme disease threaten to keep him embroiled with hearings and lawyers at the Connecticut Department of Health until the day he's forced to shutter up his office—or, if he prevails, to the end of time.

The first charge involved two siblings from Reno, Nevada, whom Jones treated partly at a distance and over the phone. The charges were initiated by a father involved in a custody dispute. Tapping a strategy commonly used in custody fights, he'd charged that his ex had Munchausen Syndrome by Proxy. When Jones disagreed, diagnosing the children with Lyme disease, the father reported him (along with many other doctors) to the medical board of his state. In Nevada, where seventeen doctors were turned in, the state tossed the complaints as "nuisance" reports. But in Connecticut, where Yale ruled the roost, the state hoped to make the charges stick.

The story (naturally) starts in the woods. During a camping trip in Oklahoma in 2000, the mother, a nurse named Robin Sparks, pulled some ticks from her children, a girl of seven and a boy of ten. According to her testimony in Hartford, it was all downhill from there. Her son, an A student before the trip, began a long descent to dysfunction, Sparks reported. By 2003, he was an F student with behavior so disruptive he was about to be expelled from school. Her daughter, meanwhile, just felt sick. Her back and joints hurt, her chest ached, she felt so exhausted that after playing for twenty minutes, she'd come inside and sob.

Lyme isn't the first diagnosis one leaps to in Reno, and Sparks said she spent years seeking other answers. It was only after exhausting possible diagnoses and recalling the Oklahoma trip that she thought of Lyme disease. She'd been diagnosed with Lyme herself. Her physician had suggested that transmission could even be congenital—perhaps her children had been *born* with it. Doctors in Nevada called the idea preposterous, so her Lyme doctor encouraged her to call Dr. Jones. In December 2003, she did.

Because Jones had such a long waiting list, it took six months from the phone call before the family could be seen. Yet perhaps because Sparks was so articulate and seemed so knowledgeable, because her children were so sick, Jones took pity on her and agreed to help from a distance before the appointment date.

At the time of that first phone call, December 2003, the boy had a cough so persistent and nagging he wasn't allowed back in school. The clinic in Reno prescribed three days of Zithromax for the cough and it started to subside. But when doctors there wouldn't authorize a refill, Sparks turned to Jones. Though he had never met the child, Jones called a pharmacy in Nevada and ordered ten more days of Zithromax, forming the basis of Connecticut's first charge.

The cough resolved but the child was still disruptive. Theorizing that the troubling behavior was rooted in Lyme disease, Sparks asked the school to call Jones. Why not place him on home-bound instruction, and treat him, allowing return to school the following year? Jones proposed.

Great, the school said, but to help with the documentation, could Jones diagnose Lyme disease?

"Not without seeing him," Jones responded. But for the purpose of school records, just to help out, he was willing to write a letter diagnosing "presumptive Lyme disease." That would work, the school felt. It used the letter to document a disability, allowing the boy to obtain accommodations and finish out the year. Connecticut used the letter to support another charge: Jones had diagnosed Lyme disease over the phone.

The allegations against Jones just escalated from there. It wasn't until May 21, 2004, that the family showed up at Jones's office in New Haven. The boy was depressed, disheveled, and suffering a grinding headache; he couldn't make conversation or look Jones in the eye. His sister was exhausted and in pain.

Following the appointment, Jones diagnosed Lyme disease (actual, not presumptive) and treatment commenced—first, amoxicillin and, when that stopped working, its stronger cousin, Augmentin. Because the mother was, after all, a nurse, and because a trip back East for three cost thousands of dollars, Jones agreed that she herself could monitor the children while Jones prescribed from afar. In Connecticut, that was a violation of the standard of care, and another charge.

By the time the children returned to New Haven on April 11, 2005, for a follow-up visit, both were back in school and appeared transformed. The little girl felt completely better: All her pain and exhaustion had left. And the boy was literally "sparkling." His headache was cured. He was able to hold direct conversations and meet Jones's eye. He was getting A's in school.

But the state had another point of view. First they brought in Eugene Shapiro, the Yale pediatrician who helped write the IDSA guidelines and saw Lyme as limited: the rash, objective signs like swollen knees, five of ten bands on a Western blot. Addressing the state's theory that the children actually suffered stress, Shapiro explained the concept of "somatoform disorder": physical complaints that originate in the psychic anxieties of life. When Robin Sparks's children reported pelvic pain, chest pain, loss of bladder control, exhaustion, it could have been due to the disturbance of their parents' divorce: "There is a very low probability that this is due to infection," Shapiro said.

Then, in keeping with Lyme's raucous side, the state flew in Jeffrey Sparks, the father who'd made the complaint. He said that during his twice-weekly visits, his son had shown none of the symptoms, not the joint pain, the night terrors, or the sensitivity to light. What's more, he told the panel, Robin had a habit of falsely claiming ailments, including a brain tumor, advanced ovarian cancer, and lupus, none of which she actually had. Once, he said, she'd told him that their son had breast cancer. He denied Robin's charges that he abused the children or failed to pay support.

In the end the panel and state regulators decided against Jones, supporting most of the allegations against him and delivering their recommendations in a hearing room in Hartford on December 18, 2007. His punishment: a $10,000 fine and two years' probation, during which time an outside monitor would review his treating practices and patient charts, effectively curtailing his ability to care for patients as before. Publicly stating it wasn't punishing Jones for practicing outside the mainstream Lyme disease guidelines, the state threw the book at him for initially treating the Nevada siblings with antibiotics sight unseen and then, after seeing them, continuing to treat for so long with negative tests. On this last count, the decision came down to the numbers. The state of Oklahoma had reported no cases of Lyme disease in years, and Nevada just a few. With risk of exposure so low, the tests so negative, and symptoms so general, they just didn't see evidence of Lyme disease. No one mentioned that other borreliosis, the Lyme-like disease studied by Ed Masters, increasingly reported in Oklahoma and causing a furor at that state's department of health.

"The most important part of the decision from my perspective," says Lorraine Johnson, one of Jones's attorneys, "is that the panel threw in a four-part test for Lyme disease *after* the trial: It can't be Lyme if there is a low risk of exposure, if the symptoms are nonspecific, if the history is nonspecific, and if the test is negative. We had no chance to defend against this during the trial, a breach of due process. Connecticut Department of Health Commissioner J. Robert Galvin has made repeated public statements that there are two standards of care and that it is too early to call the science. Then he turned around and brought an action against Jones predicated on the IDSA viewpoint. We are all entitled to know when we are violating the law *beforehand*."

Jones's lead attorney, Elliot Pollack, told the panel they'd done wrong. "Eugene Shapiro says Lyme is the rash and swollen knees and Bell's palsy. Are you now going to make this the standard? So many mavericks," he added, "have challenged and ultimately been proven right in medicine, please do not stumble here now. When is the last time this board punished a physician for curing patients?" The children had come to Jones sick, he reminded them, and now they were well.

He was answered by David Goldenberg, M.D., a member of the board. "The constant reiteration that Dr. Jones cured these patients is really obnoxious," Goldenberg literally yelled at Pollack. If the children got better during treatment, he said, it was coincidence. Connecting the two was "a complete violation of everything we know about cause and effect in disease. We don't believe Dr. Jones cured anything."

As for the suggestion that Jones was a hero, "holding up a sword and shield and needing to be put on a pedestal," Goldenberg vehemently disagreed. "You can name diseases that have been treated by mavericks," he said, "but there are others who treated outside the bounds of normal medical care and injured thousands of patients before the truth was uncovered."

The outcome was music to the ears of Lawrence Zemel, a physician at the University of Connecticut who attended part of the hearing and had been hoping for Jones's downfall for years. "With the eventual loss of Dr. Jones," he said in a letter to *Yankee* magazine, "there will *not* be a void in physicians who treat pediatric Lyme disease in Connecticut. I know of several highly qualified, board-certified specialists in infectious disease and rheumatology, myself included, who will treat not only the acute infectious complications of the illness but the noninfectious later symptoms as well. None of these physicians would abandon sick or symptomatic children, regardless of the cause." Zemel would treat their fibromyalgia, their chronic fatigue syndrome, their arthritis. For the children of Connecticut, his doors were open wide.

Parents in the room felt a chill. The descendants of Polly Murray, they had been here from the start. Many had wandered Connecticut and other Lyme zones for years under the chronic fatigue and fibromyalgia mantles, finally getting well only after being diagnosed with Lyme disease. They had fought so long and suffered so much, but for *this?*

There to bear witness was Kay Lyon, the Wenham, Massachusetts, mother I'd met in April 2000, when, in desperation myself after being shown the door by the medical powerhouses of greater New York, I'd gotten in my car and driven to Farmington, Connecticut, for a rebel conference on Lyme. Lyon was the mother whose heart-wrenching description of her daughter's fall and climb back up had at once scared me and given me hope. Before I met Kay, I'd never even heard of Dr. Jones.

"My husband and I owe our lives to Dr. Charles Ray Jones. Without him our children would not have had, and still would not have, any quality of life. In fact, our daughter would likely have died," Lyon said. "It seems evil trying to stop him at every turn. Despite being attacked he keeps on doing what he knows is right."

Kay's daughter, Meredith J. Lyon, by then eighteen years old, was healthy and whole. She'd come to Hartford, too. "Dr. Jones saved my life," she said.

By spring 2008, three other cases were pending at the Connecticut Department of Health. Two of the three involved divorced parents engaged in custody and other marital/parental disputes. In the third, Jones was accused of falsifying a child's illness to justify his absences from school, essentially colluding with the mother, who was accused of Munchausen by Proxy. "This charge, if upheld, could set a dangerous precedent for the Lyme community, endangering parents and their sick children who are accused of truancy. It must be defeated," Jones said.

Jones's attorneys, meanwhile, filed a motion asking the Connecticut Medical Examining Board to reconsider its December 2007 decision based on bias. It turned out that one of the panel members, pediatrician John Senechal, told parents of a child diagnosed with chronic Lyme disease that there was no such thing. It was a "big racket," he reportedly said, and doctors who treated it were "quacks" who were "in cahoots" with lab companies.

"Due process requires an absence of actual bias in the trial of cases," Lorraine Johnson said.

With the motion in play, a Superior Court judge put the four-part test on stay, pending appeal. "While there was still a monitor, the monitor was directed not to apply this standard," Johnson explained.

52

The Never-Ending Story:
What Happened to My Family

Stamford, Connecticut, 2005–2008

Living in downtown Stamford away from the ticks and deer, I felt enormous relief. It was bad enough having an infection without risking exposure to the very same germ again and again. How had people with our health issues stuck it out in Chappaqua for so long?

With 2005 under way, I was still off antibiotics, my good health holding strong. My head didn't hurt. My brain was clear. The buzzing had stopped and the fatigue that had stalked me fell away. I felt—there's no other way to put it—*normal.* Because I hadn't felt truly normal for most of the past decade, it seemed like a miracle, exciting, exhilarating, and new. I even did the unimaginable: I took a job, commuting by train each day from downtown Stamford to Manhattan as executive editor of *MAMM,* a magazine for women with breast and gynecological cancer. I'd always been a worker, but over the years of illness the possibility of traveling to the city on a daily, committed basis seemed as likely, given my fluctuating state of exhaustion, as flying to the moon. My waxing-waning illness had lasted so many years I imagined spending my life like that, always interrupted, perpetually at half-mast. Yet now, taking the train in the morning, working all day, and taking the train back at night, I knew I felt better. When I accepted a second gig moonlighting for *Psychology Today,* and then, finally, a full-time job acquiring and editing features for the science magazine *Discover,* I understood that I was truly well.

Mark worked in the city as executive editor for The Skin Cancer Foundation and he, too, was mostly fine—as long as he took those pills. Unlike me, he was not off antibiotics. We discussed the possibility that he try intravenous treatment as a way of curing his Lyme and getting off antibiotics for good. But the timing never suited him. His shaky memory bothered him, but taking his medication each day, he felt well enough, so why be more extreme?

Our children were a different matter. In 2005, Jason, twenty-one, and David, seventeen, were still sick. It seemed as if we'd moved David from a bed in one town to a bed in the next: He couldn't stay awake. Our plans to send him to the Harvey School fell through because he felt too fatigued to get there. By fall 2005, as a senior at Stamford High School, he was spending part of the day in class and part with home tutors, making progress toward graduation despite his health problems. As he tried to move forward, his mystery illness continued without a clue.

It was in January 2006 that Liegner called with the news. David's Western blot had finally flowered, sprouting so many bands it was positive by CDC standards, at long last. Liegner acknowledged that David was still sick despite antibiotic treatment in the past, but said, "If I were you I would put him on a few months of IV Rocephin and see if it does any good." With no indication of any other organic problem and with all the years of exposure from our tick forest in Chappaqua, we decided to bite the bullet. The fact of the matter is that up to this point, longer-term IV was something we'd never tried for either of our boys. "Sometimes," said Liegner, "nothing else works."

It wasn't Ken Liegner who ended up treating David, but Daniel Cameron, the friendly, open-minded Mount Kisco physician who had treated Jason with a second month of Rocephin at the start of our journey in Lyme. Cameron was now our primary care doctor, covered by our insurance plan. While our insurer allowed David twenty-eight days of IV Rocephin, we got around the limit by driving David to Cameron's office each day. There he received a daily infusion for the cost of a $20 co-pay, and the twenty-eight-day limit wasn't imposed. Taking time off from our jobs, Mark and I alternated getting David in for treatment. Slowly, he began to wake up. When he began traveling to Manhattan to perform stand-up comedy, I knew he was getting well, too.

The months of David's treatment were underscored by talks with Dan Cameron, a former farm boy from Minnesota who'd studied not just medicine but also epidemiology in the years before coming to New York. Diffident in speech and with an occasional stammer, Cameron had a gentle, cautious manner that belied a harder edge.

After a while I learned he could be as critical of the Lyme left as of the right. The mainstream view of Lyme was seriously at odds with Cameron's patients, people often diagnosed late who needed extra months of treatment to get well. Yet he felt many Lyme doctors were driving without a road map, using regimens so varied, empirical, and intuitive they often lacked evidence to back them up.

Cameron was trying to rectify that, one small piece at a time. In 2004, he led an ILADS team in the creation of new treatment guidelines summarizing the evidence for chronic Lyme disease and the therapies shown to work. Hoping to add to the evidence, he conducted research of his own. In one study he showed that the more delayed the diagnosis, the harder it was to cure the patient and the more days of treatment with doxycycline the patient needed to get well. In another study, this one blinded and controlled, he showed that patients who responded to treatment but later relapsed did far better with retreatment than many in the Klempner group—people who had never responded to antibiotics at all. Wasn't it a shame, Cameron commented, that those rare, nonresponding patients were setting the agenda for the rest? He was beaming the day he learned that his extensive critique of that study's flaws had been accepted for publication in *Epidemiological Perspectives and Innovations*, a prestigious journal in his field. All this in aggregate supported a second standard of care—one at odds with the mainstream view—that Cameron hoped would provide his colleagues with an evidence-based defense of their work.

Dan Cameron may have been conservative compared to many other Lyme doctors, but by treating according to the evidence-based guidelines he himself wrote for ILADS, he managed to bring David back. As David readied to leave for Vassar College in the fall, I felt certain that his Lyme disease had been dealt with, at last.

While David had gotten better, Jason was slipping away. Holed up in his room at Brown University, he made furtive calls home: He was too sick to leave his dormitory, too beat to take his test, in way too much pain to walk to the dining hall to eat his meal. His friends were bringing him food, his professors were giving him extensions. "It will work out, right?" he said.

"Take your Lyme medicine," I told him.

At first, he *did* take his antibiotics, but now they didn't seem to work. Then he couldn't focus enough to take them at all. "I can't remember, I feel too fuzzy," said Jason, "and I don't like swallowing pills."

Finally in mid-March there came a day of reckoning: He had fallen too far. He was simply too sick to go on. "Get me back to Burrascano. I'll follow his instructions now. I need to get well," Jason said in that last call home.

When I called to make the appointment, I learned that the practice was closed to new patients and even former ones. "Sorry," the receptionist said. Given Jason's condition, the news distressed me. The only Lyme doctor in New York State who'd survived trial by fire, Joe Burrascano was, by my reckoning, the only one *free* to marshal the full armamentarium and treat as he saw fit. Burrascano had gone to the mattresses for Lyme and emerged intact. So if you wanted the "to the mattresses" treatment, he was the "go-to" guy. I was strategizing what to do next when a nurse called back. "The doctor has made an exception, he's taking Jason back."

On March 30, 2006, as we drove to East Hampton to see Burrascano, I felt we'd been given a reprieve. When we arrived, the sand-and-surf mural was still on the wall, but Burrascano himself had changed. Having gone through treatment for possible prostate cancer the year before, he'd lost so much weight he had the improbable look of a reed. He was calmer and more centered, as much because he no longer had to work under the watchful eye of a monitor, I guessed, as because he had recently been certified cancer-free.

"I took you back because I felt I could fix this one," he told Jason sternly, "so let's get to work." Jason was unfinished business for Burrascano; this was a second chance for both. "Patient is seriously ill," Burrascano wrote that day in Jason's chart. His joints were swollen, his glands inflamed, and his Western blot floridly positive. His SPECT scan showed severe blood-flow problems, consistent with marked encephalopathy and Lyme. He had a dull, unpleasant, aching nausea, a whole-body itch, and his bone pain had become so overwhelming he groaned through the appointment and literally screamed in agony when Burrascano gently pressed his ribs. Sound hurt his ears and light hurt his eyes. He gasped for air. He had, he told Burrascano, given up math.

Jason had failed the last round of oral treatment and was now so sick he needed intravenous therapy to journey back to health, Burrascano said. He felt the problem was not just Lyme but also *Bartonella:* Jason was PCR positive for the *Bartonella* organism, and he had the strange, striated rash that Burrascano, in a somewhat controversial viewpoint, saw as suggestive of the disease. By the time the appointment was over, Burrascano had convinced Jason to take a semester's leave from school. If

treated over the summer and through the following fall, he felt, Jason
would get well. "You'll be filled with so much energy you'll go out dancing in the streets when we're done," Burrascano said.

Slowly but surely, by dint of aggressive therapy reserved for the sickest of his patients, Burrascano pulled Jason back up. First, to treat *Bartonella,* he prescribed the antibiotic Levaquin. But the workhorse was
doxycycline, delivered at high dose by a tube called a PICC (peripherally
inserted central catheter) directly to Jason's veins. As with David, we
couldn't afford months of a home-infusion company to deliver the IV, so
we went another route. Through an ordinary doctor's prescription, we
obtained vials of doxy powder directly from the drugstore just as one
might order pills. Our insurance company paid. We mail-ordered other
supplies from Florida, everything from saline bags and tubing to deliver
the drug to heparin locks to flush the line in Jason's arm. A visiting nurse
changed the dressing every week.

Each night Jason mixed the powdered doxy with saline and spent a
couple of hours in front of the flickering TV while the drug infused.
Two months into the regimen Burrascano added Flagyl, an oral antibiotic that he told us would burst the cysts. It was a strange, solitary life of
limbo for a twenty-two-year-old who should have been in college with
his friends. It had all been so gradual, but over the course of years, as
more modest treatments failed us and illness dogged us, we'd become
the extraterrestrial patients I'd been so shocked by at the start of our so-
journ in Lyme.

Yet our journey to the far side was paying off. David was well and off
antibiotics. And by August 2006, Jason was dramatically improved. The
nausea, bone pain, and unremitting exhaustion had lifted, his brain was
clearer. He went out for movies and meals. Once more, he saw friends.
He even felt good enough to register as a visiting student at nearby Columbia for the fall. He was better but hardly well.

Then we received a letter: "I have a major announcement to make.
After twenty-five years of medical practice, I have decided to close my
office and retire from the clinical practice of medicine," Joseph J. Burrascano Jr., M.D., wrote. "My decision comes at a good time for me
personally. I feel well, my prostate cancer seems to be in a remission,
and I have not had any bad news from the state medical board lately. In
other words, this decision has not resulted from any secret problem that
I am trying to hide. Of course, rumors will fly, but I say sincerely to all
of you that there is no hidden agenda. PLEASE try to keep the gossip
down . . ." On Lyme boards throughout the Internet, the rumors were

already flying off the charts: He'd secretly lost his license and had made a deal with the state, he just couldn't take it anymore, he was dying of cancer, who really knew. This was Lyme, after all, and no one's sense of footing was sure.

Certainly not ours. We were three months into Burrascano's eight-month treatment plan. Going for Jason's last appointment, we felt that the rug had been pulled out from under us. The noose had tightened around Lyme considerably since we got on board in 2000. Finding a doctor with Burrascano's experience and moxie had always been difficult. Finding one willing to be aggressive when nothing else worked—willing to take that risk on behalf of patients—had gotten harder, *much* harder, over the intervening years.

"You know what you need now to get better," Burrascano said to Jason, shaking his hand as we left that day in late September 2006. "Just demand your rights." Down a hallway I glimpsed a plaque that read "Lyme Warrior." In the foreground, framing Jason, was the wall-sized mural of Hawaii, by now so faded the once-green palms blended eerily into the surf.

Where would Jason demand these rights? From our insurer? From the government? From a Tijuana clinic? From Yale?

Burrascano privately fretted over such questions, too. He'd spent years in the trenches of chronic Lyme, but without clinical studies backing the empirical art he practiced, his work remained incomplete. The next part of his life would be devoted to research: Spearheading a multiyear study funded by the Turn the Corner foundation, he planned to document which treatments worked best, and for whom. It was the chance to pick up where he left off when he was unable to publish his study of 733 Lyme patients in 1988.

"Aren't you happy for me?" Burrascano asked, bubbling over with enthusiasm for his life's next adventure.

With Jason in so much need, I could hardly share his joy. "I'm not really happy about losing Jason's doctor right now," I told him bluntly. "Congratulations," I added, trying to crack a smile. We owed him a lot. But on that one day I could barely look him in the eye.

After we left the office we stopped at the Southampton Diner for dinner, but the food just stuck in my throat.

"He betrayed me," Jason complained bitterly. "He brought me back from school to treat me and now he's dumping me and doing something else."

But sipping my coffee, I regained my composure. "We have what we need from him. He gave you a treatment plan," I said. "We just have to see it through."

It wouldn't be easy finding a doctor willing to assume the months of aggressive treatment laid out before us, but following Burrascano's advice, we signed on with another doctor. It was late fall in 2006 when we drove up the Taconic to the picturesque town where the new physician worked. As we drove, we watched the deer along the highway. Some had gotten so bold they were splattered by the shoulder now, washing the parkway in red.

"I've been sick for so many years. Will I ever get well?" Jason asked as we headed for the appointment. He still had far to go.

I wanted to weep for my injured son, his lonely path, and his lost years. But my answer was upbeat. "Of course you'll get better," I said, channeling Burrascano. *I can fix this one,* he'd said, but now he'd signed on as senior vice president for a biotech firm, supervising clinical trials for drugs and devices. Once again our Lyme practitioner had left, but we were still on the journey. When would it ever end? As Jason's mother, I promised him. "I guarantee it," I said.

"Good enough," said Jason, his eyes inscrutable behind the sunglasses that filtered the light that still hurt his eyes. Then he reclined in his seat and slept for the remainder of the drive.

It was the summer of 2007 when Lyme finally smiled on us, bequeathing one small mercy in all the years of angst. My younger son, David, by then entirely well, had been off all antibiotics for almost a year and was taking a summer course at Purchase College in the heart of Westchester, New York. One night he called and said, "I've had a rash for a week. My suitemates keep saying it's Lyme disease."

"I'll be there in the morning," I said.

I arrived on campus to see David walking toward me, barefoot, across a lawn that hosted visits from rabbits, skunk, and plenty of deer. His summer had been carefree and he was not pleased to see me by his dorm. He got into my car, annoyed, and pulled his sleeve up, revealing something perfect: a large, clear nearly circular erythema migrans rash with a diameter four inches wide. The white center of this circle was surrounded by a sunburst of red.

David didn't want to leave campus with me. "I'll miss all the fun here," he complained. But I wouldn't budge, finally embarrassing him so much he came with me just to remove me from the scene.

We took a forty-minute drive to Dan Cameron's office in downtown Mount Kisco, and his physician assistant easily diagnosed a bull's-eye-shaped erythema migrans that was an archetype of the form. She prescribed a few weeks of amoxicillin and sent us on our way.

"When you get a rash so classic that everyone at college tells you it's Lyme disease, it's a beautiful thing," Dan Cameron said.

The treatment was so early and appropriate that, as promised by the mainstream doctors, David appeared to be cured easily and fast.

When I thought of all the misery, I also tallied on the plus side a bull's-eye rash as Lyme's single, merciful gift.

53

❖

Starting Over:
Don't Get Slymed Again

The labyrinthine science of Lyme disease is a brain bender. One group of studies suggests spirochetes can survive the standard treatment. An opposite set suggests the microbes always die. One set of papers shows evidence that spirochetes may hide or change form when faced with a stressor like antibiotic. Alternate papers dismiss these factors, deeming them irrelevant to the actual course of disease. Studies show, without question, that the *B. burgdorferi* spirochete regularly crosses the placenta, but many academics insist there's no evidence, whatsoever, that it impacts the unborn.

What is going on?

With the pathogenesis of Lyme disease still unclear, the truth is that mainstream experts have imposed a rigid template on an entity they don't fully understand. Because their studies flow from the disease definition, rather than the other way around, they have generated information about a "disease model," but not the disease itself. Based on the assumption that the disease definition is immutable, their studies are unable to go beyond it or push the envelope to incorporate new observations and ideas.

Evidence like this is helpful to those involved in vaccine development; without differentiating between the infected and the uninfected, it's impossible to know if a vaccine works. But oversimplifying nature's complexity is a substandard method for solving the mysteries of biomedicine. It is not the way great science is done. In the end, if one accepts as "diagnostic" the CDC's disease definition (including the two-step test from Dearborn), then the body of scientific literature codifying what we call Lyme disease provides us with "Truth." But because the definition was derived without all the evidence, and amidst so much protest from so many experts, it cannot be as immutable as boosters claim.

I have arrived at the hole in the donut, and I think of Jonas Salk, developer of the polio vaccine and one of the most celebrated medical researchers of his time. During my years as a science journalist, I had the honor of spending many hours with Salk over the course of more than a year as we worked together on an interview for a book and magazine. Scientists had to be careful, Salk told me then, lest they impose themselves too aggressively on the process of discovery and confuse their bias with the way things really work. Salk concluded there were two types of biomedical investigation. The first type of experiment sought to prove or disprove a theory or find a discrete, isolated fact. These experiments were designed narrowly, to answer just a single question, yes or no, up or down, black or white. Such experiments, Salk had said, were rote at best and, often, poised to mislead—like sand flowing through sieves at the beach, these studies were set up to discard most of the ambient data and could be manipulated to elicit the very answer the researcher wanted in advance. The second type of investigation had a more open-ended approach. Instead of simply seeking to bolster or undermine a single, discrete issue, these were experiments driven by dialog—"a dialog with nature," Salk had said, "a dialog with the ecosystem, with the genome, with the oceans or the organism or the brain," with all the levels and aspects of life. Because such experiments were designed to explore whole realms rather than answer specific questions, discarding data would be ruinous. Instead, every single data point, no matter how outrageous or seemingly anomalous, was required to complete the tapestry. Each input of information simply engendered another experiment, ad infinitum, enabling the dialog between the scientist and nature to go on.

It was the second type of investigation, said Salk, that moved science forward and shifted paradigms of thought.

This was the road not taken in Lyme.

While great science seeks to synthesize bodies of evidence to form broader concepts, in Lyme, the evidence has been chopped into narrower and narrower parts—so that one study takes no account of others unless it supports its thesis in advance. While the best science seeks to integrate new facts into extant knowledge, creating new theories, in Lyme the new facts are tossed while the old theories remain, unscathed.

In 2007, for instance, I interviewed the CDC's Ben Beard. "You have to admit," I said to him, "that the two-tier test you endorse lets many patients fall through the cracks."

"Quite to the contrary," Beard responded, "we feel this method is close to a hundred percent sensitive and a hundred percent specific for Lyme disease." My jaw dropped to the ground. After all, I'd been interviewing experts, including the most mainstream and conservative of the scientists for years by then, and had never heard a statement like that. Even the *manufacturer* of the blots told me he'd found better patterns, and that the two-tier was flawed.

"Surely you must be referring just to Lyme arthritis," I said, knowing that Allen Steere's archetypal patients set the standard the CDC liked most.

"Oh no," said Beard, "the neurological patients are virtually always positive, too." In fact, he said, the CDC had a study documenting this, published in nothing less than the prestigious and peer-reviewed *Journal of Infectious Diseases*.

Taken aback, I phoned Ken Liegner and asked for his help. Liegner took some time out of his busy, patient-filled morning to field the paper for me, and soon he was calling back.

"Pam," he said, "the study is circular. Only patients already testing positive on the two-tier were allowed in. It was an *entry requirement*."

Those are the kinds of conclusions from which epidemics are spawned, and they aren't alone.

In 2008 I sought input on the recommendation that doctors treat a tick bite with a single dose of the antibiotic doxycycline, which IDSA Guidelines claim can prevent human Lyme disease 87 percent of the time. The CDC linked to the Guidelines on its site, without qualifying at all. Imagine the dissonance I felt, then, when immunologist Nordin Zeidner, chief of the CDC's Vector-Host Laboratory in Fort Collins, Colorado, told me internal agency studies had found the strategy questionable, and definitely ineffective in mice. Zeidner's doubts were stirred after he and colleagues examined the study's math and then retested the premise experimentally, finding the single dose doxy stopped Lyme disease not in 87 percent of mice, but rather, in 20 to 30 percent at most.

But that wasn't all. With the support of his CDC colleagues, Zeidner had begun to work with industry to develop an alternative: a form of injectable doxy that could be sustained in the body for nineteen days. Trying his formulation on mice, Zeidner found that 100 percent were protected from Lyme as well as the coinfection, anaplasmosis. Instead of a single doxy dose on tick bite, this CDC scientist was developing a doxy skin patch to protect people as long as they stayed exposed.

Calling IDSA for a response, I finally got a call from New York Medical College infectious disease physician Gary Wormser, lead author of the IDSA guidelines, who I'd been trying to interview, repeatedly, since 2004, without success. Now in 2008 Wormser was on the phone, defending the one-dose doxy. Single-dose doxy should be more effective in humans than in mice because it stays in our blood longer, he said.

Yet it is hard to parse reality when the very agency supporting a practice has evidence the practice is wrong. Studies are confounding when, as in Wormser's single-dose doxy work, the disease definition is narrow and patients are followed for limited amounts of time. How could Dr. Wormser know his treatment worked in full when his patients were followed for only six weeks? How could he know, for sure, that the single dose of doxy didn't suppress the early immune response but not the disease—as other studies suggest it might?

When it comes to science, questions on methodology are crucial. Science can be flawed, it can be tricky, Jonas Salk taught me, but science is all we have. If we are ever to unravel the mysteries of Lyme disease and find a cure, it is *science*—pure and unadulterated—that will lead us home. We need science, but different science. We must travel the road not taken. Sometimes you just need to start again.

One such broad-based effort comes from Stony Brook, where infectious disease specialist Ben Luft hopes to put the old science to rest. As long ago as the early 1990s, Luft, working with the evolutionary biologist Daniel Dykhuizen, went out into the field, collecting ticks and analyzing *Borrelia*. In the course of that effort, they discovered that Lyme spirochetes appeared to be "clonal"—that is, instead of reproducing sexually, through the exchange of genetic material, each parent gave rise to clones, or replicas, of itself. Every so often a parent spirochete would mutate, and another line of clones would emerge. The mutations, when they occurred, took place largely in the genes coding for outer surface protein C (OspC), meaning that this protein, in particular, varied widely from strain to strain.

A few years later, a graduate student wearing a baseball hat—Wei-Gang Qiu—popped into Luft's office, announcing he wanted to work on Lyme disease. Soon it became Qiu's job to travel the Eastern seaboard as far north as New Hampshire and south through the Carolinas collecting ticks infected with *B. burgdorferi* spirochetes. The *Borrelie* were duly isolated and compared for differences in their genes.

Eventually the researchers focused on twenty strains, each with a different version of the changeable OspC. Working with those twenty strains, Luft learned that six didn't infect humans and ten caused only a rash. Only four of the twenty could leave the skin to invade other tissue like the heart and joints or the brain. The most virulent of the strains turned out to be the prototypical B31, the version of *B. burgdorferi* found by Jorge Benach in the original Shelter Island ticks and ultimately isolated by Burgdorfer and Barbour at the Rocky Mountain Labs in 1981.

But what made B31 and the other invasive strains different? Seeking an explanation, Luft joined with immunologist Steven Schutzer of the University of Medicine and Dentistry of New Jersey to create a team of top-notch scientists without the usual baggage in Lyme. Among their crew were such luminaries as Claire Fraser, director of the Institute for Genomic Research (TIGR) in Rockville, Maryland, one of the world's top authorities on genomics; Dick Smith, of Pacific Northwest National Laboratory, widely considered the world's top expert in proteomics (the study of proteins); and Sherwood Casjens of the University of Utah, who, along with Fraser, sequenced the genome of *B. burgdorferi* in 1998.

Working together, the team found that the invasive strains weren't just clonal—instead, they were capable of genetic exchange with each other, in other words, a form of sexual reproduction. Unlike other spirochetes, they carried negatively charged OspC molecules with an altered 3-D structure. It was the altered structure, Luft theorized, that allowed these spirochetes to travel past the skin, burrow into the host, and cause disseminated Lyme disease.

The implications are profound. One of the most important is that if just four strains of the twenty cause disseminated infection, then the roster of rash-based studies on the treatment of early Lyme disease, conducted from the 1980s to the present, would have to be reassessed. Take a moment to ponder the simple math: It would be impossible to accept results based on the assumption that 100 percent of Lyme rashes can cause invasive disease when a significant percent cannot. Some of the classic studies claim very high cure rates for early infection; yet if the causative strain were of the rash-only variety, then even orange juice would be a "cure." Are recommended treatment protocols truly curing most of those with early, invasive borreliosis? Or has noise from rash-only strains obscured less rosy results?

The answer won't be found in the twentieth-century technology of the Western blot, by today's standards crude yet still trotted out by many mainstream researchers as evidence that they are right. Instead, we must look to the science of the twenty-first century, including state-of-the-art genomics and proteomics that allow for the sequencing of every gene and protein involved in every stage of Lyme. "What we will find," says Luft, "are proteins we never tested for on our ELISAs and Western blots—proteins we were never even aware of. But they will be the critical markers for invasive, infectious Lyme disease. Perhaps people who test negative on the old tests will become positive when we look for the right markers," he adds. This new approach—a Salkian dialogue with the organism—should take the blinders off Lyme disease research, reversing the funneling of thought that has gone on for decades. "I don't want to be critical about the past, but more is possible now," Luft says of Lyme's old guard. "We have put together a team with no preconceptions about Lyme disease. We are going to move on."

And move on they have. Over the next few years, the Luft-Schutzer team will sequence every gene in every strain of *B. burgdorferi* that Wei-Gang Qiu captured along the eastern seaboard, together with many strains from Europe and the Midwest. Using recombinant biology, each gene will be made to express its individual protein in vitro, in the lab—in aggregate, every protein produced by any strain of *B. burgdorferi* in any environment, some 1,800 proteins in all.

Studying the genome and the proteins it forms has helped the scientists to see Lyme disease in a whole new light. One big discovery is that the dominant B31 strain is genetically identical in Europe and the United States, indicating a transcontinental migration of the organism in recent years. "If the organisms had been separated longer," explains Luft, "they would be different, because each would have been evolving in its own way." Indeed, the data suggest that sometime before the epidemic took off, a strain from Europe may have arrived in the United States on the back of a dog or a bird, lighting the forested suburbs like a match thrown on tinder wood, creating the perfect storm.

"When an infection becomes entrenched in an environment, when it's really socked in, you find a lot of B31," Luft notes. People may always have been infected with *Borrelia,* but when the hardy, promiscuous, virulent B31 arrived in the northeast suburbs some thirty years back, it engendered a form of Lyme that was far more infectious, and far more severe, than we'd ever seen before.

Yet it wasn't just B31 that fanned the flames of Lyme—the infection could differ from person to person and Lyme test to Lyme test, because in any given region there was a different mix of strains. In the Northeast, where Lyme was codified, there was much more uniformity, but as the team moved to the South, away from the center, strains became more variable and mixed. Different strains might cause different disease signs and symptoms in patients—and while B31 appeared to cause worse disease, it is certainly possible, says Luft, that the illness it causes is less insidious and easier to treat.

The science of the twenty-first century, it turns out, puts the two-tier diagnostic test approved in Dearborn in 1994 to shame. Indeed, as spirochetes move from tissue to tissue in the human body over time, they generate more than twice the number of proteins that it's possible to find in culture—the basis for the tests of today. "What about these other proteins? Are they the ones expressed when some people feel sick, and is that why these patients don't test positive?" asks Luft. It's all the more complicated because spirochetal proteins vary from strain to strain. "When we use B31 as the prototype for a test, that only gives us the band pattern for B31," Luft says. "What about all the other strains? How do you test positive for them?"

In the end, nothing will stop twenty-first-century genomics and proteomics from trumping the authority of the two-tier and the old-style Western blot. Still serving as the gateway to Lyme diagnosis and brandished as arbiters of Truth by Lyme's old guard, these technologies are nonetheless holdovers from a cruder, less nuanced past. Instead of testing for antibodies to ten limited proteins as the CDC suggests, the Luft team will coat all 1,800 *B. burgdorferi* proteins on a slide. "We want to test patient sera against the *entire* array of *Borrelia* proteins in all their variability," says Luft. "So if I look at a patient over time, over the course of their disease I can see whether new proteins, ones we've never noticed, might emerge."

The new genomics and proteomics are also shedding light on treatment—for instance, why the use of doxycycline might have sabotaged

Cure Unknown ◆ 352

treatment success in the Klempner study, the one so highly touted by the Infectious Diseases Society of America and used by insurers to deny claims. Examining the *B. burgdorferi* genome, the Luft team found it coded for the same kind of "efflux pump" found in *E. coli*. A virtual sump pump, the molecular apparatus literally ejected tetracycline and doxycycline out of cells before they could build concentrations high enough to stamp the infection out. "These drugs inhibit the infection," says Luft, "but cannot wipe it out."

Based on this finding, Luft, the scientist who pioneered the use of Rocephin for Lyme disease back in the 1980s, is now studying another drug—tigecycline, an intravenous antibiotic currently used for infections of the abdominal organs and skin. Its mechanism is much like that of doxycycline and tetracycline—except that its chemical structure literally inhibits the efflux pump, keeping itself from being ejected by cells. "It's a hundred times more active against the spirochete than doxycycline," says Luft. Instead of just inhibiting the spirochetes, like doxy, it kills them dead. Rocephin kills them, too, but requires a very long period of time to do the job. In the test tube, tigecycline kills *Borrelia* fast, in fact, in twenty-four hours flat.

Currently testing tigecycline in the test tube and soon, in mice and maybe dogs, Luft says he must demonstrate its efficacy in experiments before he unleashes it on us. "The only way I can be of service is by being as rational and methodical as possible, so that my work will be reproducible," he says.

"We're at a critical point," says Luft. "We have powerful new tools and a fundamental understanding of the biology of the *Borrelia*. We know every gene in that organism. We know all the variations of those genes. We know what's in the human genome. So when someone gets sick we've got to put this together, in context, and ask what's going on."

For years, he says, his colleagues have asked irrelevant questions and looked at Lyme disease *out* of context. For instance, despite the known fact that few actively infected neuroborreliosis patients have spirochetal DNA in their spinal fluid, scientists are constantly looking for DNA in the spinal fluid as proof or disproof of infection. It's an approach born of prejudice because people know, in advance, that it will support their point of view.

"Now we have the opportunity to understand this disease," Luft said, and listening to him talk, I knew Jonas Salk would be proud. "Some researchers have thrown down their gloves and retreated to their corners, leaving patients out in the cold. But despite what they say, the patients are still sick. It's a question of doing right by them—it's not a question of whether you might have to eat crow. We've got to go in and do the right experiments, and then we can look truth in the eye."

54

❖

And the Bands Play On

The wisecracking, high-energy Alan MacDonald appeared like a vision at a meeting of Lyme doctors in the fall of 2006. Tall and thin and almost totally bald, the heretic who dared report spirochetes in Alzheimer's brains was altered, but he was back. Living in Texas, remarried, and working under the radar as a bench pathologist at a Quest lab, MacDonald had tried to forget about Lyme disease. But in his fifteenth year of exile, the mysteries unsolved and the patients still sick drew him back. So he told his wife about his Lyme years and together they moved east.

Eventually settling in as pathologist for the St. Catherine of Siena Medical Center in Smithtown, Long Island, New York, he reviewed his former list: ALS, Parkinson's, Alzheimer's, dementia of any sort. For some of these patients, he fervently believed, Lyme could be the true root cause.

Fifteen years earlier, he'd received Alzheimer's brains from a brain bank and searched them for spirochetes with silver stain and monoclonal antibodies. That was suggestive—but with the spirochete genome deciphered, MacDonald could now hunt for something more definite, *Borrelia* DNA itself. First, he ordered ten Alzheimer's brains from the Harvard McLean brain bank. Then, drawing from the hippocampus, the center of learning and memory, he made each brain into slides. Finally, searching the slides with special, molecular probes, he found something literally monstrous: In the cells of seven of those brains, he tracked a

DNA sequence apparently part human, part spirochete, a deadly ungodly hybrid combining *Borrelia* and us. What he has found, MacDonald asserts, is evidence of a "transfection," in which the proteins causing illness are no longer manufactured by *B. burgdorferi* spirochetes but by the genes of the patients themselves. "The DNA of the spirochete combined with the human chromosome, and the site of the linkage was the same in seven of ten brains," he said. "Once it's in your DNA and you're churning it out yourself, you're cooked."

Reporting his findings in a six-article series in the journal *Medical Hypotheses,* MacDonald says he has found the hybrid DNA in areas of the brain rich in the plaque causing Alzheimer's. "Alzheimer's plaques in those brains lit up like lights on a Christmas tree, but the areas around the plaques were dark." The targets inside the plaques were literally round, he adds, suggesting the motif of cysts. Extrapolating the find, he notes that diseases causing dementia, from Lewy body to Parkinson's to ALS, have been associated with spheres inside neurons. "These could be cystic forms of the spirochete, killing the cells from the inside out," MacDonald suggests. He further theorizes that infection might jump across the synapse between nerve cells, infecting entire neural circuits of the brain. This phenomenon, he says, would explain the progression of Alzheimer's from early disease to late.

In a twist that is almost unbelievable, MacDonald now suggests his transfections may be the autoimmune trigger that his nemesis, Steere, has been seeking with such futility for so long. While MacDonald has found only short snippets of *Borrelia* DNA inside human cells thus far, he says that "if a *Borrelia* DNA segment of sufficient length were inserted into a human cell," that cell would start producing *B. burgdorferi* proteins, setting the stage for a situation in which the immune system attacked the self. "Occult intracellular infection equals autoimmunity," MacDonald states.

Across the cosmos, in the other Lyme universe, the Infectious Diseases Society of America published its updated *Clinical Practice Guidelines* for Lyme disease in October 2006. The august body, including most infectious disease doctors in the United States, had, commendably, shimmied to the left on coinfections. For a decade the Lyme doctors had been hammered for treating babesiosis and ehrlichiosis, but now the mainstream was climbing aboard, and in an open-minded sense. The *Babesia* section, written by Peter Krause of the University of Connecticut, said that infection could be chronic and treatment, in extreme cases, open-ended until signs of the disease were gone. Discussing ehrlichiosis, pathologist J. Stephen Dumler of Johns Hopkins advised treating the infection based on suspicion and symptoms, without awaiting the results of a test. These were laudable additions to the narrow script. In 2000, when my family was first diagnosed, the idea of testing symptomatic patients for these coinfections was, to primary care practitioners, not just foreign but absurd. A couple of years later, Eugene Shapiro of Yale told me that in his set of patients, at least, coinfections were insignificant, and virtually never involved. Yet here was Shapiro's name on the guidelines putting coinfections on the map. It was progress, and I took note.

But when it came to Lyme itself, the new guidelines were more restrictive than ever in limiting the scope of treatment and the patients who could be diagnosed. Taking an ever-harder line in response to what it saw as patient extremism on the ground, IDSA came out against clinical discretion in determining whether or not patients had Lyme disease. Drawing a line in the sand between the classic disease described in the textbooks and patients outside the paradigm, IDSA imposed a Lyme formula so narrow it excluded large numbers of the ill. As before, those with the dread "minor" symptoms of fatigue, confusion, and pain were cast out of the Lyme fold unless they also had a physician-diagnosed EM rash or one of the late, "major manifestations" like swollen knees or meningitis, followed by passage of the two-tiered Dearborn series. The narrow strictures meant that at any stage of illness, many patients could be missed. It wasn't much of an issue, said the authors, because late-stage Lyme was rarely seen but was virtually always cured, usually with simple doxycycline, in twenty-eight days.

Citing the Klempner study, IDSA portrayed even the possibility of persistent infection as nonsense and rejected treatments used by Lyme doctors: any form of empirical or long-term antibiotic therapy, any drug combination, even the standard vitamins and mineral supplements typically used for patients (Lyme or not) when exhausted and run-down. IDSA did not mention the heretic ILADS guidelines at all.

Endorsed by the CDC, IDSA's *Clinical Practice Guidelines* became the latest weapon in the Lyme inquisition, geared to quash the patient movement the way a daisy bomb might pulverize a village of tents.

On a cool crisp day at the end of November 2006, hundreds of Lyme patients rallied outside the Westchester Medical Center in Valhalla, New York, where Gary Wormser, the lead author of the IDSA guidelines, was the chief of infectious disease. They waved a sea of green-paper faces (representing patients too sick to attend) and a multitude of banners and signs. "Don't blame ticks. Chronic Lyme is a nightmare created by the

IDSA authors," one typical poster read. The crowd was visible from the road, and, this being Lyme country, drivers nodded encouragement and slowed through the afternoon to give them the thumbs-up.

Pat Smith of the LDA stepped up to the podium with a clock—one that moved counterclockwise, back in time. "Just like this clock, the IDSA guidelines are taking us back to the dark ages," she said, throwing the clock and a copy of the guidelines in the trash. "Chronic Lyme disease has been scrubbed." With a name, chronic Lyme could be studied, treated, and eventually even cured, she concluded. But by marginalizing the illness and defining it out of existence, the guidelines had consigned its unwilling victims to debilitating lives of progressive illness and pain. The problem, she said, was that IDSA had rejected alternate opinions or any peer-reviewed research that didn't align with its views.

Moved by the ruckus, and what he saw as real transgressions, Richard Blumenthal, the attorney general of Connecticut, launched an antitrust investigation into IDSA and its guidelines, charging abuse of monopoly power and exclusion of other points of view. The authors were key opinion leaders who also held extensive commercial interests in Lyme-related projects and ventures, and had too much to gain by maintaining the status quo, Blumenthal felt—from stature in their professions to the payoff from patents to the constant flow of grants. He found the conflicts of the IDSA authors to be profound: They consulted for big pharma and owned Lyme-related patents; they received fees as expert witnesses in medical-malpractice, civil, and criminal cases related to Lyme disease; and they were paid by insurance companies to field—and help reject—Lyme-related claims. Of the fourteen authors, nine received money from vaccine manufacturers and four were funded to create test kits, products that would be more likely to reap profit if the definition of Lyme disease remained essentially unchanged.

"These guidelines were set by a panel that essentially locked out competing points of view. Presumably, the IDSA is a nonprofit-making organization, but such organizations can still be used for anticompetitive purposes," said Blumenthal. "This is not theoretical. It will come down to dollars and cents."

In Lyme, this was a nuclear assault.

By May 2007, another set of guidelines, this time from the American Academy of Neurology and published in the journal *Neurology,* came from many of the same authors and repeated virtually the same IDSA script. The Connecticut attorney general duly subpoenaed documents from the AAN and its authors as well.

It was October 2007 when the guideline authors lobbed a blistering response in the august pages of the *New England Journal of Medicine,* reaching doctors nationwide. Their article dismissed even the possibility of chronic infection after treatment and called the devastating minor manifestations of fatigue, pain, and cognitive confusion "mild and self-limiting." The patients just weren't that sick, the authors insisted, and studies suggesting they were had been "preordained."

When symptomatic patients requested more antibiotic, the authors told doctors they must refuse. "Explaining that there is no medication, such as an antibiotic, to cure the condition is one of the most difficult aspects of caring for such patients. Nevertheless, failure to do so in clear and empathetic language leaves the patient susceptible to those who would offer unproven and potentially dangerous therapies," the authors said.

Daniel Cameron, our doctor, and the new president of ILADS, went through the paper's flaws: It based its conclusions on 221 patients in three clinical trials, a cohort much too small and rarefied to extend to the whole of Lyme. "Applying the findings to Lyme patients with different characteristics may limit the options of those who would benefit more," he said. Anyway, the studies in question hadn't been completely negative as the IDSA authors implied: Patients in one of them had shown significant permanent improvement in fatigue, and in another, fatigue and pain.

There was too much contention in medicine, Cameron pointed out, and the stakes were too high, for this kind of article to run without a nod to opposing points of view. Why had the authors dismissed, as irrelevant, the ILADS treatment guidelines? "It is only by airing different positions that the medical and scientific community can reach a better understanding," Cameron said. He implored the *Journal* to present all reasoned positions so that a dialogue could ensue.

It's doubtful that his plea will end the thirty-year-old Lyme war, which rages on. Three decades after Polly Murray rang the alarm, patients with Lyme disease, even forms so classic they belong in a textbook, often seek diagnosis for months or years without resolve. Lyme patients have fought valiantly for their voices to be heard, but the defanging of their doctors has taken a heavy toll. Sitting around dinner one night with Pat Smith and her lieutenants following Jones's testimony at his hearing in Hartford, I commented on Burrascano's retirement. His aggressive style of treatment, I said, was increasingly difficult to obtain, even from seasoned Lyme doctors who had treated this way in the past.

"It is only because of who we are and what we do," responded a woman at the table, someone high up in the patient movement, "that *our own* children are taken care of, and aren't left disabled like the rest." It was a brutal observation, but true. Even the Lyme doctors had become more conservative. You often had to be a "made person"—a leader in the movement or the author of a book—to access the kind of therapy that brought Jason back to Earth.

In 2008, oral antibiotics, especially low-dose orals, are the regimen most often prescribed by Lyme doctors, even when patients may need more. The doctors know what works for the sickest patients, but many now take the risk only for a vaunted few.

In writing this book I have traveled the lands of Lyme, from the wooded suburbs of Boston and the windswept beaches of Long Island to the Coast Range in California. I have been to Cape Girardeau, Missouri, along the Mason-Dixon Line, and driven north to Michigan in a single, sleepless stretch. These are beautiful lands, where homes are nestled into forests and cantilevered over oceans and sprawled along spacious river-banks and around the shores of lakes. Wildlife, especially deer and field mice, but also squirrels and raccoons and skunk, freely roam the bounty of these lands, and birds of many species fly overhead.

But the most radiant of all the Lymelands could be Lyme, Connecti-cut, where the story began. Famous not only for Lyme disease but also as the birthplace of impressionist art in America, Lyme is visually thrilling, from wide-open vistas of the Long Island Sound, south and west, to the looming Nehantic State Forest on the east. As a sign over the Interstate attests, Lyme is an American art mecca, home to the renowned Lyme Art Colony and the Florence Griswold Museum.

Out of money and out of luck in 1899, Florence Griswold was forced to open her Georgian-style mansion to boarders. One of them happened to be the landscape artist Henry Ward Ranger, who, while riding past on a train, looked out the window and exclaimed, "This is a place just wait-ing to be painted!" Ranger got off the train and booked a room with Miss Florence, eventually convincing other artists, including the great impressionist Childe Hassam, to follow suit.

Driving into Lyme myself, I understand. On the day I arrive, the leaves are changing color, boats are bobbing in the marina, and vintage New England houses give way to the Atlantic's blue immensity beyond. The light in Lyme is so clear, the sky so transparent, I realize that up un-til now, I have been viewing my landscapes through fog. It is on a whim that I decide to visit Polly Murray's street, unbeknownst to her, so that I can take some private time to look around. Joshuatown Road is a sharp left off the highway, a leisurely loop through gorgeous countryside and woods. My drive down this road will be a journey back in time, I tell myself. But the farther I go, the more uncomfortable I feel.

The classic country homes on Joshuatown Road are ensconced in nature, as their creators intended, each family residence nestled beneath the trees and surrounded by forest. Stone-wall perimeters, natural havens for ticks, separate one family residence from the next. I must drive slowly, very slowly, because big brown bucks, graceful does, and spindly fawns are everywhere. Despite the discovery of Lyme disease on this very road, the residents—who were among the first subjects of the earliest studies at Yale—have thrown caution to the wind. No one could live more enmeshed in nature, more at one with the ecosystem and the spirochete, than these folks, unless one were to live on the forest floor itself.

Here at ground zero, the residents remain vulnerable to the disease named after them. You couldn't pay me to get out of my car and walk around, I think to myself as I drive along the thickly forested curves saturated with deer. *I have never seen so many in one small place.*

There is just a single house on Joshuatown Road with the trees cleared back and the bulk of a stone wall replaced by a white picket fence. There is just one house on this winding rural road situated not within the woods in the shadow of trees, but in a wide open clearing, on a sunlit expanse of lime green lawn. This is Polly Murray's house. Luminous in the sun, as if caught in a spotlight, Murray's white colonial is a beacon and anomaly in these woods. Polly Murray, alone, has taken the precautions the experts have suggested for residents of the Lymelands—clearing the trees away from the places children play and people live, reducing stone walls beloved by ticks. After all this community has suffered, only Polly Murray has taken the lessons home. And even Murray has deer as sentinels at her front gate, even Murray's house sits just a few dozen feet from the edge of woods.

Making my way into town, I find an outdoor mall with a bookstore, and notice a wall of shelves devoted to local authors—but Murray's volume is not among them. I ask the proprietor to check. She hasn't heard of Polly Murray and must look in the computer to see. "We sold a copy six months ago," she tells me, "but we haven't reordered because there haven't been any requests."

Perhaps we enjoy living recklessly. Perhaps we feel invulnerable, and thus immune to dangers and risks. We don't like to ponder bad news before it happens. Despite Leonard Sigal's suggestion that Lyme can be a harbor when life gets too tough, I've found that few who are healthy care to give much thought to disease—I know that I didn't. We welcome the messenger who tells us not to worry, not to think about it—I know that I did.

In this context, the idea that the residents of the Lymelands are a population in search of a disease (lest they have to work too hard or endure too much stress) defies credibility. If this were so, wouldn't the paranoia on Joshuatown Road be rocking off the charts? If the residents of Joshuatown Road, where it all began, have failed to take precautions in lifestyle, have failed to acknowledge the risk—if they do not even request Polly Murray's book, much less stock it on their shelves—then what about the rest of us?

I have been writing this book for years, and for years I couldn't wrap it up. *I'm waiting for a better ending,* I told myself in honest moments, but dared not mention that to others: my editors, my agent, my husband, my kids. I put the manuscript down for many months at a time. Year after year my children were sick. Year after year more Lyme patients were misdiagnosed, mistreated, then meanly hung out to dry. Every year more doctors—*my doctors*—were put out of business or reported to medical boards for the way they treated Lyme. Every year I met more patients turned away not just by the mainstream but also by the very Lyme doctors who'd helped me and mine. Ever the optimist, I hoped something would break—official admission that patients were infected, better treatments, a cure for Jason, my son. I waited years for a better ending, but it never came.

"You have to end on a positive note, Pam, you have to give us hope," people told me. I've found that hard. I'm still optimistic that science will give us answers and patients will then get well. But *today* I live in the Lymelands. Caught in Lyme's gravity, I pray it will loosen its grip and let me fly away.

Epilogue

I write this note from the stoop of my walk-up in downtown Brooklyn. We live one flight up in a cramped, pricey warren of rooms, surrounded by brownstones and bistros as far as the eye can see. There are cobblestones underfoot. The local park is concrete. I can walk to the water's edge and touch the Brooklyn Bridge. The big city, Manhattan, beckons just ten minutes and a few short subway stops away. Castaways from a careless move to the suburbs that derailed our lives for a decade, we have washed up here in this urban oasis, dazed but still breathing, safe from the deer and the ticks, from new exposure to the disease.

Lyme still touches our lives. It was summer 2008 when, suffering from an ear infection, I received antibiotics. In a few days the ear was better, but that familiar malaise—the buzzing and numbness, the headache and nausea, the stilted speech and stupor—all returned in force. Something had roused the monster, sending my immune system into overdrive and stirring the vortex of Lyme. *Never really gone*, I thought at the time. As in years past, I stayed on the antibiotics until my head cleared, the numbness receded, and the immune storm washed back to sea.

Not long after, Mark had reached a low. His memory was so poor that he lost the train of conversation and had trouble staying on track just watching TV. He needed the big gun—Rocephin—to reach his brain and push his infection away. Over three months of treatment, his improvement was marked, but one night his fever soared and he started shaking with the chills. We rushed him to the ER, to find his IV line infected. It was removed and Mark, decidedly less symptomatic, flew antibiotic-free like me.

Our children were not as fortunate—sicker than we were from the start, they were sick still. With Joe Burrascano out of the picture, we took Jason to Richard Horowitz, a Lyme doctor in the graceful Hudson Valley hamlet of Hyde Park, New York, famous for its hiking trails, its river views, and the Roosevelt and Vanderbilt estates. By Burrascano's reckoning, Horowitz was one of the few Lyme doctors pushing pedal to metal, wielding antibiotics, treating the coinfections, boosting the immune system, addressing sleep issues, detoxing metals—using the whole armamentarium at once.

A meeting with Richard Horowitz is not for the faint of heart. A rapid-fire talker with laser-focused thoughts, he parses every detail of your medical history, reviews past treatment, then critiques, dissects, moves on. Whatever your last doctor did, Horowitz has a broader, more nuanced and far more complex plan. Miss your doses? Horowitz is unhappy. Mangle his instructions? His eyes flash such displeasure it's hard to meet his gaze. A physician who lives and breathes medicine but also dances and acts, Horowitz has filled his office with Tibetan tapestries, little statues of Buddha, and blessings from the monks who help him keep on track. Since he practices in Lyme country, his windows face the woods.

Richard Horowitz grew up in Queens, New York, "with a strong connection to God." At Bayside High, he played the leads in *Plaza Suite*, *Barefoot in the Park*, and *Arsenic and Old Lace*. At Northwestern University, biology and theater formed the yin and yang of his life. He did his medical training at the Free University of Brussels, in Belgium, where classes were conducted in French.

Perhaps because medical school was so uniquely stressful, Horowitz took up meditation at a center just four blocks from his Brussels apartment. Under the tutelage of Buddhist teachers from Tibet, he not only relaxed but also explored the deep spiritual questions: What was the meaning of life? Why were we here at all?

"What is the most important thing you can teach me?" the American doctor-in-training asked his Tibetan mentors one day.

"Exchange yourself with the other. Have compassion," they said.

After medical school, Horowitz returned to New York City, ultimately becoming an internist. But when it came to setting up his practice in 1987, he chose the Hudson Valley, a place of spectacular natural beauty and home to a Buddhist retreat center where he could meditate and train.

As a board-certified internist associated with the well-known Vassar hospital, it didn't take Horowitz long to fill his practice with patients suffering from heart disease, asthma, diabetes, and stroke. But you couldn't practice in Lyme country for long before Lyme patients walked through your door. Some patients got better after just thirty days of treatment with antibiotics like amoxicillin, which worked by attacking the cell wall, says Horowitz. "However, it was obvious there was a group for whom all the symptoms came back." Why were these patients relapsing? he wanted to know, and what could be done?

By the early nineties he'd hit upon one answer, babesiosis, caused by the malaria-like parasite the powers that be insisted could not exist in the Hudson Valley. (Laboratory testing by Thomas Mather, professor of entomology at the University of Rhode Island, ultimately proved Horowitz correct.) "A lot of Lyme patients started getting better when I treated their *Babesia* with Mepron and Zithromax," Horowitz says. But many were still sick.

That is when Horowitz began, in earnest, to modify his treatments one strategy at a time, seeking always to get at the root cause of the disease—and lift more patients off the floor.

Like Burrascano he raised doses and treated longer, but that was just the start. For instance, one of his patients suffered joint pain and fatigue, but also ulcers. Horowitz treated the ulcer, caused by infection with the spiral bacterium *H. pylori*, with standard therapy of bismuth and tetracycline, eventually adding Flagyl. In response to Flagyl, the ulcer patient experienced a Lyme-like herx, and the fatigue and joint pain resolved.

Horowitz later conducted a study among his patients, finding that some of the most intractable responded to Flagyl, reclaiming their lives after years. In the aftermath of this work, other researchers found that Flagyl could break Lyme cysts apart in culture and Flagyl became part of the Horowitz arsenal—but still, so many stayed ill.

As the years passed, Richard Horowitz went through every possible reason for treatment failure, addressing them one by one. Was infection trapped in the brain? His treatments crossed the blood-brain barrier. Were spirochetes hiding inside cells? Horowitz made sure to offer an intracellular antibiotic. Did one intracellular antibiotic fail? The patient might need two at once.

For the chronically ill, sometimes only combination treatments worked. "I might add Biaxin, an intracellular antibiotic, to amoxicillin, a cell wall antibiotic." Was the patient still sick? Intracellular antibiotics had different mechanisms—the quinolines like Levaquin attacked DNA, for instance, while tetracycline interfered with protein synthesis in the cells' tiny ribosomes. With so many strains and varying patient reactions, two intracellulars could sometimes work better than one.

By the year 2000, Horowitz was pushing the envelope—treating with cell wall, cystic, and intracellular antibiotics simultaneously and finding a much higher rate of success. The combinations and rotations took on meaning as Horowitz looked beyond Lyme and *Babesia* to other intracellular pathogens—*Anaplasma*, *Bartonella*, and *Mycoplasma*, to name three. Operating way outside the narrow guidelines, he rejected cookie-cutter treatments, instead tailoring therapies to clinical response. When a patient plateaued he would rotate the medicines, coming at the infection from a whole different angle, lifting the patient again.

Yet after all this, some patients failed his treatments—so Horowitz looked further: Some 20 percent of the still-sick, he found, had heavy-metal poisoning and needed detox. "Metals suppressed their immune systems, and they could not clear the Lyme," he states. Still others had chronic inflammation triggered by infection. Their bodies were awash in inflammatory cytokines, and treatments like glutathione, which lowered inflammation, helped them improve. The barriers to cure could be myriad: adrenal dysfunction, lack of B or D vitamins, imbalance of hormones, suppression of the immune system so infection could not be cleared.

"Every year I found another piece of the puzzle," says Horowitz, and more patients were lifted up or went into remission, able to subsist without antibiotics, on herbs and supplements alone.

The waiting list was endless, but with Burrascano gone and Jason so sick, I picked up the phone and—once more—begged. "Please tell doctor Horowitz this is Pam Weintraub," I told the front desk. It took a couple of months, but Jason was in.

From 2007 to the present, using the range of his strategies, Richard Horowitz has finished, for Jason, the job Joe Burrascano began. He has treated Jason's Lyme and babesiosis with a combination of oral antibiotics; he has boosted his immune system, supplemented his vitamins, addressed his sleep problems, and helped him sustain his newfound health with antimicrobial herbs. Jason is a success story—the teen once so sick he could not leave the bathtub, the boy who could barely walk, the young man thrown away by the medical establishment, is now so strong he's finished Brown University and heads for film school in the fall.

In the end it isn't Jason, but David who Lyme has destroyed. I'd rejoiced in the summer of 2007 when David was treated for his classic bull's-eye rash—to me a thing of beauty, early, treatable, uncomplicated Lyme. But defying the IDSA's guidelines, David failed their treatment. Perhaps the problem was *Babesia*, an infection confirmed by Quest Labs—or the overlay of new Lyme strains impinging on the old. Whatever the reason for the treatment failure, by 2008, back at Vassar College, David was falling down the Lyme hole—couldn't stay awake, couldn't focus on work, couldn't remember or think. On top of it all, his ears had started to vibrate, every few seconds going into spasm and causing him shocks of pain. David couldn't go on at Vassar. We had to bring him home.

As he had with Jason, Horowitz lifted David up. In fact, by summer 2009 there was one enduring problem—the spasming, painful ears. The Lyme had been so devastating, the ear pain had seemed minor, but with most of the Lyme in remission, the ear pain loomed large. "With so much pain in my ears, I still can't think," David said.

The Lyme had damaged David's cranial nerves, our Manhattan otoneurologist finally told us, causing middle-ear myoclonus, a rare condition with few known causes. One cause was a brain tumor. (David did not have one.) Another was Lyme disease.

For us the journey continues, and we are not alone. With tick-borne disease spreading throughout the country, with diagnosis so restrictive and doctors in retreat, patients have fewer options. Rejected by insurers, the Lyme doctors take their sizable fees in cash, keeping Lyme families strapped. Even for cash payers, the wait to get in can take months.

Filling the gap for the sick and the broke: An online emporium of self-help books, Internet sites, and pyramid schemes passing for therapy. From countless herbs (some quite helpful) to outright poisons to the laying on of hands, from light to sound to intravenous ozone, from pet-catalog antibiotics to clinics in Mexico, patients without doctors or money are forced to treat themselves in the heartbreaking outback of Lyme.

Rejection by the Infectious Diseases Society and its powerful team of doctors flows freely from the journals, where IDSA members tend to staff the ad hoc review committees, standing as gatekeepers for Lyme. Of particular concern are the publications, more prominent in recent months, suggesting that uncured patients are not really sick with Lyme disease, but with a strange psychiatric malaise. "Psychiatric comorbidity and other psychological factors distinguished [chronic Lyme disease] patients from other patients commonly seen in Lyme disease referral centers, and were related to poor functional outcomes," Leonard Sigal wrote in the journal *Arthritis and Rheumatism* in 2008.

Gary Wormser and Eugene Shapiro, authors of the 2006 IDSA Guidelines, follow a similar train of thought in the *Journal of Women's Health* in 2009: " 'Post-Lyme disease syndrome' refers to prolonged subjective symptoms after antibiotic treatment and resolution of an objective manifestation of *Borrelia burgdorferi* infection (Lyme disease). 'Chronic Lyme disease' is a vaguely defined term that has been applied to patients with unexplained prolonged subjective symptoms, whether or not there was or is evidence of *B. burgdorferi* infection," they wrote. The object of their study: "To determine if the population of patients with chronic Lyme disease differs from the populations of patients with either Lyme disease or post-Lyme disease syndrome by examining the gender of patients with these diagnoses." Their conclusion: "Illnesses with a female preponderance, such as fibromyalgia, chronic fatigue syndrome, or depression, may be misdiagnosed as chronic Lyme disease."

To some, this is the future: "We definitely need to move in another direction for sure. Some have proposed having a conference on medically unexplained syndromes (MUS), which would include conditions such as chronic Lyme disease, fibromyalgia, chronic fatigue syndrome, etc. These would be looked at in a new, broad, and fresh way, with no assumptions or preconceived ideas as to their cause and/or treatment," Phil Baker states.

But I see it differently: While new approaches are needed to help the sick get well, lumping Lyme patients in with others sets things back to the stone age—before we understood Lyme as an infection at all. Conflating chronic Lyme patients with chronic fatigue patients and fibromyalgia patients means tossing them all into the psychosomatic basket with the disordered and depressed. Forevermore such patients—many of them women—would be seen through the psychiatric lens, the etiology of their illness ignored.

This approach only flies if one accepts, without question, the IDSA view of Lyme disease, including the restrictive testing and the insistence that treatment cannot fail. The premise that chronic patients are actually psychiatric patients requires that we blindly discount what science reveals about borrelial strains, seronegativity, and widespread treatment failure for the late-diagnosed. Dismissing the patients and disappearing the disease demands that we buy into the dogma that Lyme is hard to catch, easy to cure, and diagnosed without issue virtually 100 percent of the time.

Despite a hardening inside parts of academia, the mood on the street has changed. Part of it is the publicity. The action of the Connecticut attorney general and the debut of a frightening, heartfelt documentary,

Under Our Skin, has garnered news and media coverage never before seen for this disease. And in its own, quieter way, *Cure Unknown* has helped, too—from five printings in hardcover and a new life in paperback to magazine excerpts to national radio interviews on high-profile shows like Leonard Lopate and Diane Rehm to reads from congressmen and doctors and scientists, it, too, has changed the dialogue in the wider world. Word has gotten out: The disease is complex, the conflicts are rife, the patients are left out in the cold.

The tone in the press has changed as well because of something often unstated—the epidemic is spreading. More often now, the journalists who call me have Lyme disease themselves, and they find what I found: It is hard to write a story invalidating your own experience. When you yourself have been misdiagnosed, when you have failed the treatment, when your spouse or children are sick, you dig deeper and find more.

Things have changed in science, too. Here in New York State, four teaching hospitals focus on Lyme disease. One, New York Hospital, houses the IDSA doctors, those dismissive of broader diagnostic standards and the notion of chronic Lyme disease.

But at three other New York teaching hospitals—Columbia Presbyterian, New York University, and SUNY Stony Brook, a more open-minded view has taken hold.

The work on strains at places from Stony Brook to Berkeley to UC Irvine "could alter how we diagnose and treat the disease in the years to come," says Alan Barbour, director of the Pacific-Southwest Regional Center of Excellence for Biodefense and Emerging Infectious Diseases at the University of California Irvine and one of the world's foremost spirochete experts. "If some strains are more likely than others to spread in the blood, and by that route to other tissues, then identification of the strain a person is infected with could help guide therapy," Barbour explains. "Some strains may call for a longer course of antibiotics. The problem is isolating the microbe out of the patient to see what strain it is. This could be done by a Polymerase Chain Reaction (PCR) test of the blood or a skin biopsy, when there is a rash. Isolating the microbe is harder when the illness has been going on for longer than a few weeks, but any isolate of *Borrelia burgdorferi* from a patient would mean a diagnosis of Lyme disease."

At New York University (NYU) Langone Medical Center, a new Lyme disease program will integrate basic medical parasitology, neurology, neuroradiology, and neuropathology. Led by neurologist David S. Younger, the program will open its arms to chronically ill patients and their treating doctors, wielding science to get a handle on the disease. Younger and team will offer a service currently unavailable anywhere else in the world: Collaborating with community doctors to treat infection that may be chronic, while at the same time reversing the neurological damage caused by an immune system gone awry.

"We are going to err on the side of treating aggressively," states Younger, whose patients may receive aggressive antibiotics for their infection along with immunomodulatory therapies like intravenous immunoglobulin (IVIG) to restore damaged portions of the nervous system by giving the immune system a boost.

But that's just the start. The extensive patient base expected to seek NYU's expertise will help fuel a wide-ranging research effort aimed at curing the disease by studying animal models and applying results in the human realm.

The first project, already launched, comes from NYU medical parasitologist and veterinarian Ute Frevert, whose mouse model will track the spirochete from the moment it penetrates the skin, through the body to junctures at the blood-nerve and blood-brain barriers, where damage is often extreme. Frevert's field of view will be exceptional, thanks to spirochetal colonies, donated by Yale, that have been engineered to glow when exposed to green fluorescent protein. By tracking the glowing spirochetes, the researchers will be able to locate their exact location in any organ, including the brain.

At the same time, the NYU scientists will seek similar information in the human subjects they treat. In one experimental technique, neuroscientist Oded Gonen will use whole brain proton magnetic resonance spectroscopy (H+–MRS) best known for its precision in diagnosing multiple sclerosis (MS). This technique is far more sensitive than conventional neuroimaging like SPECT and MRI, says Younger, because it is analyzed in three dimensions, instead of just two, and because it measures damage to nerve cells and myelin by tracking markers of oxidative stress. One of those markers will help the researchers track damage through the entire gray and white matter of the brain.

Finally, NYU neuropathologist David Zagzag will be studying fusin, a chemokine (small inflammatory protein) that appears to regulate the immune cells needed to clear the infection for good. T cells specific to *Borrelia burgdorferi* have already been demonstrated in the cerebrospinal fluid of patients with central nervous system Lyme disease, says Younger. Zagzag and Younger hypothesize that the Lyme-specific T cells are formed when the spirochete interacts with fusin and its receptors in the body. By following the inflammatory proteins, receptors, and immune cells associated with fusin in the patients they treat, they hope to develop biological assays that will monitor every stage of active central nervous system Lyme disease from early infection to late stage disease all the way to cure.

At Columbia, the new Lyme and Tick-borne Diseases Research Center, established to help answer the questions surrounding chronic Lyme disease, continues to focus its energies on the development of new diagnostic assays, the identification of immune and imaging biomarkers that may predict treatment outcome, and the exploration of a range of potential therapies, from antibiotics to neuropharmacotherapies to immune modulators, says Brian Fallon, who has begun collaborating with scientists around the world. Of particular importance is Fallon's specimen bank, including tissue samples from patients with chronic Lyme. Without these types of specimens, nobody would be able to find new diagnostic assays for patients with chronic symptoms. These new studies may bring to the U.S. a much more sensitive and specific diagnostic test," Fallon states. In fact, data collected from prior Lyme neuroimaging work will soon be used to help measure alterations in the brain's immune functioning directly. "This can best be accomplished at a world-class neuroscience center like the one at Columbia. We now know that the brain has both local and systemic control of the immune response. A better understanding of this process will lead to more targeted and effective treatments for chronic Lyme," he states.

At UC Davis Steven Barthold (in collaboration with Ben Luft) strives to see whether he can stop Lyme persistence in mice. From special antibiotics to experimental nanoparticles, the strategies at Davis are diverse.

In an extraordinary act of conciliation, the CDC in Atlanta last summer hosted a three-day workshop on Lyme disease in the South.

And at the University of Colorado, immunologist M. Karen Newell is researching a treatment that seems to get to the very heart of the problem for many patients—the nexus where infection and immunity meet. As important studies from UC Davis, Tulane, and the University of Utah indicate, pockets of persistent infection may incite massive inflammation through interaction with molecules called Toll-like receptors. That inflammation is a required and important part of the innate immune response to infection—one of the ways we have of killing invaders and beating back disease. In some people, a failure to control the inflammation leads to *chronic* illness, including autoimmune disease.

And this is where Newell comes in. Based on her theoretical model, she is designing a series of peptides that stop the process cold. The novel, computer-designed peptides, matched to each individual's immune system, are double edged. First they alter immune cells (B lymphocytes) caught in the fruitless inflammatory process so that other immune cells (T cells) can recognize and kill them. With the offending B cells gone, the immune system rights itself.

The initial inflammation is generally followed by a more specific antibody response. But failure to control that inflammation "may trigger chronic hyper-immune activation," Newell explains. "Once the inflammation is stopped, then the specific anti-pathogen immune response should be able to clear the infection without antibiotics at all."

In 2009—despite the freeze from the IDSA—researchers who believe the patients are real search for answers, and science moves on.

The march of science is slow and often fairly quiet, but politics in Lyme are loud. In Connecticut, where patients have fought the longest, the drama is profound. On a sunny day in May I get in my car and one last time head for New Haven and the office of Charles Ray Jones. At first I don't recognize it—the grimy brick building has been power-washed, its color somehow lighter, and the rusting steel terrace rails replaced with burnished beams. Jones's office itself has new chairs, new rugs, new toys. The facilities have been renovated but Jones is drained to the bone.

We cross the street for lunch at a small Korean place—Jones walks slowly now—and his nightmare spills out: More charges are pending, and each seems crazier than the last. The first new case involves the grandchild of a woman Jones knows. Based on the grandmother's description, the child appeared symptomatic, so Jones ordered a Lyme disease test in anticipation of an appointment. The parents canceled the appointment, and Jones never saw the child. But the state took issue, charging Jones with ordering tests before doing a physical exam.

Two more cases were triggered by fathers involved in the bitter throes of divorce. In one of them Jones took a history over the phone, finding the girl had an erythema migrans rash diagnosed at the hospital emergency department, bone pain, headaches, light sensitivity, and night sweats, symptoms compatible with Lyme disease and babesiosis. Running labs, he found the child tested positive for the infections. Because his waitlist was six months long, he commenced treatment in conjunction with the girl's family doctor, and the girl got better. But as in the Nevada case, the state has charged Jones with treating over the phone.

The last case involves a Lyme patient who also had tonsillitis. When the mother arranged for a needed tonsillectomy, the father, in a power play, tried to block it—so Jones reported him to the Connecticut Department of Children and Families. The father retaliated that very same day, reporting Jones to the licensing board of the Health Department for treating his daughter's Lyme disease.

Even the physician monitor brought in to review Jones's patient charts while the Nevada case goes through appeal has turned Jones in. He reported him to the licensing board based on patient files culled from his court-ordered quarterly reviews. Despite the fact that the monitor was told to refrain from judging Jones based on his off-guideline treatments, the doctor, an expert in pediatric fibromyalgia, has done just that. "He told me every child I treat is another Tuskegee experiment," Jones reports.

The Jones drama plays out against the backdrop of Lyme politics in Connecticut, where the state's attorney general launched the investigation that unseated the IDSA guidelines panel, including Gary Wormser of New York Medical College and Eugene Shapiro of Yale. Now a new panel has been seated to reexamine the evidence, and their judgments will prevail. It behooves the new panel to go beyond the work of the old panel in their examination of the science—as this update goes to press the new team is getting to work.

Will the new panel tweak the guidelines issued by its predecessors? Time will tell.

"Is it hopeless?" Jones asks me as our lunch concludes.

"Not hopeless, just endless," I respond.

The Connecticut Department of Health might go after Jones until the day he dies, but a broader inquisition has been stanched, for now. On June 21, 2009, Governor M. Jodi Rell signed a bill allowing Connecticut doctors to prescribe long-term antibiotics in the treatment of persistent Lyme disease—outside of standard guidelines—without fear of sanctions from the state. "Doctors in Connecticut—the absolute epicenter of Lyme disease—can continue to do what is best for their patients suffering from this complex illness," Rell said.

The political struggle over Lyme disease is likely to rage for years, but it is ultimately science, not politics, that will rule the day. In defending its turf, the old guard has continually pitched its case against the anecdotal stories of very sick patients, as if the antiseptic "objectivity" of one trumps the sheer desperation of the other, proving they must be right. As someone who has traveled the country for almost eight years now interviewing scientists to write my book, I can state unequivocally: This is a cop-out. No matter what the new IDSA panel decides many of the top researchers at the top institutions in the world do not think the original panel got it right.

While you can limit the evidence in your guidelines and dismiss the experiences of patients, you can't stop the march of research; in the end, you can't dumb down complexity no matter how many journals you staff and how many committees you chair. You can try to disappear a disease—but in the face of a burgeoning epidemic with ever more people sick, would you really want to succeed?

As for me and mine, you can find us in Brooklyn, still waiting for that exit visa, that get-out-of-jail-free card—still praying for passage from Lyme.

Brooklyn, New York
2009

Notes and References

This is a work of investigative journalism based on interviews with others, on many documents and correspondences, on articles in the peer-reviewed literature, on video- and audiotapes of past events, and on personal attendance at many meetings. The research was conducted from 2001 to fall 2009. This book is also partly a memoir of my individual experience, with those sections based on personal memory, perceptions, notes, and physician records. Except in a few instances, where I was asked to protect patient privacy, the names used are real.

INTRODUCTION: NAVIGATING BY LYMELIGHT

1 *Starting in the early 1990s:* The narrative here is based largely on personal and family recollections, on medical records, and on notes from meetings. Most of this chapter is a summary of material documented, extensively, throughout the body of the book. Where material appears here only I note the source.

4 *Lyme or not Lyme?:* In-person interviews with Betty Gross, founder of the Westchester Lyme Disease Support Group, 2003–2004, and with Leonard Sigal, M.D., at the time director of the Lyme Disease Center at the Robert Wood Johnson Hospital in New Jersey, January 2, 2003. Also: "Lyme neuroborreliosis manifesting as an intracranial mass lesion." *Neurosurgery.* May 1992; 30 (5): 769–73.

5 *a number the CDC estimates:* Telephone interview with C. Ben Beard, Ph.D., chief of the Bacterial Diseases Branch of the Division of Vector-Borne Infectious Diseases of the CDC, 2007.

5 *more than an estimated 270,000:* www.cdc.gov/ncidod/dvbid/lyme/resources/Lyme07Cases.pdf.

PROLOGUE: SECOND JOURNEY OUT

This section describes my trajectory as a journalist as I began and then continued to investigate Lyme disease and its coinfections. It explains my internal thought process in conducting this research. Where discrete facts are introduced, I reference them.

8 *2006 guidelines:* Wormser, G. P., Dattwyler, R. I., Shapiro, E. D., Halperin, J. I., Steere, A. C., Klempner, M. S., Krause, P. I., Bakken, I. S., Strle, F., Stanek, G., Bockenstedt, I., Fish, D., Dumler, J. S., Nadelman, R. B. "The clinical assessment, treatment, and prevention of Lyme disease, human granulocytic anaplasmosis, and babesiosis: clinical practice guidelines by the Infectious Diseases Society of America." *Clinical Infectious Diseases.* November 1, 2006; 43 (9): 1089–1134. Epub October 2, 2006.

9 *people like C. Ben Beard:* Telephone interview with C. Ben Beard, 2007.

9 *Brian Fallon, a psychiatrist:* In-person interview with Brian Fallon, New York Psychiatric Institute, 2004.

9 *"If a doctor asks the patient":* Excerpted from extensive e-mail sent by Harold Smith, M.D., May 3, 2004.

10 *a conference in Dearborn:* Association of State and Territorial Public Health Laboratory Directors (ASTPHLD). Proceedings of the second national conference on the serological diagnosis of Lyme disease, October 27–29, 1994. Dearborn, MI. ASTPHLD, 1995.

10 *pattern was determined:* Interviews with Kenneth B. Liegner, Nick Harris, and dozens of others.

10 *Antibodies can stick:* Schutzer, S. E., Coyle, P. K., Reid, P., Holland, B. "*Borrelia burgdorferi*-specific immune complexes in acute Lyme disease." *Journal of the American Medical Association.* November 24, 1999; 282 (20): 1942–46.

11 *suppress the antibody:* Dattwyler, R. J., Volkman, D. J., Luft, B. J., Halperin, J. J., Thomas, J., Golightly, M. G. "Seronegative Lyme disease. Dissociation of specific T- and B-lymphocyte responses to *Borrelia burgdorferi.*" *New England Journal of Medicine.* December 1, 1988; 319 (22): 1441–46.

11 *Even Immunetics:* In-person interview with Andrew Levin, president of Immunetics, in Cambridge, MA, in July 2003.

11 *Where the rash was required:* Gerber, M.A., Shapiro, E. D., Burke, G. S., Parcells, V. J., Bell, G. L. "Lyme disease in children in southeastern Connecticut. Pediatric Lyme Disease Study Group." *New England Journal of Medicine.* October 24, 1996; 335 (17): 1270–74. Also: Sigal, L. H., Zahradnik, J. M., Lavin, P., Patella, S. J., Bryant G., Haselby, R., Hilton, E., Kunkel, M., Adler-Klein, D., Doherty, T., Evans, J., Molloy, P. J., Seidner, A. L., Sabetta, J. R., Simon, H. J., Klempner, M. S., Mays, J., Marks, D., Malawista, S. E. "A vaccine consisting of recombinant *B. burgdorferi* outer-surface protein A to prevent Lyme disease. Recombinant Outer-Surface Protein A Lyme Disease Vaccine Study Consortium." *New England Journal of Medicine.* July 23, 1998; 339 (4): 216–22.

11 *Where patients were diagnosed:* Steere, A. C., Dhar, A., Hernandez, J., Fischer, P. A., Sikand, V. K., Schoen, R. T., Nowakowski, J., McHugh, G., Persing, D. H. "Systemic symptoms without erythema migrans as the presenting picture of early Lyme disease." *American Journal of Medicine.* January 2003; 114 (1): 58–62.

11 *most of them agreed I had pegged it right:* Concept discussed in interviews with about a dozen university-based researchers specializing in Lyme disease. The individual I discussed this with most thoroughly was infectious disease

specialist Benjamin Luft of the State University of New York at Stony Brook, in two in-person interviews in 2002. Also Peter Krause, M.D., University of Connecticut.

12 *The conflict was distilled for me:* Burling, Stacey. "Shining a light on medically unexplained symptoms." *Philadelphia Inquirer.* August 19, 2003.

12 *article sparked the ire of:* Stone, Alan. *Philadelphia Inquirer.* Letter to the editor, August 27, 2003.

12 *counterpunch:* Ehrlich, George E., M.D. *Philadelphia Inquirer.* Letter to the editor, August 27, 2003.

12 *Skeptical of chronic:* Sigal, L. H. "Summary of the first 100 patients seen at a Lyme disease referral center." *American Journal of Medicine.* June 1990; 88 (6): 577–81. Also: Sigal, L. H., Patella, S. J. "Lyme arthritis as the incorrect diagnosis in pediatric and adolescent fibromyalgia." *Pediatrics.* October 1992; 90 (4): 523–28.

13 *A survey by the New York State Legislature:* In-person interview with pharmacologist Ardith Bondi, Ph.D., who is spearheading the New York Legislature Lyme Disease Survey. September 23, 2003.

13 *Perez-Lizano decided to alert Geneva-based Lee Jong-wook:* Perez-Lizano, Miguel. Letter to Lee Jong-wook, director general, WHO, September 3, 2003.

13 *"We perfectly understand your concern":* Pang, Tikki, director, Research Policy and Cooperation, WHO. Letter to Miguel Perez-Lizano, October 9, 2003.

14 *The devastating consequence of untreated Lyme was undeniable:* Telephone and in-person interviews with Benjamin Luft, M.D., Stony Brook; Raymond Dattwyler, M.D., New York Medical College; Kenneth Liegner, M.D., of Armonk, New York; and Joseph Burrascano, M.D., of East Hampton, 2003–7. Also: Shadick, N. A., Phillips, C. B., Logigian, E. L., Steere, A. C., Kaplan, R. F., Berardi, V. P., Duray, P. H., Larson, M. G., Wright, E. A., Ginsburg, K. S., et al. "The long-term clinical outcomes of Lyme disease. A population-based retrospective cohort study." *Annals of Internal Medicine.* October 15, 1994; 121 (8): 560–67. Also: Asch, E. S., Bujak, D. I., Weiss, M., Peterson, M. G., Weinstein A. "Lyme disease: an infectious and postinfectious syndrome." *Journal of Rheumatology.* March 21, 1994; 21 (3): 454–61.

14 *One day, sitting with Peter Krause, a pediatrician:* In-person interview with Peter Krause, M.D., University of Connecticut, Hartford, 2004.

15 *You can't train doctors:* In-person interview with Leonard Sigal.

15 *Eugene Shapiro of Yale:* In-person interview with Eugene Shapiro, Yale University, 2002.

16 *Dattwyler picked up a marker:* In-person interviews with Raymond Dattwyler, who is an infectious disease specialist, Stony Brook, 2002.

16 *superbugs:* Telephone interview with Phillip J. Baker, Lyme Disease Program Officer, National Institutes of Health, 2004.

17 *Robyn Greco:* Telephone interview with Robyn Greco, February 2004.

17 *Profiled in an article entitled "Stalking Dr. Steere":* Grann, David. "Stalking Dr. Steere over Lyme disease." *New York Times Magazine,* June 17, 2001.

19 *One night after a conference:* Lyme Disease Foundation Conference, Farmington, CT, 2003.

1. INTO THE WOODS

25 *In the year 1993, I spread a map:* The personal narrative is based on personal and family recollections, and on medical records.

27 *One study:* Steere, A. C., Taylor, E., McHugh, G. L., Logigian, E. L. "The over-diagnosis of Lyme disease." *Journal of the American Medical Association.* April 14, 1993; 269 (14): 1812–16.

27 *tinge of worry:* Barbour, A. G., Fish, D. "The biological and social phenomenon of Lyme disease." *Science.* June 11, 1993; 260 (5114): 1610–16; and Barbour, A. G. "Biological and social determinants of the Lyme disease."

29 *The CDC required:* Association of State and Territorial Public Health Laboratory Directors (ASTPHLD). *Proceedings of the second national conference on the serological diagnosis of Lyme disease.* October 27–29, 1994. Dearborn, MI. Washington, DC: ASTPHLD, 1995. Plus phone interviews with C. Ben Beard and Barbara Johnson, chief of the molecular biology section at Arbovirus Diseases Branch, Division of Vector-Borne Infectious at the CDC, 2007.

29 *changing band patterns:* Telephone interview with Maria Aguero-Rosenfeld, laboratorian at New York Medical College, 2003.

2. A PLACE IN THE WHIRLWIND

I interviewed Sheila Statlender in July 2003 in Framingham, MA, and again in August 2007, in Falmouth, MA. Additional details provided by e-mail during October, November, and December 2007.

3. SON OF A PREACHER MAN

I interviewed David Martz in Colorado Springs, Colorado, in August 2007. Additional details provided by e-mail in November 2007.

4. CONNECTICUT GENESIS

43 *In the spring of 1956:* Murray, Polly. *The Widening Circle.* New York: St. Martin's Press, 1999.

44 *another mother:* Mensch, Judith. "Lyme Disease." *Maryland Medical Journal.* July 1985; 34: 691–92.

45 *the researchers William E. Mast and William M. Burrows:* Mast, W. E., Burrows, W. M. "Erythema chronicum migrans and Lyme arthritis." *Journal of the American Medical Association.* November 22, 1976; 236 (21): 2392; Mast, W. E., Burrows, W. M., Jr. "Erythema chronicum migrans in the United States." *Journal of the American Medical Association.* August 16, 1976; 236 (7): 859–60.

45 *a doctor in Hamden:* In-person interviews with Charles Ray Jones in 2002 at his office in New Haven, CT.

46 *biomedical juggernaut:* I confirmed Jones's employment at Memorial Sloan–Kettering by speaking with Esther Carver of the hospital's personnel department in 2003. Additional evidence came from the medical database pubmed. I checked the pubmed database at www.ncbi.nih.gov/entrez/query.fcgi. Cited articles include: Lieberman, P. H., Jones, C. R., Steinman, R. M., Erlandson, R. A., Smith, J., Gee, T., Huvos, A., Garin-Chesa, P., Filippa, D. A., Urmacher, C., Gangi, M.D., Sperber, M. "Langerhans cell (eosinophilic) granulomatosis. A clinicopathologic

study encompassing 50 years." *American Journal of Surgical Pathology.* May 1996; 20 (5): 519–52; and Lieberman, P. H., Jones, C. R., Filippa, D. A. "Langerhans cell (eosinophilic) granulomatosis." *Journal of Investigative Dermatology.* July 1980; 75 (1): 71–72. Charles Ray Jones was also listed by the American Medical Association. Listing is on the AMA Web site, at AMA Physician select: www.ama-assn.org/aps/amahg.htm.

47 *first salvo:* Murray, Polly. *The Widening Circle.*

5. A NEW DISEASE AND A RING OF FIRE

48 *A student at Columbia:* School of Medicine Class Day address, Yale Medical School, New Haven, CT, May 27, 1990. The transcript of this talk was provided by Allen Steere as representative of his experience and views. He did, however, decline to be interviewed by me for this book or to participate in a fact check despite several requests. Also relevant to the chronology of this chapter: "Catching the bug: How scientists found the cause of Lyme disease and why we're still not out of the woods yet," an article by Joel Lang published in *Connecticut Medicine.* June 1989; 53 (6). *Connecticut Medicine* reprinted this article from the May 11, 1986, issue of *Northeast Magazine,* published by the *Hartford Courant.* Dr. Allen Steere recommended this article as an especially accurate rendition of historical events, and suggested that I follow this chronology in describing the sequence of his early research.

48 *he played with Itzhak Perlman:* Grann, David. "Stalking Dr. Steere." *New York Times Magazine.*

49 *EIS was established:* See EIS Web site at www.cdc.gov/eis/.

49 *"the heretical idea":* Steere, Allen C. "Epidemiology and the elucidation of Lyme disease: Excerpts from the 1995 Langmuir Lecture." *EIS Bulletin.* Summer 1995. Sent to me by Dr. Steere for use in communicating his story. Also: France, David. "Scientist at work: Lyme expert developed big picture of tiny tick." *New York Times.* May 16, 1999.

49 *mode of transmission:* Steere, A. C., Malawista, S. E., Snydman, D. R., Shope, R. E., Andiman, W. A., Ross, M. R., Steele, F. M. "Lyme arthritis: an epidemic of oligoarticular arthritis in children and adults in three Connecticut communities." *Arthritis & Rheumatism.* January–February 1977; 20 (1): 7–17.

50 *describing the European:* Fitzpatrick, Thomas B. *Fitzpatrick's Dermatology in General Medicine.* New York: McGraw Hill, 1971.

50 *But this didn't convince:* Steere, A. C., Hardin, J. A., Malawista, S. E. "Lyme arthritis: a new clinical entity." *Hospital Practice.* April 1978; 13 (4): 143–58. Also: Aronowitz, Robert A. "Lyme Disease: The social construction of a new disease and its social consequences." *The Millbank Quarterly.* 1991; 69 (1).

50 *"enlarging clinical spectrum,":* Steere, A. C., Malawista, S. E., Hardin, J. A., Ruddy, S., Askenase, W., Andiman, W. A. "Erythema chronicum migrans and Lyme arthritis. The enlarging clinical spectrum." *Annals of Internal Medicine.* June 1977; 86 (6): 685–98.

50 *But could patients from Connecticut:* Material in this paragraph was drawn from the material sent to me by Allen Steere, and is detailed above. Steere refused to grant me an interview.

51   *He rejected for the children and adults:* Steere, A. C., Malawista, S. E.,
     Newman, J. H., Spieler, P. N., Bartenhagen, N. H. "Antibiotic therapy in Lyme
     disease." *Annals of Internal Medicine.* July 1980; 93 (1): 1–8; Steere, A. C.,
     Gibofsky, A., Patarroyo, M. E., Winchester, R. J., Hardin, J. A., Malawista, S.
     E. "Chronic Lyme arthritis. Clinical and immunogenetic differentiation from
     rheumatoid arthritis." *Annals of Internal Medicine.* June 1979; 90 (6): 896–901;
     Steere, A. C., Hardin, J. A., Ruddy, S., Mummaw, J. G., Malawista, S. E. "Lyme
     arthritis: correlation of serum and cryoglobulin IgM with activity, and serum
     IgG with remission." *Arthritis and Rheumatism.* May 1979; 22 (5): 471–83;
     Hardin, J. A., Walker, L. C., Steere, A. C., Trumble, T. C., Tung, K. S.,
     Williams, R. C., Jr., Ruddy, S., Malawista, S. E. "Circulating immune com-
     plexes in Lyme arthritis. Detection by the 125I-C1q binding, C1q solid phase,
     and Raji cell assays." *Journal of Clinical Investigation.* March 1979; 63 (3):
     468–77; Steere, A. C., Hardin, J. A., Malawista, S. E. "Erythema chronicum
     migrans and Lyme arthritis: cryoimmunoglobulins and clinical activity of skin
     and joints." *Science.* June 1977; 196 (4294): 1121–22; Steere, A. C., Malawista,
     S. E., Hardin, J. A., Ruddy, S., Askenase, W., Andiman, W. A. "Erythema
     chronicum migrans and Lyme arthritis. The enlarging clinical spectrum."
     Annals of Internal Medicine. June 1977; 86 (6): 685–98; Steere, A. C.,
     Malawista, S. E., Snydman, D. R., Shope, R. E., Andiman, W. A., Ross, M. R.,
     Steele, F. M. "Lyme arthritis: an epidemic of oligoarticular arthritis in children
     and adults in three Connecticut communities." *Arthritis and Rheumatism.*
     January/February 1977; 20 (1): 7–17.

51   *It was only in 1980:* Steere, A. C., Hutchinson, G. J., Rahn, D. W., Sigal, L. H.,
     Craft, J. E., DeSanna, E. T., Malawista, S. E. "Treatment of the early manifesta-
     tions of Lyme disease." *Annals of Internal Medicine.* July 1983; 99(1): 22–26.

52   *It was a rheumatologist's view:* Interviews with Raymond Dattwyler and Ben
     Luft of SUNY Stony Brook, 2002–4.

52   *steroids:* In-person interviews with Ken Liegner, M.D., 2001–3. In-person interview
     with Dr. R. Straubinger, summer 2002. Also: Straubinger, R. K., Straubinger, A. F.,
     Summers, B. A., Jacobson, R. H. "Status of *Borrelia burgdorferi* infection after
     antibiotic treatment and the effects of corticosteroids: An experimental study."
     Journal of Infectious Diseases. March 2000; 181 (3): 1069–81; and Straubinger, R.
     K., Straubinger, A. F., Summers, B. A., Jacobson, R. H., Erb, H. N. "Clinical man-
     ifestations, pathogenesis, and effect of antibiotic treatment on Lyme borreliosis in
     dogs." *Wiener Klinische Wochenschrift.* December 23, 1998; 10 (24): 874–81.

52   *multisystemic infectious disease that impacts many organs:* In-person interview
     with Raymond Dattwyler, 2002.

53   *failed to factor in a hundred years of research from Europe:* Robert Aaronowitz,
     plus extensive references listed for chapter 13.

6. FINDING LYME'S COUNTERCULTURE

I spent two days speaking with presenters and attendees at the 13th International
Scientific/Medical Conference, sponsored by the Lyme Disease Foundation in a Marriott in
Farmington, CT, March 25–26, 2000. The description of the conference is based on the notes
I took during and after the event.

7. HIDE IN PLAIN SIGHT

Interviews with Sheila Statlender, 2003 and 2007.

8. THE EPIDEMIC SPREADS

64 *bittersweet:* Interview with Charles Ray Jones in New Haven, CT, 2002.

65 *Today in her sixties:* I interviewed Phyllis Mervine on her 600-acre ranch in Ukiah, CA, on December 9 and December 11, 2002, and throughout the summer of 2007 by telephone.

67 *a young doctor named Joe Burrascano:* In-person interview with Joe Burrascano at the Southampton Hospital in May 2002.

67 *Another local doctor:* Roueche, Berton. *The Medical Detectives.* New York: E. P. Dutton, 1985. Also: "Annals of medicare: The foulest and . . . ," *New Yorker.* September 12, 1988; 64 (30): 83.

9. CROSSING THE LINE

We set off for New Haven. The narrative here is based on visits to New Haven in 2000, including personal notes and medical records.

10. THE ROCKY ROAD

Personal memoir of the period.

11. THEN THERE WERE THREE

Interviews with Sheila Statlender, 2003 and 2007, and e-mail correspondence, 2007.

12. NIGHT FALLS FAST

Interview with David Martz in Colorado Springs, Colorado, August 2007.

13. DISCOVERING THE SPIROCHETE

This chapter is based largely on in-person interviews. These include two in-person interviews with microbiologist and entomologist Willy Burgdorfer at the Rocky Mountain Laboratories in Hamilton, Montana, on October 15 and October 16, 2002; an in-person interview with Jorge Benach, director of the Center for Infectious Diseases, professor, Department of Molecular Genetics, and professor, Department of Pathology, State University of New York, Stony Brook, November 1, 2002; an in-person interview with physician and microbiologist Alan Barbour, M.D., at the University of California, Irvine, in 2001; and an in-person interview with molecular biologist Russell Johnson at the University of Minnesota in Minneapolis, 2003. Some information has been drawn from an interview with Dr. Burgdorfer conducted by Deidre Boggs for the NIH in the summer of 2001. The NIH provided me with a transcript for use in this book.

82 *the German physician Alfred Buchwald:* Buchwald, A. "Ein Fall von diffuser idiopathischer Haut-Atrophie." *Archives of Dermatology and Syphilis.* 1883; 15: 553–56.

82 *in 1902:* Herxheimer, K., and Hartmann, K. "Über Acrodermatitis chronica atrophicans." *Archives of Dermatology and Syphilis.* 1902; 61: 57–76, 255–300.

82 *in 1909:* Afzelius, A. "Verhandlungen der dermatologischen Gesellschaft zu Stockholm." *Archives of Dermatology and Syphilis.* 1910; 101: 404.

82   *many times over:* Lipschutz B. "Über eine seltene Erythemform (Erythema chronicum migrans)." *Archives of Dermatology and Syphilis.* 1913; 118: 349–56.

82   *in 1930:* Hellerström, S. "Erythema chronicum migrans Afzelius." *Acta
dermato-venereologica* (Stockholm). 1930; 11: 315–21.

82   *published in the* Southern Medical Journal: Hellerström, S. "Erythema chronicum migrans Afzelius with Meningitis." *Southern Medical Journal.* 1950; 43:
330–35.

82   *in 1955:* Binder, E., Doepfmer, R., Hornstein, O. "Experimentelle Übertragung
des erythema chronicum migrans von Mensch zu Mensch." *Hautarzt.* 1955; 6:
494–96.

83   *first American:* Scrimenti, R. J. "Erythema chronicum migrans." *Archives of
Dermatology and Syphilis.* July 1970; 102: 104–105.

83   *admired the work:* Scrimenti, R. J., Scrimenti, M. "Lyme disease redux: the legacy
of Sven Hellerström." *Wisconsin Medical Journal.* January 1993; 92 (1): 20–21.

      The chapter has been supplemented, where necessary, by the following
sources: Burgdorfer, W. "How the discovery of *Borrelia burgdorferi* came
about." *Clinics in Dermatology.* 1993; 11: 335–38; Benach, J. L., White, D. J.,
Burgdorfer, W., et al. "Changing patterns in the incidence of Rocky Mountain
spotted fever on Long Island (1971–1976)." *American Journal of Epidemiology.*
1977; 106: 380–87; Burgdorfer, W., Barbour, A. G., Hayes, S. F., Benach, J. L.,
Grunwaldt, F., Davis, J. P. "Lyme Disease—A Tick-borne Spirochetosis?"
Science. June 18, 1982; 216 (4552): 1317–19; Barbour, A. G. "Isolation and
Cultivation of Lyme Disease Spirochetes." *Yale Journal of Biology and Medicine.*
1984; 57: 521–25; Berger, B. W., Clemmensen, O. J., Ackerman, A. B. "Lyme
disease is a spirochetosis. A review of the disease and evidence for its cause."
American Journal of Dermatopathology. April 1983; 5(2): 111–24; Berger, B.
W., Clemmenson, O. J., and Gottlieb, G. J. "Spirochetes in lesions of erythema
migrans." *American Journal of Dermatopathology.* April 1983; 5 (2); Berger, B.
W. "Erythema chronicum migrans of Lyme disease." *Archives of Dermatology.*
August 1984; 120 (8): 1017–21; Berger, B. W., Kaplan, M. H., Rothenberg, I. R.,
Barbour, A. G. "Isolation and characterization of the Lyme disease spirochete
from the skin of patients with erythema chronicum migrans." *Journal of the
American Academy of Dermatology.* September 1985; 13 (3): 444–49; Benach,
J. L., Bosler, E. M., Hanrahan, J. P., Coleman, J. L., Habicht, G. S., Bast, T. F.,
Cameron, D. J., Ziegler, J. L., Barbour, A. G., Burgdorfer, W., Edelman, R.,
Kaslow, R. A. "Spirochetes isolated from the blood of two patients with Lyme
disease." *New England Journal of Medicine.* March 31, 1983; 308 (13): 740–42;
Steere, A. C., Grodzicki, R. L., Kornblatt, A. N., Craft, J. E., Barbour, A. G.,
Burgdorfer, W., Schmid, G. P., Johnson, E., Malawista, S. E. "The spirochetal
etiology of Lyme disease." *New England Journal of Medicine.* March 31, 1983;
308 (13): 733–40; Burgdorfer, W. "Arthropod-borne spirochetoses: a historical
perspective." *European Journal of Clinical Microbiology and Infectious Disease.*
January 2001; 20 (1): 1–5; Lubke, L. I., and Garon, C. F. "The Lyme disease
spirochete, *Borrelia burgdorferi,* forms spheroblasts in the presence of spin-
golipid analogue PPMP." *Proceedings of Microscopy and Microanalysis.* 1999;
5, Supplement 2: 1136–37.

14. THE CHASM WIDENS

89 *validated in his hunch:* In-person interviews with Charles Ray Jones at his office in New Haven, CT, 2001.

91 *went back to the drawing board:* Steere, A. C., Hutchinson, G. J., Rahn, D. W., Sigal, L. H., Craft, J. E., DeSanna, E. T., Malawista, S. E. "Treatment of the early manifestations of Lyme disease." *Annals of Internal Medicine.* July 1983; 99 (1): 22–26.

91 *were disturbed:* Brenner, C. "Emergence," 2004. Unpublished manuscript. Plus in-person and telephone interviews with Carl Brenner, 2002–2007.

93 *even scientists at Stony Brook:* In-person interviews with Raymond Dattwyler and Benjamin Luft, 2002 and 2003, at the Health Sciences Center, State University of New York at Stony Brook.

94 *organisms would survive:* Dattwyler, R. J., Halperin, J. J. "Failure of tetracycline therapy in early Lyme disease." *Arthritis & Rheumatism.* April 1987; 30 (4): 448–50.

95 *Using amoxicillin:* Luft, B., Mariuz, P. "Use of third-generation cephalosporins. Spirochetes." *Hospital Practice.* 1991; 26 Suppl 4: 34–39, discussion, 53–54; Dattwyler, R. J., Luft, B. J. "Antibiotic treatment of Lyme borreliosis." *Biomed Pharmacother.* 1989; 43 (6): 421–26.

95 *greatest achievement:* Dattwyler, R. J., Halperin, J. J., Volkman, D. J., Luft, B. J. "Treatment of late Lyme borreliosis—randomised comparison of ceftriaxone and penicillin." *Lancet.* May 28, 1988; 1 (8596): 1191–94; Luft, B. J., Volkman, D. J., Halperin, J. J., Dattwyler, R. J. "New chemotherapeutic approaches in the treatment of Lyme borreliosis." *Annals of the New York Academy of Science.* 1988; 539: 352–61; Dattwyler, R. J., Halperin, J. J., Pass, H., Luft, B. J. "Ceftriaxone as effective therapy in refractory Lyme disease." *Journal of Infectious Diseases.* June 1987; 155 (6): 1322–25.

95 *some 15 or 20 percent:* Luft, B. J., Gorevic, P. D., Halperin, J. J., Volkman, D. J., Dattwyler, R. J. "A perspective on the treatment of Lyme borreliosis." *Reviews of Infectious Diseases.* September–October 1989; 11 Suppl 6: S1518–25.

15. HOW THE LYME WORLD SPLIT IN TWO

This chapter is based on a series of in-person and telephone interviews with Joseph Burrascano, M.D., Alan MacDonald, M.D., and Jorge Benach, M.D. I interviewed Dr. Burrascano at Southampton Hospital in Southampton, NY, and at his office in East Hampton, NY, in 2002 and 2003, and over the telephone and by e-mail in 2007. I interviewed Dr. Benach at his office at SUNY Stony Brook in 2002. I interviewed Dr. MacDonald in a series of telephone interviews in 2006 and 2007.

Also of relevance: MacDonald, A. B. "*Borrelia* in the brains of patients dying with dementia." *Journal of the American Medical Association.* October 1986; 24–31; 256 (16): 2195–96; MacDonald, A. B., Miranda, J. M. "Concurrent neocortical borreliosis and Alzheimer's disease." *Human Pathology.* July 1987; 18 (7): 759–61; MacDonald, A. B. "Concurrent neocortical borreliosis and Alzheimer's disease. Demonstration of a spirochetal cyst form, Lyme Disease and Related Disorders," *Annals of the New York Academy of Science.* August 26, 1988; vol. 539.

16. LOST IN THE RUINS: THE INFESTATION OF THE SUBURBS

105   *Before I realized:* Personal memoir.

105   *outside Ithaca, New York:* Personal description of a car-deer collison we were involved in while on our way to visit Niagara Falls. We passed through Ithaca, which is in Tompkins County, NY, in 2002.

106   *The explosion of deer:* In-person interview with Dr. Andrew Spielman at the Harvard School of Public Health, Boston, MA, July 2003. Also: Matuschka, F. R., Spielman, A. "The emergence of Lyme disease in a changing environment in North America and central Europe." *Experimental and Applied Acarology.* December 1986; 2 (4): 337–53; Spielman, A. "The emergence of Lyme disease and human babesiosis in a changing environment." *Annals of the New York Academy of Science.* December 15, 1994; 740: 146–56.

108   *The white-tailed deer:* In-person interview with Kirby Stafford, Connecticut Agricultural Station, Lockwood Farm, Hamden, CT, March 23, 2003.

108   *in Maryland:* Maryland Department of Natural Resources.

108   *Pennsylvania, a whopping 1.3 million:* Revkin, A. C. "States seek to restore deer balance." *New York Times.* December 29, 2002.

109   *The same woods contained:* Brisson, D., Dykhuizen, D. E., Ostfeld, R. S. "Conspicuous impacts of inconspicuous hosts on the Lyme disease epidemic." *Proceedings. Biological Sciences/The Royal Society.* January 22, 2008; 275 (1631): 227–35.

Also: Riehlman, D., Suprock, L., and Hesselton, W. "White-tailed deer population management." New York State Department of Conservation, 2003. In Ithaca, where our car crashed, a measurement of deer density: New York State Department of Environmental Conservation (DEC) wildlife biologist Dave Riehlman, *Cornell University News,* March 2, 2000. www.news.cornell.edu/releases/March00/deer_count.hrs.html.

17. MUTTS LIKE US: LYME TESTS AND TRIBULATIONS

The chapter starts as a personal memoir, but then segues into coverage of the standard Lyme disease tests and their lack of specificity and sensitivity—and overall inability to rule Lyme disease in or out. The issues are integrated, narratively, into our personal story, but for the technical reader, relevant articles supporting the section include:

Golightly, M. G., Viciana A. L. "ELISA and immunoblots in the diagnosis of Lyme borreliosis: sensitivities and sources of false-positive results." In *Lyme disease: molecular and immunologic approaches.* Edited by Steven E. Schutzer. Plainview, NY: Cold Spring Harbor Laboratory Press, 1992; Dattwyler, R. J., Volkman, D. J., Luft, B. J., Halperin, J. J., Thomas J., Golightly, M. G. "Seronegative Lyme disease. Dissociation of specific T- and B-lymphocyte responses to *Borrelia burgdorferi.*" *New England Journal of Medicine.* December 1, 1988; 319 (22): 1441–46; *Proceedings of the second national conference on the serological diagnosis of Lyme disease.* October 27–29, 1994, in Dearborn, MI. Washington DC: ASTPHLD, 1995; Engstrom, S. M., Shoop, E., and Johnson, R. C. "Immunoblot interpretation criteria for serodiagnosis of early Lyme disease." *Journal of Clinical Microbiology.* 1995; 33: 419–27; Aguero-Rosenfeld, M. E., Nowakowski, J., McKenna, D. F., Carbonaro, C. A., Wormser, G. P. "Serodiagnosis in early Lyme disease." *Journal of Clinical Microbiology.* 1993;

3090–3195; Aguero-Rosenfeld, M. E., Nowakowski, J., McKenna, D. F., Carbonaro, C. A., Wormser, G. P. "Evolution of the serologic response to *Borrelia burgdorferi* in treated patients with culture-confirmed erythema migrans." *Journal of Clinical Microbiology.* 1996; 34: 1–9; Bakken, L. L., Callister, S. M., Wand, P. J., Schell, R. F. "Interlaboratory comparison of test results for detection of Lyme disease by 516 participants in the Wisconsin State Laboratory of Hygiene/College of American Pathologists proficiency testing program." *Journal of Clinical Microbiology.* 1997; 35: 537–43; Luger, S. W., Krauss, E. "Serologic tests for Lyme disease: interlaboratory variability." *Archives of Internal Medicine.* 1990; 15: 761–63; Golightly, M. G., Thomas, J. A., Viciana, A. L. "The laboratory diagnosis of Lyme Borreliosis." *Laboratory Medicine.* 1990; 21: 299–304; Ma, B., Christen, B., Leung, D., Vigo-Pelfry, C. "Serodiagnosis of Lyme Borreliosis by Western immunoblot: reactivity of various significant antibodies against *Borrelia burgdorferi.*" *Journal of Clinical Microbiology.* 1992; 30: 370–76; Magnarelli, L. A., Anderson, J. F., Johnson, R. C. "Cross-reactivity in serological tests for Lyme disease and other spirochetal infections." *Journal of Infectious Disease.* 1987; 56: 183–88; Mitchell, P. D., Reed, K. D., Aspeslet, T. L., Vandermause, M. F., Melski, J. W. "Comparison of four immunoserologic assays for detection of antibodies to *Borrelia burgdorferi* in patients with culture-positive erythema migrans." *Journal of Clinical Microbiology.* 1994; 32: 1958–62; Harris, N. S., Harris, S. J., Joseph, J. J., Stephens, B. G. "*Borrelia burgdorferi* antigen levels in urine and other fluids during the course of treatment for Lyme disease: a case study." Presented at the VII International Congress of Lyme Borreliosis, June 16–21, 1996, San Francisco, CA; Craft, J. E., Fischer, D. K., Shimamoto, G. T., Steere, A. C. "Antigens of *Borrelia burgdorferi* recognized during Lyme disease: appearance of a new immunoglobulin M response and expansion of the immunoglobulin G response late in the illness." *Journal of Clinical Investigation.* 1997; 78: 934–39; Jain, V. K., Hilton, E., Maytal, J., Dorante, G., Ilowite, N. T., Sood, S. K. "Immunoglobulin M immunoblot for diagnosis of *Borrelia burgdorferi* infection in patients with acute facial palsy." *Journal of Clinical Microbiology.* 1996; 34: 2033–35; Sivak, S. L., Aguero-Rosenfeld, M. E., Nowakowski, J., et al. "Accuracy of IgM immunoblotting to confirm the clinical diagnosis of early Lyme disease." *Archives of Internal Medicine.* 1996; 156: 2105–9; Goodman, J. L., Bradley, J. F., Ross, A. E., et al. "Bloodstream invasion in early Lyme disease: results from a prospective, controlled, blinded study using the polymerase chain reaction." *American Journal of Medicine.* 1995; 9: 6–12.

117 *Stony Brook researchers:* Telephone interview with Ben Luft, May 2009. Also: Luft, B. J., Dattwyler, R. J., Johnson, R. C., Luger, S. W., Bosler, E. M., Rahn, D. W., Masters, E. J., Grunwaldt, E., Gadgil, S. D. "Azithromycin compared with amoxicillin in the treatment of erythema migrans. A double-blind, random-ized, controlled trial." *Annals of Internal Medicine.* May 1, 1996; 124 (9): 785–91.

118 *Insight comes from Phillip Baker:* E-mail from Phillip Baker, April 24, 2009.

119 *According to the peer-reviewed journal* Mayo Clinic Proceedings: Bratton, R. L., Whiteside, J. W., Hovan, M. J., Engle, R. L., Edwards, F. D. "Diagnosis and

treatment of Lyme disease." *Mayo Clinic Proceedings.* May 2008; 83(5): 566–71.

119 *The most comprehensive review:* Coulter, P., Lema, C., Flayhart, D., Linhardt, A. S., Aucott, J. N., Auwaerter, P. G., Dumler, J. S. "Two-year evaluation of *Borrelia burgdorferi* culture and supplemental tests for definitive diagnosis of Lyme disease." *Journal of Clinical Microbiology.* October 2005; 43 (10): 5080–4.

119 *Even Andrew Levin:* In-person interview with Andrew Levin, Cambridge, MA, 2003.

18. PATIENTS DISPOSSESSED

122 *The patients who failed:* Based on interviews with and the writings of early Lyme activists, including Betty Gross, Mona Marcus, Barbara Goldklang, Karen Forschner, Phyllis Mervine, Pat Smith, and others.

123 *Among the hardest hit:* Karen Forschner testimony. Oversight Hearing, Lyme Disease: A Diagnostic and Treatment Dilemma, Senate Committee on Labor and Human Resources, 430 Dirksen, 10:00 A.M. to 12:00 P.M., August 5, 1993. Public Hearing on Insurance Coverage of Lyme Disease, Legislative Office Building, State of Connecticut, Room 2, February 24, 1999.

124 *Karen even posted signs:* Waldman, Hillary. "Conflict shadows couple's Lyme disease crusade." *Hartford Courant.* July 13, 1997.

126 *living in a fantasyland:* Interview with Leonard Sigal, 2002.

126 *no Lyme disease in Missouri:* Interview with Andrew Spielman, 2003.

126 *blamed the publicity:* In-person interview with Alan Barbour, 2001; telephone interview with Durland Fish, 2001. Also: Barbour A. G., Fish, D. "The biological and social phenomenon of Lyme disease." *Science.* June 11, 1993; 260 (5114): 1610–16; and Barbour, A. G. "Biological and social determinants of the Lyme disease." *Infectious Agents and Disease.* February 1992; 1 (1): 50–61.

126 *consult letter:* Steere, Allen C., M.D. Letter to a fellow physician, a report on a patient consult, 1991.

126 *most outspoken:* Many of the mainstream scientists I spoke with brought up the issue of Jamie Forschner without my asking, and declared he had never had Lyme disease.

19. THE SCOURGE OF "LIME" DISEASE

127 *Leonard Sigal is a small, wiry, bearded man:* The chapter is based largely on an in-person interview with Leonard Sigal, M.D., at the time director of the Lyme Disease Center at the Robert Wood Johnson Hospital in New Jersey, January 2, 2003.

130 *publishing a study:* Sigal, L. H. "Summary of the first 100 patients seen at a Lyme disease referral center." *American Journal of Medicine.* June 1990; 88 (6): 577–81.

130 *American College of Rheumatology:* 1990 Criteria for the Classification of Fibromyalgia. Report of the Multicenter Criteria Committee. *Arthritis & Rheumatism.* February 1990; 33 (2): 160–72.

130 *Copenhagen Declaration:* Csillag, C. "Conference: Fibromyalgia: The Copenhagen Declaration." *Lancet.* September 12, 1992; 340 (8820): 663.

131   *chronic fatigue syndrome:* Johnson, Hillary. *Osler's Web: Inside the labyrinth of the chronic fatigue syndrome epidemic.* New York: Crown Publishing Group, 1996.

131   *humor columnist:* Lettau, L. "Lime vs. Lyme disease." *Annals of Internal Medicine.* 1991; 115: 157.

132   *skepticism:* Robbins, J. M., Kirmayer, L. J., Kapusta, M. A. "Illness worry and disability in fibromyalgia syndrome." *The International Journal of Psychiatry in Medicine.* 1990; 20 (1). Also: Cohen, M. L., Quintner, J. L. "Fibromyalgia syndrome, a problem of tautology." *Lancet.* October 9, 1993; 342 (8876): 906–9; Quintner, J. L., Cohen, M. L. "Fibromyalgia falls foul of a fallacy." *Lancet.* March 27, 1999; 353 (9158): 1092–94.

132   *"therapeutic domain":* Hazemeijer, I., Rasker, J. J. "Fibromyalgia and the therapeutic domain. A philosophical study on the origins of fibromyalgia in a specific social setting." *Rheumatology.* April 2003; 42 (4): 507–15.

20. PEELING THE ONION

134   *a different lens:* This section is based largely on in-person interviews with Kenneth Liegner, M.D., in his office in Armonk, New York, through 2002 and 2003. Followed by updates by e-mail and telephone through 2007.

138   *Gary Wormser:* I requested interviews with Wormser three times over the course of four years. He repeatedly declined to speak with me.

139   *The spirochetes in culture:* Liegner, K. B., Rosenkilde, C. E., Campbell, G. L., Quan, T. J., and Dennis, D. T. "Culture-confirmed treatment failure of cefotaxime and minocycline in a case of Lyme meningoencephalomyelitis in the United States." Abstract 63, p. A10. Program abstract of the 5th International Conference of Lyme Borreliosis, 1992.

140   *Ken Liegner declared his position:* Liegner, K. B. "Lyme disease: the sensible pursuit of answers." *Journal of Clinical Microbiology.* August 1993; 31 (8): 1961–63.

21. FAMILY THERAPY

This chapter recounts my family's experience with the Chappaqua School District, and especially, the Horace Greeley High School.

22. BICYCLE BOY AND OTHER LYMEBRAINS

145   *first time:* Personal experience, 2000.

145   *Some of those early:* Reik, Louis, Jr., M.D. *Lyme Disease and the Nervous System.* New York: Thieme Medical Publishers, 1991. Also: Reik, L., Steere, A. C., Bartenhagen, N. H., et al. "Neurologic abnormalities of Lyme disease." *Medicine.* 1979; 58:281–94. For those interested in the earliest research beyond that presented here, go to: Garin, C., Bujadoux, D. "Paralysie par les tiques." *Journal de Médecine de Lyon.* 1922; (77): 765–67; Bannwarth, A. "Chronische lymphocytare meningitis, entzundliche polyneuritis and Ôrheumtisums." *Archiv für Psychiatrie and Nervenkrankheiten.* 1941; 113: 284–376.

146   *When these devastating:* Pachner, A. R., Steere, A. C. "The triad of neurologic manifestations of Lyme disease: meningitis, cranial neuritis, and radiculoneuri-

tis." *Neurology*. January 1985; 35 (1): 47–53. Also: Logigian, E. "Peripheral Nervous System Lyme Borreliosis." *Seminars in Neurology*. March 1997; 25–29.

146 *At Stony Brook:* Telephone interview with John J. Halperin, April 22, 2004. Also: Halperin, J. J., Little, B. W., Coyle, P. K., Dattwyler, R. J. "Lyme disease: cause of a treatable peripheral neuropathy." *Neurology*. November 1987; 37 (11): 1700–6.

146 *Could the intermittent:* Halperin, J., Luft, B. J., Volkman, D. J., Dattwyler, R. J. "Lyme neuroborreliosis. Peripheral nervous system manifestations." *Brain* (Oxford University Press). 1990; 113 (4): 1207–21.

146 *caused psychiatric disease:* Reik, I., Jr., Smith, L., Khan, A., Nelson, W. "Demyelinating encephalopathy in Lyme disease." *Neurology*. February 1985; 35 (2) 267–69. Also: Pachner, A. R., Duray, P., Steere, A. C. "Central nervous system manifestations of Lyme disease." *Archives of Neurology*. July 1989; 46 (7): 790–95. Some of the narrative details come from Raven, Neil. "Bicycle Boy." *The Washingtonian*. January 1991.

147 *The German neurologist:* Horstrup, P., Ackermann, R. "Durch zecken übertragene Meningopolyneuritis (Garin-Bujadoux, Bannwarth)." *Fortschritte der Neurologie Psychiatrie*. 1973; 41: 583–606.

147 *seizures:* Reik, Louis, Jr., M.D. *Lyme Disease and the Nervous System*.

147 *"the new great imitator":* Pachner, A. R. "Neurologic manifestations of Lyme disease, the new 'great imitator.'" *Review of Infectious Diseases*. September–October 1989; 11 Suppl 6: S1482–26.

147 *group from Stanford:* Stein, S. L., Solvason, H. B., Biggart, E., Spiegel, D. "A 25-year-old woman with hallucinations, hypersexuality, nightmares, and a rash." *American Journal of Psychiatry*. April 1996; 153 (4): 545–51.

147 *Tourette's syndrome:* Riedel, M., Straube, A., Schwarz, M. J., Wilske, B., Muller, N. "Lyme disease presenting as Tourette's syndrome." *Lancet*. February 7, 1998; 351 (9100): 418–19.

147 *catatonia:* Pfister, H. W., Preac-Mursic, V., Wilske, B., Rieder, G., Forderreuther, S., Schmidt, S., Kapfhammer, H. P. "Catatonic syndrome in acute severe encephalitis due to *Borrelia burgdorferi* infection." *Neurology*. February 1993; 43 (2): 433–35.

147 *and even schizophrenia:* Hess, A., Buchmann, J., Zettl, U. K., Henschel, S., Schlaefke, D., Grau, G., Benecke, R. "*Borrelia burgdorferi* central nervous system infection presenting as an organic schizophrenialike disorder." *Biological Psychiatry*. March 15, 1999; 45 (6): 795.

147 *Parkinson's:* Cassarino, D. S., Quezado, M. M., Ghatak, N. R., Duray, P. H. "Lyme-associated parkinsonism: A neuropathologic case study and review of the literature." *Archives of Pathology and Laboratory Medicine*. September 2003; 127 (9): 1204–6.

147 *Alzheimer's:* Miklossy, J. "Alzheimer's disease—a spirochetosis?" *Neuroreport*. September 1993; 4 (9): 1069. Also: Hammond, R. R., Gage, F. H., Terry, R. D. "Alzheimer's disease and spirochetes; a questionable relationship." *Neuroreport*. July 1993; 4 (7): 840.

148 *stroke:* Romi, F., Krakenes, J., Aarli, J. A., Tysnes, O. B. "Neuroborreliosis with vasculitis causing stroke-like manifestations." *European Neurology*. 2004; 51(1):

49–50. Epub November 21, 2003; Heinrich, A., Khaw, A. V., Ahrens, N., Kirsch, M., Dressel, A. "Cerebral vasculitis as the only manifestation of *Borrelia burgdorferi* infection in a 17-year-old patient with basal ganglia infarction." *European Neurology*. 2003; 50(2): 109–12; Akhvlediani, R., Mogilevskii, A., Kontan, S. ["Clinical thinking in neurological diagnosis (French experience)."] *Zhurnal neurologii i psikhiatrii imeni S.S. Korsakova*. 2003; 103 (7): 62–66; Scheid, R., Hund-Georgiadis, M., von Cramon, D. Y. "Intracerebral haemorrhage as a manifestation of Lyme neuroborreliosis?" *European Journal of Neurology*. January 2003; 10 (1): 99–101; Klingebiel, R., Benndorf, G., Schmitt, M., von Moers, A., Lehmann, R. "Large cerebral vessel occlusive disease in Lyme neuroborreliosis." *Neuropediatrics*. February 2002; 33 (1): 37–40; Seijo Martínez, M., Grandes Ibáñez, J., Sánchez Herrero, J., García-Moncó, J. C. "Spontaneous brain hemorrhage associated with Lyme neuroborreliosis." *Neurologia*. January 2001; 16 (1): 43–45; Deloizy, M., Devos, P., Stekelorom, T., Testard, D., Belhadia, A. "Left-sided sudden hemiparesis linked to a central form of Lyme disease." *Revue Neurologique* (Paris). December 2000; 156 (12): 1146–54; Wilke, M., Eiffert, H., Christen, H. J., Hanefeld, F. "Primarily chronic and cerebrovascular course of Lyme neuroborreliosis: case reports and literature review." *Archives of Disease in Childhood*. July 2000; 83 (1): 67–71; Zhang, Y., Lafontant, G., Bonner, F. J., Jr. "Lyme neuroborreliosis mimics stroke: a case report." *Archives of Physical Medicine and Rehabilitation*. April 2000; 81 (4): 519–21; Laroche, C., Lienhardt, A., Boulesteix, J. "Ischemic stroke caused by neuroborreliosis." *Archives of Pediatrics*. December 1999; 6 (12): 1302–5; Schmitt, A. B., Kuker, W., Nacimiento, W. "Neuroborreliosis with extensive cerebral vasculitis and multiple cerebral infarcts." *Nervenarzt*. February 1999; 70 (2): 167–71; Hausler, M. G., Ramaekers, V. T., Reul, J., Meilicke, R., Heimann, G. "Early and late onset manifestations of cerebral vasculitis related to varicella zoster." *Neuropediatrics*. August 1998; 29 (4): 202–7; Seinost, G., Gasser, R., Reisinger, E., Rigler, M. Y., Fischer, L., Keplinger, A., Dattwyler, R. J., Dunn, J. J., Klein, W. "Cardiac manifestations of Lyme borreliosis with special reference to contractile dysfunction." *Acta Medica Austriaca*. 1998; 25 (2): 44–50; Henriksen, T. B. "Lyme neuroborreliosis in a 66-year-old woman. Differential diagnosis of cerebral metastases and cerebral infarction." *Ugeskrift for Laeger*. May 19, 1997; 159 (21): 3175–77; Keil, R., Baron, R., Kaiser, R., Deuschl, G. "Vasculitis course of neuroborreliosis with thalamic infarct." *Nervenarzt*. April 1997; 68 (4): 339–41; Corral, I., Quereda, C., Guerrero, A., Escudero, R., Marti-Belda, P. "Neurological manifestations in patients with sera positive for *Borrelia burgdorferi*." *Neurologia*. January 1997; 12 (1): 2–8. Spanish. Erratum in: *Neurologia*. May 1997; 12 (5): 200. Gasser, R., Fruhwald, F., Schumacher, M., Seinost, G., Reisinger, E., Eber, B., Keplinger, A., Horvath, R., Sedaj, B., Klein, W., Pierer, K. "Reversal of *Borrelia burgdorferi* associated dilated cardiomyopathy by antibiotic treatment?" *Cardiovascular Drugs Therapy*. July 1996; 10 (3): 351–60; Riikonen, R., Santavuori, P. "Hereditary and acquired risk factors for childhood stroke." *Neuropediatrics*. October 1994; 25 (5): 227–33; Reik, I., Jr. "Stroke due to Lyme disease." *Neurology*. December 1993; 43 (12): 2705–7; Hammers-Berggren, S., Grondahl, A., Karlsson, M., von Arbin, M., Carlsson, A., Stiernstedt, G.

"Screening for neuroborreliosis in patients with stroke." *Stroke.* September 1993; 24 (9): 1393–96; Defer, G., Levy, R., Brugieres, P., Postic, D., Degos, J. D. "Lyme disease presenting as a stroke in the vertebrobasilar territory: MRI." *Neuroradiology.* 1993; 35 (7): 529–31; Gasser, R., Dusleag, J., Fruhwald, F., Klein, W., Reisinger, E. "Early antimicrobial treatment of dilated cardiomyopathy associated with *Borrelia burgdorferi.*" *Lancet.* October 1992; 17, 340 (8825): 982; May, E. F., Jabbari, B. "Stroke in neuroborreliosis." *Stroke.* August 1990; 21 (8): 1232–35; Olsson, J. E., Zbornikova, V. "Neuroborreliosis simulating a progressive stroke." *Acta Neurologica Scandinavica.* May 1990; 81 (5): 471–74; Brogan, G. X., Homan, C. S., Viccellio, P. "The enlarging clinical spectrum of Lyme disease: Lyme cerebral vasculitis, a new disease entity." *Annals of Emergency Medicine.* May 1990; 19 (5): 572–76; Zbornikova, V., Olsson, J. E. "Progressive cerebral infarction caused by borrelia infection." *Läkartidningen.* April 6, 1988; 85 (14): 1235–36; Uldry, P. A., Regli, F., Bogousslavsky, J. "Cerebral angiopathy and recurrent strokes following *Borrelia burgdorferi* infection." *Journal Neurology Neurosurgery & Psychiatry.* December 1987; 50 (12): 1703–4.

148   *work done on ALS:* Waisbren, B. A., Cashman, N., Schell, R. F., Johnson, R. "*Borrelia burgdorferi* antibodies and amyotrophic lateral sclerosis." *Lancet.* August 8, 1987; 2 (8554): 332–33.

148   *nineteen ALS patients:* Halperin, J. J., Kaplan, G. P., Brazinsky, S., Tsai, T. F., Cheng, T., Ironside, A., Wu, P., Delfiner, J., Golightly, M., Brown, R. H., et al. "Immunologic reactivity against *Borrelia burgdorferi* in patients with motor neuron disease." *Archives of Neurology.* May 1990; 47 (5): 586–94.

148   *measured deficits:* Halperin, J. J., Pass, H. L., Anand, A. K., Luft, B. J., Volkman, D. J., Dattwyler, R. J., "Nervous system abnormalities in Lyme disease." *Annals of the New York Academy of Sciences.* 1988; 539: 24–34. Also: Telephone interview with John J. Halperin, April 19, 2004.

149   *One of the first to enter the fray:* In-person interviews with Brian Fallon, New York Psychiatric Institute, 2004 and 2007.

149   *focus on hypochondria:* Fallon, B. A., Javitch, J. A., Hollander, E., Liebowitz, M. R. "Hypochondriasis and obsessive compulsive disorder: overlaps in diagnosis and treatment." *Journal of Clinical Psychiatry.* November 1991; 52 (11): 457–60.

149   *the German researcher Kohler:* Kohler, J. "Lyme borreliosis in neurology and psychiatry." *Fortschrift Medicine.* April 10, 1990; 108 (10): 191–93, 197.

150   *structured clinical interviews:* Fallon, B. A., Nields, J. A., Parsons, B., Liebowitz, M. R., Klein, D. F. "Psychiatric manifestations of Lyme borreliosis." *Journal of Clinical Psychiatry.* July 1993; 54(7): 263–68.

150   *Surveying 193:* Fallon, B. A., Nields, J. A., Burrascano, J. J., Liegner, K., DelBene, D., Liebowitz, M. R. "The neuropsychiatric manifestations of Lyme borreliosis." *Psychiatry Quarterly.* Spring 1992; 63 (1): 95–117.

150   *As for children:* Tager, F. A., Fallon, B. A., Keilp, J., Rissenberg, M., Jones, C. R., Liebowitz, M.R. "A controlled study of cognitive deficits in children with chronic Lyme disease." *Journal of Neuropsychiatry and Clinical Neuroscience.* Fall 2001; 13 (4): 500–7.

153 *In 2009:* Fallon, B. A., Lipkin, R. B., Corbera, K. M., Yu, S., Nobler, M. S., Keilp, J. G., Petkova, E., Lisanby, S. H., Moeller, J. R., Slavov, I., Van Heertum, R., Mensh, B. D., Sackeim, H. A. "Regional cerebral blood flow and metabolic rate in persistent Lyme encephalopathy." *Archives of General Psychiatry.* May 2009; 66 (5): 554–63.

150 *a traumatic brain expert:* Telephone interviews with Leo Shea, May 2009 and June 2009.

153 *Taking note:* In-person interview with Robert Bransfield in his office in Redbank, NJ, June 2002, and telephone interview, June 29, 2004.

154 *Bransfield described the case:* Fallon, B. A., Schwartzberg, M., Bransfield, R., Zimmerman, B., Scotti, A., Weber, C. A., Liebowitz, M. R. "Late-stage neuropsychiatric Lyme borreliosis. Differential diagnosis and treatment." *Psychosomatics.* May–June 1995; 36 (3): 295–300.

154 *Lyme disease and autism:* Bransfield, R. C., Wulfman, J. S., Harvey, W. T., Usman, A. I. "The association between tick-borne infections, Lyme borreliosis and autism spectrum disorders." *Medical Hypotheses.* November 1, 2007.

155 *22 percent:* Vojdani, A. "Immunology of Lyme disease and associated disorders." Lyme-induced Autism Conference, 2007.

155 *30 percent:* Nicholson, G. "The Role of Chronic Intracellular Infections in ASD." Lyme-induced Autism Conference, 2007.

155 *immune molecules produce:* Bransfield, Robert C. "Preventable cases of autism: relationship between chronic infectious diseases and neurological outcome." *Pediatric Health.* April 2009; 3 (2): 125–40.

155 *Virginia Sherr:* In-person interview with Virginia Sherr at her home and office in Holland, PA, January 22, 2003. Also: Sherr, V. T. "The Physician as a Patient: Lyme Disease, Ehrlichiosis, and Babesiosis: A Recounting of a Personal Experience with Tick-Borne Diseases." *Practical Gastroenterology.* January 2000; 24(1), online at www.ilads.org/sherr2.htm.

156 *have psychiatric disorders instead:* In-person interview with Leonard Sigal, 2003.

156 *Fallon explains:* In-person interview with Brian Fallon, 2004.

23. A DEVASTATING REALIZATION

Interview with Sheila Statlender, 2003 and 2007.

24. LONGING FOR LYME

Interview with David Martz, 2007.

25. A NANTUCKET BURNING: I'M DIAGNOSED WITH BABESIOSIS

162 *sometime after the new year:* Personal memoir and medical records.

162 *Andrew Spielman, a tropical medicine expert:* In-person interview with Andrew Spielman, M.D., at the Harvard School of Public Health, Boston, MA, July 2003.

163 *wealthy Nantucket woman:* Western, K. A., Benson, G. D., Gleason, N. N., et al. "Babesiosis in a Massachusetts resident." *New England Journal of Medicine.* 1970; 283: 854–56.

163 *Observing the cycles:* Spielman, A. "Human babesiosis on Nantucket Island: transmission by nymphal Ixodes ticks." *American Journal of Tropical Medicine and Hygiene.* November 1976; 25 (6): 784–87. Also: Spielman, A., Clifford, C.

M., Piesman, J., Corwin, M. D. "Human babesiosis on Nantucket Island, USA: description of the vector, *Ixodes (Ixodes) dammini,* n. sp. *(Acarina: Ixodidae)."* *Journal of Medical Entomology.* March 23, 1979; 15 (3): 218–34; Piesman, J., Spielman, A., Etkind, P., Ruebush, T. K., 2nd, Juranek, D. D. "Role of deer in the epizootiology of babesia microti in Massachusetts, USA." *Journal of Medical Entomology.* September 4, 1979; 15 (5–6): 537–40.

163   *identified by Willy:* Interview with Spielman, 2003.

164   *in retrospect:* Personal memoir and hypothesis.

164   *classic acute babesiosis:* Signs and symptoms were described for me during an in-person interview with Peter Krause, M.D., University of Connecticut, Hartford, 2003. Krause is one of the world experts on this disease.

26. PHOTO SAFARI

Interview with David Martz, 2007.

27. TICK MENAGERIE: THE COINFECTIONS OF LYME DISEASE

168   *first sliced open:* In-person interview with Willy Burgdorfer, 2002.

168   *Richard Ostfeld:* In-person interview with Richard Ostfeld at the Institute for Ecosystem Studies in Millbrook, NY, 2004.

168   *Eva Sapi:* Sapi, Eva. University of New Haven Annual Lyme Symposium, 2007. Also: e-mail correspondence, 2007.

169   *Some of those coinfections:* In-person interviews with John Anderson, director, and Louis Magnarelli, chief scientist, Connecticut Agricultural Experiment Station, New Haven, CT, March 26, 2003. Also: Thompson, C., Spielman, A., Krause, P. J. "Coinfecting deer-associated zoonoses: Lyme disease, babesiosis, and ehrlichiosis." *Clinical Infectious Diseases.* September 1, 2001; 33 (5): 676–85.

169   *One of the first:* In-person interview with Peter Krause, M.D., University of Connecticut, 2003.

169   *resembled that of malaria:* Krause, P. J., Daily, J., Telford, S. R., Vannier, E., Lantos, P., Spielman, A. "Shared features in the pathobiology of babesiosis and malaria." *Trends in Parasitology.* December 23, 2007; 12: 605–10.

169   Babesia *was spreading:* Krause, P. J., Telford, S. R., III, Pollack, R. J., Ryan, R., Brassard, P., Zemel, L., Spielman, A. "Babesiosis: an underdiagnosed disease of children." *Pediatrics.* June 1992; 89 (6 Part 1): 1045–48.

169   *on Long Island:* Benach, J. L., Coleman, J. L., Habicht, G. S., MacDonald, A., Grunwaldt, E., Giron, J. A. "Serological evidence for simultaneous occurrences of Lyme disease and babesiosis." *Journal of Infectious Diseases.* September 1985; 152 (3): 473–77.

169   *reported in 2003:* Krause, P. J., McKay, K., Gadbaw, J., Christianson, D., Closter, L., Lepore, T., Telford, S. R., III, Sikand, V., Ryan, R., Persing, D., Radolf, J. D., Spielman, A. "Increasing health burden of human babesiosis in endemic sites." *American Journal of Tropical Medicine and Hygiene.* April 2003; 68 (4): 431–36.

169   *Lyme and* Babesia *together:* Krause, P. J., Telford, S. R., III, Spielman, A., Sikand, V., Ryan, R., Christianson, D., Burke, G., Brassard, P., Pollack, R., Peck, J.,

Persing, D. H. "Concurrent Lyme disease and babesiosis. Evidence for increased severity and duration of illness." *Journal of the American Medical Association.* June 5, 1996; 275 (21): 1657–60.

170   Babesia microti *is persistent:* Krause, P. J., Spielman, A., Telford, S. R., III, Sikand, V. K., McKay, K., Christianson, D., Pollack, R. J., Brassard, P., Magera, J., Ryan, R., Persing, D. H. "Persistent parasitemia after acute babesiosis." *New England Journal of Medicine.* July 16, 1998; 339 (3): 160–65.

170   *programmed by evolution:* Allred, David R. Talk, Lyme Disease Foundation Meeting, June 2003.

170   *donate blood:* Leiby, D. A. "Babesiosis and blood transfusion: flying under the radar." *Vox Sanguinis.* April 2006; 90 (3): 157–65. Also: Perdrizet, G. A., Olson, N. H., Krause, P. J., Banever, G. T., Spielman, A., Cable, R. G. "Babesiosis in a rental transplant recipient acquired through blood transfusion." *Transplantation.* July 15, 2000; 70 (1): 205–8. And: Raju, M., Salazar, J. C., Leopold, H., Krause, P. J. "Atovaquone and azithromycin treatment for babesiosis in an infant." *Pediatric Infectious Diseases Journal.* February 2007; 26 (2): 181–83.

170   *Recrudescence:* Krause, P. J., Spielman, A., Telford, S. R., III, Sikand, V. K., McKay, K., Christianson, D., Pollack, R. J., Brassard, P., Magera J., Ryan, R., Persing, D. H. "Persistent parasitemia after acute babesiosis." *New England Journal of Medicine.* July 16, 1998; 339 (3): 160–65.

170   *Mepron and Zithromax:* Krause, P. J., Lepore, T., Sikand, V. K., Gadbaw, J., Jr., Burke, G., Telford, S. R., III, Brassard P., Pearl, D., Azlanzadeh, J., Christianson, D., McGrath, D., Spielman, A. "Atovaquone and azithromycin for the treatment of babesiosis." *New England Journal of Medicine.* November 16, 2000; 343 (20): 1454–58.

170   *transfusion:* Krause, P. J. "Babesiosis diagnosis and treatment." *Vector-Borne Zoonotic Diseases.* Spring 2003; 3 (1): 45–51.

170   *Lyme zones nationwide:* Homer, M. J., Bruinsma, E. S., Lodes, M. J., Moro, M. H., Telford III, S., Krause, P. J., Reynolds, L. D., Mohamath, R., Benson, D. R., Houghton, R. L., Reed, S. G., Persing, D. H. "A polymorphic multigene family encoding an immunodominant protein from *Babesia microti.*" *Journal of Clinical Microbiology.* January 2000; 38 (1): 362–68; Yabsley, M. J., Romines, J., Nettles, V. F. "Detection of *Babesia* and *Anaplasma* species in rabbits from Texas and Georgia, USA." *Vector Borne Zoonotic Diseases.* Spring 2006; 6 (1): 7–13.

170   *New Jersey:* Eskow, E. S., Krause, P. J., Spielman, A., Freeman, K., Aslanzadeh, J. "Southern extension of the range of human babesiosis in the eastern United States." *Journal of Clinical Microbiology.* June 1999; 37 (6): 205–52.

170   *Maryland:* Coan, M. E., Stiller, D. "*Ixodes dammini (Acari: Ixodidae)* in Maryland, USA, and a preliminary survey for *Babesia microti.*" *Journal of Medical Entomology.* July 28, 1986; 23 (4): 446–53.

170   *Westchester and Dutchess:* Moreno, C. X., Moy, F., Daniels, T. J., Godfrey, H. P., Cabello, F. C. "Molecular analysis of microbial communities identified in different developmental stages of *Ixodes scapularis* ticks from Westchester and Dutchess Counties, New York." *Environmental Microbiology.* May 2006; 8 (5): 761–72.

170   WA-1: Persing, D. H., Herwaldt, B. L., Glaser, C., Lane, R. S., Thomford, J. W.,
      Mathiesen, D., Krause, P. J., Phillip, D. F., Conrad, P. 'A. "Infection with
      Babesia-like organism in northern California." *New England Journal of
      Medicine.* February 2, 1995; 332 (5): 298–303.

170   MO-1: Gelfand J. A., Callahan, M. V. "Babesiosis: An Update on Epidemiology
      and Treatment." *Current Infectious Disease Report.* February 2003; 5 (1):
      53–58.

170   Babesia *strains have been found worldwide:* Leeflang, P., Oomen, J. M., Zwart, D.,
      Meuwissen, J. H. "The prevalence of *Babesia* antibodies in Nigerians."
      International Journal of Parasitology. April 1976; 6 (2): 159–61; Bonnet, S.,
      Jouglin, M., L'Hostis, M., Chauvin, A. "*Babesia sp.* EU1 from roe deer and trans-
      mission within *Ixodes ricinus.*" *Emerging Infectious Diseases.* August 2007; 13
      (8): 1208–10; Wielinga, P. R., Fonville, M., Sprong, H., Gaasenbeek, C.,
      Borgsteede, F., Giessen, J. W. "Persistent detection of *Babesia EU1* and *Babesia
      microti* in *Ixodes ricinus* in the Netherlands during a 5-year surveillance:
      2003–2007." *Vector Borne Zoonotic Diseases.* August 30, 2008; Hunfeld, K. P.,
      Brade, V. "Zoonotic *Babesia*: possibly emerging pathogens to be considered for
      tick-infested humans in Central Europe." *International Journal of Medical
      Microbiology.* April 2004; (293) 37: 93–103. Review; Häselbarth, K., Tenter, A.
      M., Brade, V., Krieger, G., Hunfeld, K. P. "First case of human babesiosis in
      Germany—Clinical presentation and molecular characterisation of the pathogen."
      International Journal of Medical Microbiology. June 2007; 297 (3): 197–204;
      Hunfeld, K. P., Hildebrandt, A., Gray, J. S. "Babesiosis: recent insights into an
      ancient disease." *International Journal of Parasitology.* September 2008; 38 (11):
      1219–37; Hunfeld, K. P., Lambert, A., Kampen, H., Albert, S., Epe, C., Brade, V.,
      Tenter, A. M., "Seroprevalence of *Babesia* infections in humans exposed to ticks in
      midwestern Germany." *Journal of Clinical Microbiology.* July 2002; 40 (7):
      2431–36; Saito-Ito, A., Takada, N., Ishiguro, F., Fujita, H., Yano, Y., Ma, X. H.,
      Chen, E. R. "Detection of Kobe-type *Babesia microti* associated with Japanese
      human babesiosis in field rodents in central Taiwan and southeastern mainland
      China." *Parasitology.* May 2008; 135 (6): 691–99; Saito-Ito, A., Kasahara, M.,
      Kasai, M., Dantrakool, A., Kawai, A., Fujita, H., Yano, Y., Kawabata, H., Takada,
      N. "Survey of *Babesia microti* infection in field rodents in Japan: records of the
      Kobe-type in new foci and findings of a new type related to the Otsu-type."
      Microbiol Immunol. 2007; 51 (1): 15–24; Tsuji, M., Wei, Q., Zamoto, A., Morita,
      C., Arai, S., Shiota, T., Fujimagari, M., Itagaki, A., Fujita, H., Ishihara, C.
      "Human babesiosis in Japan: epizootiologic survey of rodent reservoir and isola-
      tion of new type of Babesia microti-like parasite." *Journal of Clinical
      Microbiology.* December 2001; 39 (12): 4316–22; Kim, J. Y., Cho, S. H., Joo, H.
      N., Tsuji, M., Cho, S. R., Park, I. J., Chung, G. T., Ju, J. W., Cheun, H. I., Lee, H.
      W., Lee, Y. H., Kim, T. S. "First case of human babesiosis in Korea: detection and
      characterization of a novel type of *Babesia sp. (KO1)* similar to ovine babesia."
      Journal of Clinical Microbiology. June 2007; 45 (6): 2084–87; Tampieri, M. P.,
      Galuppi, R., Bonoli, C., Cancrini, G., Moretti, A., Pietrobelli, M. "Wild ungulates
      as *Babesia* hosts in northern and central Italy." *Vector Borne Zoonotic Diseases.*
      October 2008; 8 (5): 667–74; Zamoto, A., Tsuji, M., Kawabuchi, T., Wei, Q.,

Asakawa, M., Ishihara, C. "U.S.-type *Babesia microti* isolated from small wild mammals in Eastern Hokkaido, Japan." *Journal of Veterinary Medical Science.* August 2004; 66 (8): 919–26; Duh, D., Jelovsek, M., Avsic-Zupanc, T. "Evaluation of an indirect fluorescence immunoassay for the detection of serum antibodies against *Babesia divergens* in humans." *Parasitology.* 2007; 134: 179–85; Gorenflot, A., Moubri, K., Précigout, E., Carcy, B., Schetters, T. P. "Human babesiosis." *Ann Trop Med Parasitol.* 1998; 92: 489–501; Gray, J. S. "Identity of the causal agents of human babesiosis in Europe." *International Journal of Medical Microbiology.* 2006; 296 (40): 131–36; Herwaldt, B. L., Cacciò, S., Gherlinzoni, F., Aspöck, H., Slemenda, S. B., et al. "Molecular characterization of a non-*Babesia divergens* organism causing zoonotic babesiosis in Europe." *Emerging Infectious Diseases.* 2003; 9: 942–48; Hildebrandt, A., Tenter, A. M., Straube, E., Hunfeld, K. P. "Human babesiosis in Germany: Just overlooked or truly new?" *International Journal of Medical Microbiology* 2007.

172   *ehrlichiosis:* Relevant sources include: Bakken, J. S. "The discovery of human granulocytotropic ehrlichiosis." *Journal of Laboratory and Clinical Medicine.* September 1998; 132 (3): 175–80; Chen, S. M., Dumler, J. S., Bakken, J. S., Walker, D. H. "Identification of a granulocytotropic ehrlichia species as the etiologic agent of human disease." *Journal of Clinical Microbiology.* May 1994; 32 (3): 589–95; Bakken, J. S., Dumler, J. S., Chen, S. M., Eckman, M. R., Van Etta, L. L., Walker, D. H. "Human granulocytic ehrlichiosis in the upper Midwest United States. A new species emerging?" *Journal of the American Medical Association.* July 20, 1994; 272 (3): 212–18; Dumler, J. S., Bakken, J. S. "Human granulocytic ehrlichiosis in Wisconsin and Minnesota: a frequent infection with the potential for persistence." *Journal of Infectious Diseases.* April 1996; 173 (4): 1027–30; Dumler, J. S., Madigan, J. E., Pusterla, N., Bakken, J. S. "Ehrlichoses in humans: epidemiology, clinical presentation, diagnosis, and treatment." *Journal of Clinical Infectious Diseases.* July 15, 2007; 45 Suppl 1: S45–51.

172   *rod-shaped bacterium:* Eskow, E., Rao, R. V., Mordechai, E. "Concurrent infection of the central nervous system by *Borrelia burgdorferi* and *Bartonella henselae:* evidence for a novel tick-borne disease complex." *Archives of Neurology.* September 2001; 58 (9): 1357–63.

172   *In California:* Chang, C. C., Chomel, B. B., Kasten, R. W., Romano, V., Tietze, N. "Molecular evidence of bartonella spp. in questing adult *Ixodes pacificus* ticks in California." *Journal of Clinical Microbiology.* April 2001; 39 (4): 1221–26.

172   *Burrascano of the Hamptons says:* In-person talk with Joseph Burrascano, East Hampton, NY, 2006.

172   *genetic diversity:* Bemis, D. A., Kania, S. A. "Isolation of *Bartonella* sp. from sheep blood." *Emerging Infectious Diseases.* October 2007. Available from www.cdc .gov/EID/content/13/10/1565.htm. Also: Chang, C. C., Chomel, B. B., Kasten, R. W., Heller, R., Kocan, K. M., Ueno, H., et al. "*Bartonella* spp. isolated from wild and domestic ruminants in North America. *Emerging Infectious Diseases.* 2006; 6: 306–11. And: Dehio, C., Lanz, C., Pohl, R., Behrens, P., Bermond, D., Piemont, Y., et al. "*Bartonella schoenbuchii* sp. nov., isolated from the blood of wild roe deer." *International Journal of Systematic and Evolutionary Microbiology.* 2001; 51: 1557–65.

172 *foxes and dogs:* Henn, J. B., Gabriel, M. W., Kasten, R. W., Brown, R. N., Theis, J. H., Foley, J. E., Chomel, B. B. "Gray foxes (*Urocyon cinereoargenteus*) as a potential reservoir of a *Bartonella clarridgeiae*-like bacterium and domestic dogs as part of a sentinel system for surveillance of zoonotic arthropod-borne pathogens in northern California." *Journal of Clinical Microbiology.* August 2007; 45 (8): 2411–18.

173 Mycoplasma: Sapi, Eva. University of New Haven Lyme Symposium, 2007. Also: Eskow, E., Adelson, M. E., Rao, R. V., Mordechai, E. "Evidence for disseminated Mycoplasma fermentans in New Jersey residents with antecedent tick attachment and subsequent musculoskeletal symptoms." *Journal of Clinical Rheumatology.* April 2003; 9 (2): 77–87.

173 *"bigger than Lyme":* In-person talk with Joseph Burrascano, 2006.

173 *the jury:* Fallon, Brian. Lyme Disease Association Conference, 2004.

173 *Alone and in combination:* In-person interview with insect microbiologist Timothy J. Kurtti and entomologist Ulrike Munderloh at the University of Minnesota in Minneapolis, 2003.

28. HOLE IN THE DONUT: THE FIGHT OVER SOUTHERN LYME

I interviewed Dr. Edwin Masters over the course of three days in Hartford, CT, in June 2003, and in Cape Girardeau, MO, in July 2003. Where Dr. Masters is quoted or referred to, I draw from these interviews. Dr. Masters also provided me with original copies of letters he wrote to and received from the Centers for Disease Control, the Missouri Department of Health, the Illinois Department of Health, and various political representatives and scientific experts. He also provided me with a series of CDC-produced drafts of a paper, stamped with the CDC seal, that the agency sent him over the course of years from 1992 to 1994. He provided me with extensive documentation of his history with the CDC, including letters, facsimiles, and internal draft reports and memos from the Centers for Disease Control and the Missouri Department of Health. Masters provided results on his study patients (with patient names blacked out) from various reference and pathology labs, including those within the CDC. He provided data collected by the State University of New York at Stony Brook for a National Institutes of Health study in which Masters's patients were enrolled. I reconstruct historical events almost totally from documentary evidence, and reference individual documents where they apply, throughout the text. In addition, I interviewed Dr. Andrew Spielman of Harvard and Dr. Robert Lane of University of California at Berkeley in person on these issues in 2003.

175 *a brand-new tick:* Spielman, A., et al. "Human babesiosis on Nantucket Island, USA."

176 *Spielman eventually saw:* In-person interview with Spielman, 2003.

176 *Lyme out West:* In-person interview with Robert Lane at his office at the University of California at Berkeley, March 2009.

177 *The California disease was different:* Brown, R. N., Lane, R. S. "Lyme disease in California: a novel enzootic transmission cycle of *Borrelia burgdorferi*." *Science.* June 1992; 256 (5062): 1439–42.

177 *discovered a microbe:* Burgdorfer, W., Lane, R. S., Barbour, A. G., Gresbrink, R. A., Anderson, J. R. "The western black-legged tick, Ixodes pacificus: a vector of *Borrelia burgdorferi*." *American Journal of Tropical Medicine and Hygiene.* September 1985; 34 (5): 925–30.

177   *western gray squirrel:* Salkeld, D. J., Leonhard, S., Girard, Y. A., Hahn, N., Mun, J., Padgett, K. A., Lane, R. S. "Identifying the reservoir hosts of the Lyme disease spirochete *Borrelia burgdorferi* in California: the role of the western gray squirrel *(Sciurus griseus)*." *American Journal of Tropical Medicine and Hygiene.* October 2008; 79 (4): 535–40.

177   *The western Lyme strains and species:* Lane, R. S., Lennette, E. T., Madigan, J. E. "Interlaboratory and intralaboratory comparisons of indirect immunofluorescence assays for serodiagnosis of Lyme disease." *Journal of Clinical Microbiology.* August 1990; 28 (8): 1774–79.

177   *began studying Phyllis Mervine:* Lane, R. S., Manweiler, S. A., Stubbs, H. A., Lennette, E. T., Madigan, J. E., Lavoie, P. E. "Risk factors for Lyme disease in a small rural community in northern California." *American Journal of Epidemiology.* December 1992; 136 (11): 1358–68.

177   *a breakthrough paper:* Clover, J. R., Lane, R. S. "Evidence implicating nymphal *Ixodes pacificus* (Acari: Ixodidae) in the epidemiology of Lyme disease in California." *American Journal of Tropical Medicine and Hygiene.* December 1995; 53: 237–40.

177   *Western Fence Lizard:* Lane, R. S., Quistad, G. B. "Borreliacidal factor in the blood of the western fence lizard *(Sceloporus occidentalis)*." *Journal of Parasitolology.* February 1998; 84 (1): 29–34. Also: Kuo, M. M., Lane, R. S., Giclas, P. C. "A comparative study of mammalian and reptilian alternative pathway of complement-mediated killing of the Lyme disease spirochete *(Borrelia burgdorferi)*." *Journal of Parasitology.* December 2000; 86 (6): 1223–28.

178   *spirochetal forms in local ticks:* Kerry Clark, University of North Florida, telephone interview, June 2009.

181   *upcoming NIH study:* Luft, B. J., Dattwyler, R. J., Johnson, R. C., Luger, S. W., Bosler, E. M., Rahn, D. W., Masters, E. J., Grunwaldt, E., Gadgil, S. D. "Azithromycin compared with amoxicillin in the treatment of erythema migrans: A double-blind, randomized, controlled trial." *Annals of Internal Medicine.* May 1, 1996; 124 (9): 785–91.

181   *By 1991:* Rosenthal, Elizabeth. "Rise in Lyme Disease Cases Creates Mystery." *New York Times.* March 21, 1991.

181   B. burgdorferi *spirochetes:* Gubler, Duane J. Letter to Edwin J. Masters, M.D., July 22, 1992.

181   *quote from William Harvey:* Edwin Masters's poster, accepted by peer review and presented at the Fifth International Conference on Lyme Borreliosis, in Washington, DC, June 1992.

182   *almost two years later:* Centers for Disease Control. Fax transmittal to Denny Donnell, Missouri Department of Health, May 22, 1993.

183   *Wisconsin study:* Melski, J. W., Reed, K. D., Mitchell, P. D., Barth, G. D. "Primary and secondary erythema migrans in central Wisconsin." *Archives of Dermatology.* June 1993; 129 (6): 709–16.

183   *dermatologist Bernard Berger:* Berger, B. "Dermatologic manifestations of Lyme disease." *Review of Infectious Diseases.* 1989; 11 (Supplement 6): 1475–81.

183   *inexplicable mistakes:* Masters, Edwin J. "The CDC, Missouri, and Lyme

Disease." Reference #24. Color photographs of rashes for patient #'s: NC-21, 121, 133, and 144, taken in 1990. July 20, 1993.

183 *three days later:* Campell, Grant L., M.D., Ph.D., et al. "CDC Draft Document #930513, Epidemiologic and Diagnostic Studies of Patients with Suspected Early Lyme Disease, Missouri, 1990–1992." May 1993.

184 *stop-and-start dates:* Medical record of patient #107, August 11, 1991.

185 *complained passionately:* Masters, Edwin J. Letter to Phillip R. Lee, M.D., Assistant Secretary for Health. December 16, 1993.

185 *dismissed laboratory work:* Duray, F., M.D., and Ross, J., M.D. Department of Pathology and Laboratory Medicine, Division of Anatomic Pathology, Albany Medical Center, Albany, NY. Also: dismissal of spirochetes documented in patients #131, # 133, #134, and #138. Cordes, Paul, M.D., Southeast Missouri Hospital, Cape Girardeau, MO.

185 *rejected dozens of positive blood tests performed at its own lab:* Quan, Thomas J., Ph.D., M.P.H., Diagnostic and Reference Section, CDC. Letter to Edwin J. Masters, M.D., October 31, 1991. And ELISA report for patient blood tests. Also: Report of Serologic Tests, Bacterial Zoonoses Branch, CDC, Accession #: MO-91-0021, January 10, 1992; Accession #: 1193, July 31, 1992; Table of optical density ratio of Masters's patients, whole cell sonicate ELISA vs. FLA-ELISA.

185 *CDC kept changing:* Dennis, David, M.D., Letter to Edwin J. Masters, M.D., August 19, 1994.

185 *When you biopsied a Lyme rash:* Telephone interview with Duane Gubler, 2004.

186 *Masters and Donnell had resigned:* Masters, Edwin J., M.D. Letter and fax to Roy Campbell, David Dennis, and Duane Gubler, August 10, 1994. Also: Donnell, H. Denny, Jr., M.D., M.P.H. Letter to David Dennis, Bacterial Zoonoses Branch, Division of Vector-Borne Infectious Disease, CDC, August 11, 1994.

186 *They were so efficient that their article*: Masters, E. J., Donnell, H. D. "Lyme and/or Lyme-like disease in Missouri." *Missouri Medicine.* 1995; 92: 346–53.

186 *When the CDC article came out:* Campbell, G. L., Paul, W. S., Schriefer, M. E., Craven, R. B., Robbins, K. E., Dennis, D. T. "Epidemiologic and diagnostic studies of patients with suspected early Lyme disease, Missouri, 1990–1993." *Journal of Infectious Diseases.* 1995; 182: 470–80.

186 *world-class entomologist:* Magnarelli, L. A., Oliver, J. H., Jr., Hutcheson, H. J., Boone, J. L., Anderson, J. F. "Antibodies to *Borrelia burgdorferi* in rodents in the eastern and southern United States." *Journal of Clinical Microbiology.* June 1992; 30(6): 1449–52.

186 *Sapelo Island:* Oliver, J. H., Jr., Chandler, F. W., Jr., Luttrell, M. P., James, A. M., Stallknecht, D. E., McGuire, B. S., Hutcheson, H. J., Cummins, G. A., Lane, R. S. *Proceedings of the National Academy of Sciences.* August 1, 1993; 90 (15): 7371–75.

186 *merely a subset:* Oliver, J. H., Jr., Owsley, M. R., Hutcheson, H. J., James, A. M., Chen, C., Irby, W. S., Dotson, E. M., McLain, D. K. "Conspecificity of the ticks *Ixodes scapularis* and *I. dammini (Acari: Ixodidae)*." *Journal of Medical Entomology.* January 1993; 30 (1): 54–63.

187 *Nothing is ever so simple:* Felz, M. W., Durden, L. A., Oliver, J. H., Jr. "Ticks parasitizing humans in Georgia and South Carolina." *Journal of Parasitology.*

June 1996; 82 (3): 505–8; Oliver, J. H., Jr. "Lyme borreliosis in the southern United States: a review." *Journal of Parasitology*. December 1996; 82(6): 926–35; Felz, M. W., Chandler, F. W., Jr., Oliver, J. H., Jr., Rahn, D. W., Schriefer, M. E. "Solitary erythema migrans in Georgia and South Carolina." *Archives of Dermatology*. November 1999; 135 (11): 1398–400.

187 *Adding nuance:* Telephone interview with Kerry Clark, June 2009.

187 *the South was complex:* Oliver, J. H., Clark, K. L., Chandler, F. W., Jr., Tao, L., James, A. M., Banks, C. W., Huey, L. O., Banks, A. R., Williams, D. C., Durden, L. A. "Isolation, cultivation, and characterization of *Borrelia burgdorferi* from rodents and ticks in the Charleston area of South Carolina." *Journal of Clinical Microbiology*. January 2000; (38) 1: 120–24.

187 *As for the vector:* Clark, K. L., Oliver, J. H., Jr., Grego, J. M., James, A. M., Durden, L. A., Banks, C. W., "Host associations of ticks parasitizing rodents at *Borrelia burgdorferi* enzootic sites in South Carolina." *Journal of Parasitology*. December 2001; 87 (6): 1379–86.

188 *diversity in the . . . strains:* Lin, T., Oliver, J. H., Jr., Gao, L., Kollars, T. M., Jr., Clark, K. L. "Genetic heterogenity of *Borrelia burgdorferi sensu lato* in the southern United States based on restriction fragment length polymorphism and sequence analysis." *Journal of Clinical Microbiology*. July 2001; (39) 7: 2500–7.

188 *one objection relates to lizards:* Clark, K., Hendricks, A., Burge, D. "Molecular identification and analysis of *Borrelia burgdorferi sensu lato* in lizards in the southeastern United States." *Applied Environmental Microbiology*. May 2005; 71 (5); 2616–25.

189 *a new kind of* Borrelia: Telephone interview with Durland Fish, 2001.

189 *Montana scientists:* Merriam, Ginny. "Health officials search for illness as warm weather brings out ticks." *Missoulian*. March 30, 2004.

189 *"Zones of borreliosis":* Telephone interview with Joe Piesman, August 2003.

189 *no one was clearer:* Telephone interview with Ed Masters, 2007. Also: Masters, E. J. "STARI or Masters Disease: Lone Star Tick-Vectored Lyme-Like Illness." *Infectious Disease Clinics of North America*. 2008; and Masters, E. J. "Lyme-like Illness Currently Deserves Lyme-like Treatment." Letter. *Clinical Infectious Diseases*. February 15, 2006.

190 *In 2009, a CDC study:* Murphree, R., Hackwell, N., Mead, P. S., Bachand, A., Stromdahl, E. Y. "Prospective health assessment of Fort Campbell, Kentucky patrons bitten by ticks." *Military Medicine*. April 2009; 174 (4); 419–25.

190 *"Until studies indicate otherwise":* Dennis, D. T. "Rash decisions: Lyme disease, or not?" *Clinical Infectious Diseases*. October 1, 2005; 41 (7): 966–68. Also: telephone interview with David Dennis, 2004.

29. RESTRICTING DIAGNOSIS AND KEEPING THE RIFFRAFF OUT OF LYME

193 *a child's death: Lyme in Our Own Backyard*. Video. July 31, 1991.

194 *The death unleashed a firestorm:* In-person interviews with Ken Fordyce, chairman for the State of New Jersey Governor's Lyme Disease Advisory Council, and Kerry Fordyce, president of the Lyme Disease Association of New Jersey during the 1990s. Additional invaluable information came from Pat Smith, current president of the national Lyme Disease Association, and Leonard Sigal, M.D.

194   *front and center in the effort to debunk the claims:* In-person interview, 2002, plus Leonard M. Sigal, M.D., letter to colleagues, retrieved from the Lyme disease files of Neill B. Varner, D.O., M.P.H., Saginaw County Department of Public Health. Letter, fall 1990.

194   *had barely heard of Lyme disease:* In-person interview with Pat Smith, Wall Township, NJ, 2003.

197   *Munchausen Syndrome by Proxy:* Sigal, Leonard H. "Long-term consequences of Lyme disease." In *Lyme Disease, Key Diseases Series, 1.* edited by Daniel Rahn and Janine Evans. Philadelphia: American College of Physicians, 1998.

197   *hotly disputed:* Weintraub, Pamela. "Unusual Suspects." *Psychology Today.* July/August 2007. Also: Pankratz, L. "Persistent problems with the Munchausen Syndrome by Proxy label." *Journal of the American Academy of Psychiatry Law.* 2006; 34 (1): 90–95; Allison, David B., Roberts, Mark S. *Disordered Mother or Disordered Diagnosis? Munchausen by Proxy Syndrome.* Hillsdale, NJ: Analytic Press, 1998; Mart, Eric. "Problems with the Diagnosis of Factitious Disorder by Proxy in Forensic Settings." *American Journal of Forensic Psychology.* 1999; 17 (1). Mart, Eric. *Munchausen's Syndrome by Proxy Reconsidered.* Manchester, NH: Bally Vaughan Publishing, 2002.

197   *Chris Smith requested that she talk:* In-person interview with Pat Smith. Also: "An Angry Constituent." *Asbury Park Press.* March 29, 1992; and Smith, Chris. "Top Health Officials Focus on New Jersey Lyme Cases." *Congressman Chris Smith Reports Home.* March 1992.

199   *congressional Lyme Disease Forum:* In-person interview with Pat Smith, 2003. In addition: Kaplan, Lois S. "Teen Tells of Lyme Distress." *Wall Herald.* October 1992.

200   *There were many speakers:* Videotape of congressional Lyme Disease Forum in Wall Township, October 9, 1992.

200   *Of the sixty-five children studied:* Dennis, David. Videotape of congressional Lyme Disease Forum in Wall Township, October 9, 1992. Also: CDC write-up of "School Children Study," September 9, 1992.

201   *Before anyone could blink:* Interviews with Pat Smith, Ken Fordyce, Kerry Fordyce, Duane Gubler. Also: "Ceftriaxone-associated biliary complications of treatment of suspected disseminated Lyme disease—New Jersey, 1990–1992." *MMWR Morbidity and Mortality Weekly Report.* January 22, 1993; 42 (2): 39–42. And "Ceftriaxone-associated biliary complications of treatment of suspected disseminated Lyme disease—New Jersey, 1990–1992." *Journal of the American Medical Association.* February 24, 1993; 269 (8): 979–80.

201   *"The study hammered doctors":* Telephone interview with Pat Smith, August 2004.

202   *to do only with methodology:* Telephone interview with Duane Gubler, former director, Division of Vector-Borne Infectious Diseases, CDC, and currently director, Asian-Pacific Institute of Tropical Medicine and Infectious Diseases, University of Hawaii School of Medicine, Honolulu. August 3, 2004.

202   *Brian Fallon, the Columbia psychiatrist:* Written testimony of Brian Fallon, M.D., for the Committee on Labor & Human Resources, U.S. Senate, entered into record August 5, 1993.

202   *His notes on the encounter:* Notes taken by Ken Fordyce during his meeting with the CDC in Atlanta, March 1993.

203   *"I am the parent of one of the fourteen young patients":* Garvilla, Lorraine. Wantage, NJ. Letter to Kenneth Fordyce, January 26, 1993.

204   JAMA *ran another article:* Steere, A. C, Taylor, E., McHugh, G. L., Logigian, E. L. "The overdiagnosis of Lyme disease." *Journal of the American Medical Association.* April 14, 1993; 269 (14): 1812–16.

204   *The patient community was alarmed:* Interview with Pat Smith, 2002.

204   *responses poured in:* Brenner, Carl, Gabriel, Marc C., O'Donnell, John S. "Response to the overdiagnosis of Lyme disease." The Lyme Disease Network. *LymeNet Newsletter.* May 4, 1993; 1 (10).

204   *complained that Steere ignored guidelines:* Burrascano, J. J., Jr. "The overdiagnosis of Lyme disease." Letter to the Editor. *Journal of the American Medical Association.* December 8, 1993; 270 (22): 2682.

205   *forced to retrace Polly Murray's footsteps:* Interviews and discussions with many patients and doctors from 2000 to 2007.

205   *without an accurate test:* Blank, E. C., Quan, T. J., Mayer, L. W., Craven R. B., Bailey, R. E., Dennis, D. T., Campbell, G. L., Gubler, D. J. "Lyme disease serology test kit evaluations." In *Proceedings of the First National Conference on Lyme Disease Testing.* November 1–2, 1990, in Dearborn, MI. Washington, DC: ASTPHLD, 1991; 79–89. Also: Bakken, L. L., Case, K. L., Callister, S. M., et al. "Performance of 45 laboratories participating in a proficiency testing program for Lyme disease serology." *Journal of the American Medical Association.* 1992; 268: 891–95.

205   *Second National Conference:* Association of State and Territorial Public Health Laboratory Directors (ASTPHLD). *Proceedings of the Second National Conference on the Serological Diagnosis of Lyme Disease.* October 27–29, 1994, in Dearborn, MI. Washington, DC: ASTPHLD, 1995.

206   *missed 20 to 30 percent:* Bakken, L. L., Callister, S. M., Wand, P. J., Schell, R. F. "Interlaboratory comparison of test results for detection of Lyme disease by 516 participants in the Wisconsin State Laboratory of Hygiene/College of American Pathologists proficiency testing program." *Journal of Clinical Microbiology.* 1997; 35: 537–43; Luger, S. W., and Krauss, E. "Serologic tests for Lyme disease: interlaboratory variability." *Archives of Internal Medicine.* 1990; 15: 761–63; Golightly, M. G., Thomas, J. A., Viciana, A. I. "The laboratory diagnosis of Lyme Borreliosis." *Laboratory Medicine.* 1990; 21: 299–304.

206   *microbiologist Russell Johnson:* In-person interview with Russell Johnson, University of Minnesota, 2003. Also: Engstrom, S. M., Shoop, E., Johnson, R. C. "Immunoblot interpretation criteria for serodiagnosis of early Lyme disease." *Journal of Clinical Microbiology.* February 1995; 33 (2): 419–27.

206   *in collaboration with:* Dressler, F., Whalen, J. A., Reinhardt, B. N., Steere, A. C. "Western blotting in the serodiagnosis of Lyme disease." *Journal of Infectious Diseases.* 1993; 167: 392–400.

206   *one more slap in the face:* In-person interview with Nick Harris, Ph.D., president of IGeneX, Palo Alto, CA, 2003. In-person interviews with Kenneth Liegner, M.D., and Daniel Cameron, M.D., 2002–2007. Also see: International Lyme and

Associated Diseases Society, "Position Paper on the CDC's Statement Regarding Lyme Diagnosis." www.ilads.org/cdc_paper.htm.

206 *In 1986:* Craft, J. E., Fischer, D. K., Shimamoto, G. T., Steere, A. C. "Antigens of *Borrelia burgdorferi* recognized during Lyme disease. Appearance of a new immunoglobulin M response and expansion of the immunoglobulin G response late in the illness." *Journal of Clinical Investigation.* October 1986; 78 (4): 934–39.

207 *worked against some of the sickest patients:* Interviews with Nick Harris and Kenneth Liegner.

207 *its levels increased:* In-person interview with Tom Schwan, Ph.D., Rocky Mountain Laboratory, Hamilton, Montana, winter 2002. Also: Schwan, T. G. "Temporal regulation of outer surface proteins of the Lyme-disease spirochaete *Borrelia burgdorferi.*" *Biochemical Society Transactions.* February 2003; 31 (Part 1): 108–12; Schwan, T. G., Piesman, J. "Temporal changes in outer surface proteins A and C of the lyme disease-associated spirochete, *Borrelia burgdorferi,* during the chain of infection in ticks and mice." *Journal of Clinical Microbiology.* January 2000; 38 (1): 382–88.

207 *he wrote a letter to Marc:* Liegner, Kenneth. Letter to Marc Golightly, 1994.

208 *But in its second role:* In-person interviews with Benjamin Luft and Patricia Coyle, SUNY Stony Brook, 2003.

209 *fashionable new name:* Sigal, L. H. "Pseudo-Lyme disease." *Bulletin on the Rheumatic Diseases.* December 1995; 44 (8): 1–3.

209 *In 1996, Yale Medicine:* Wortman, Marc. "Special Report on Lyme Disease." *Yale Medicine.* May 15, 1996.

210 *fit to be tied:* Telephone interview with Tom Grier, 2003.

210 *"I am writing to you as someone who is in the trenches":* Smith, Patricia. Letter to Duane J. Gubler, Sc.D., director, Division of Vector-Borne Infectious Diseases, CDC, Fort Collins, CO, February 11, 1999.

211 *"Do not feel":* Gubler, Duane, Sc.D. Letter to Patricia Smith, president, Lyme Disease Association of New Jersey, February 25, 1999.

211 *As Patricia Smith pondered the outcome:* Telephone interview with Pat Smith, July 30, 2004.

30. THE LONG ROAD HOME
Interview with Sheila Statlender, 2003 and 2007.

31. REPORTING OUR PEDIATRICIAN
215 *placed a call to Ned Hayes:* Telephone interview with Ned Hayes, 2001.

216 *I registered a complaint:* Weintraub, Pamela. Complaint form, Office of Professional Medical Conduct, New York State Department of Health. March 28, 2001.

217 *"completed its review of your complaint":* Biski, Patricia, R. N., medical conduct investigator, Office of Professional Medical Management, New York State Department of Health, 2001.

32. THE LYME INQUISITION: DOCTORS ON THE RUN
219 *"I think it is unfortunate":* Steere, Allen C. Letter to George Kraus, M.D., director of health, Department of Health, Milford, CT, July 30, 1990.

220 *patients were in a bind:* In-person interviews with Ken Fordyce and Kerry Fordyce, Denver.

220 *husband-and-wife:* Kim Uffleman, Pat Smith, Barbara Goldklang.

220 *scheduled a hearing:* Nusbaum, Kenneth E. "Science to circus: enter Lyme disease." In *From the Lab to the Hill: Essays Celebrating 20 Years of Congressional Science and Engineering Fellows.* Edited by Anthony Fainberg. Washington, DC: American Association for the Advancement of Science, 1994.

221 *There is a core group:* Burrascano, Joseph, M.D. Testimony before the Committee on Labor and Human Resources, U.S. Senate, August 5, 1993.

222 *Those in the audience:* In-person interview with Barbara Goldklang and Carl Brenner, 2003–2004.

222 *When Allen Steere spoke:* Testimony before the Committee on Labor and Human Resources, U.S. Senate, August 5, 1993.

223 *got a whiff of the future:* "GAO Investigation Called—Probe Targets DHHS Agency." *LymeLight.* Posted on the Web site of the Lyme Disease Foundation, www.lyme.org/lymelight/gao_investigation.html.

223 *William Brown of Portland, Oregon:* Mervine, Phyllis. "Threat of disciplinary action creates tense atmosphere for Lyme docs." *Lyme Times.* October 1994.

224 *Zemel reported Watsky:* Zemel, Lawrence, M.D. Letter to Donna Brewer, Department of Public Health and Addiction Services, Hearing Office, Hartford, CT, September 14, 1993.

224 *by the summer of 1995:* "Charges against CT doctor dropped." *LymeLight.* 1996; 1.

225 *Brewer sent Watsky a written warning:* Waldman, Loretta. "City doctor cleared in Lyme disease case." *Bristol Press.* February 2, 1996.

225 *backed off from the treatment of Lyme disease:* Ramp, Stephanie. "The dirty truth about Lyme disease research." *Westchester County Weekly.* October 14, 2000.

225 *Natole's disastrous journey:* In-person interview with Jane Huegel, Saginaw, MI, July 15, 2002, and in-person interview with Sharon Smith of the Lyme Alliance, Saginaw, MI, July 16, 2002. Also: Mervine, Phyllis. "Threat of disciplinary action creates tense atmosphere for Lyme docs." *Lyme Times.* October 1994.

227 *The testimony against him came from Allen Steere:* State of Michigan Department of Commerce, Bureau of Occupational & Professional Regulation, Board of Medicine. Deposition of Allen C. Steere, M.D., Boston, MA, July 26, 1994.

228 *license had been temporarily suspended:* Kaczmarek, Honorable Robert L., Circuit Judge. "Opinion and Order of the Court." State of Michigan in the Circuit Court for the County of Saginaw, Joseph Natole Jr., M.D., Petitioner, versus File No. 96-15560-AA-2. Michigan Board of Medicine Respondent. Also: Amicus Brief of Lyme Alliance of South Central Michigan. State of Michigan in the Circuit Court for the County of Saginaw in the Matter of Joseph Natole Jr., M.D., Case No. 96-15560-AA, Hon. Robert Kaczmarek, Petitioner vs. Michigan Board of Medicine, Respondent. Also: Smith, Sharon. "Appeal denied: judge hands down decision in Dr. Natole's appeal." www.Lymealliance.com. February 1998.

228 *he'd been indicted:* Kelly, Fred. "Lyme disease alleged to be false diagnosis." *Ann Arbor News.* June 19, 1998.

228   *Joe Burrascano was finally interviewed:* This section is based on an in-person interview with Joseph Burrascano at his office in East Hampton, NY, in 2004 and on transcripts of his hearing before the Office of Professional Medical Management at the New York Department of Health. It is also based on numerous other documents, interviews with dozens of patients and doctors, and my personal presence at legislative hearings, demonstrations, and meetings in Albany, in Westchester, and in New York City. Deep background for the reader can be obtained through the Foundation for the Advancement of Innovative Medicine: www.faim.org/lyme.htm#DrB.

228   *the Lyme scene in New York State:* As a Lyme patient and the mother of a Lyme patient who resided in Chappaqua, New York, I personally lived through these events and participated fully in them.

228   *OPMC had written back:* Marks, Ansel R., executive secretary, New York State Board for Professional Medical Conduct. Letter to anonymous patient, December 23, 1999; and Osten, Wayne M., director, Office of Health Systems Management, New York State. Letter "To Senator Daniel Patrick Moynihan," September 13, 1999. For the interested reader, more letters from New York State officials and responses by Lyme advocates and their legislators surrounding these events are posted on the Internet. They span the years 1999–2000 and can be seen at www .angelfire.com/ny5/lymelinks/index.html.

228   *To the state legislature:* The New York State Legislature held two hearings on these issues. I attended both. Sponsored by the Standing Committee on Health was a public hearing on chronic Lyme disease and long-term antibiotic treatment. November 27, 2001; and sponsored by the Joint Assembly Standing Committee on Health, the Assembly Standing Committee on Higher Education, and the Assembly Standing Committee on Codes was a public hearing on OPMC reform and the disciplinary process of physicians and physician assistants. January 21, 2002. Full transcripts can be found on the Internet at www.lymeinfo.net/hearings.html.

229   *On November 9, 2000:* I was present in New York City during this rally. In addition, see Noble, Holcomb B. "Lyme doctors rally behind a colleague under inquiry." *New York Times.* November 10, 2000.

229   *Burrascano's trial commenced:* Joseph Burrascano gave me access to the full transcripts of these proceedings.

229   *even Burrascano's enemies:* Top-level source, identity off the record.

232   *delivered its decision:* New York State Department of Health. "Re: In the Matter of Joseph Burrascano, M.D., Determination and Order No. 01-265." The full documentation regarding the OPMC's decision is linked from its Web site at http://w3 .health.state.ny.us/opmc/factions.nsf/physiciansearch?openform. In "keyword," type in the name "Burrascano," and you'll find the documentation.

233   *"I'll give it to you":* Peter Welch to me in February 2000, upon diagnosing Jason, my son, with Lyme disease.

33. A NOTE FROM THE UNDERGROUND
Interview with David Martz, 2007.

228   *Then, in December:* Miller, Robert. "Patients Grapple with Lyme Disease." *News-Times.* Danbury, CT. May 12, 2003.

34. SECOND-CHANCE KIDS
Interview with Sheila Statlender, 2004 and 2007.

35. ONCE BITTEN: ACCEPTING THE SPIROCHETE'S ENDLESS LOVE
Personal memoir.

36. SECRETS OF AN EVIL GENIUS: THE EVIDENCE FOR PERSISTENCE

247   *Vicki Logan:* Liegner, K. B., Rosenkilde, C. E., Campbell, G. L., Quan, T. J., and Dennis, D. T. "Culture-confirmed treatment failure of cefotaxime and minocycline in a case of Lyme meningoencephalomyelitis in the United States." Abstr. 63, p. A10. Program abstract, 5th International Conference on Lyme Borreliosis, 1992.

247   *patient studied by Pat Coyle:* Lawrence, C., Lipton, R. B., Lowy, F. D., Coyle, P. K. "Seronegative chronic relapsing neuroborreliosis." *European Neurology.* 1995; 35 (2): 113–17.

247   *spirochetes have been recovered:* Preac-Mursic, V., Weber, K., Pfister, W., Wilske, B., Gross, B., Bauman, A., Prokop, J. Survival of *B. burgdorferi* antibiotically treated patients with Lyme borreliosis." *Infection.* 1989; 17: 355.

247   *rashes:* Weber, K. "Treatment failure in erythema migrans—a review." *Infection.* January–February 1996; 24(1): 73–75.

247   *irises:* Preac-Mursic, V., Pfister, H. W., Spiegel, H., Burk, R., Wilske, B., Reinhardt, S., Bohmer, R. "First isolation of *Borrelia burgdorferi* from an iris biopsy." *Journal of Clinical Neuroophthalmology.* September 1993; 13 (3): 155–61. Discussion, p. 162.

247   *spleens:* Cimmino, M. A., Azzolini, A., Tobia, F., Pesce, C. M. "Spirochetes in the spleen of a patient with chronic Lyme disease." *American Journal of Clinical Pathology.* January 1989; 91 (1): 95–97.

247   *many such cases:* Oksi, J., Marjamaki, M., Nikoskelainen, J., Viljanen, M. K. "*Borrelia burgdorferi* detected by culture and PCR in clinical relapse of disseminated Lyme borreliosis." *Annals of Medicine.* June 1999; 31 (3): 225–32; Malawista, S. E., Barthold, S. W., Persing, D. H. "Fate of *Borrelia burgdorferi* DNA in tissues of infected mice after antibiotic treatment." *Journal of Infectious Diseases.* November 1994; 170 (5): 1312–16; Häupl, T., Hahn, G., Rittig, M., Krause, A., Schoerner, C., Schönherr, U., Kalden, J. R., Burmester, G. R. "Persistence of *Borrelia burgdorferi* in ligamentous tissue from a patient with chronic Lyme borreliosis." *Arthritis & Rheumatism.* November 1993; 36 (11): 1621–26.

247   *First Straubinger placed infected:* Straubinger, R. K., Summers, B. A., Chang, Y. F., Appel, M. J. "Persistence of *Borrelia burgdorferi* in experimentally infected dogs after antibiotic treatment." *Journal of Clinical Microbiology.* January 1997; 35 (1): 111–16.

247   *In a follow-up of the work:* Straubinger, R. K. "PCR-based quantification of *Borrelia burgdorferi* organisms in canine tissues over a 500-day post-infection period." *Journal of Clinical Microbiology.* June 2000; 38 (6): 2191–99.

248   *Elegant experiments with mice:* Telephone interview with Stephen Barthold, January 7, 2008. Also: Hodzic, E., Feng, S., Freet, K. J., Barthold, S. W.

"Attenuation of *Borrelia burgdorferi* by antibiotic treatment in mice." *Antimicrobial Agents and Chemotherapy*. In press, 2008. See also: Bockenstedt, L. K., Mao, J., Hodzic, E., Barthold, S. W., Fish, D. "Detection of attenuated, noninfectious spirochetes in *Borrelia burgdorferi*–infected mice after antibiotic treatment." *Journal of Infectious Diseases*. November 15, 2002; 186 (10): 1430–37.

251   *"How can you say"*: In-person interview with Leonard Sigal, 2002.

251   *A possible answer*: Interview with Stephen Barthold.

252   *"pro-inflammatory effects"*: deSouza, M. S., Fikrig, E., Smith, A. L., Flavell, R. A., Barthold, S. W. "Nonspecific proliferative responses of murine lymphocytes to *Borrelia burgdorferi* antigens." *Journal of Infectious Diseases*. 1992; 165: 471–78. Also: Ebnet, K., Brown, K. D., Siebenlist, U. K., Simon, M. M., Shaw, S. "*Borrelia burgdorferi* activates nuclear factor-KB and is a potent inducer of chemokine and adhesion molecule gene expression in endothelial cells and fibroblasts." *Journal of Immunology*. 1997; 158: 3285–92; Giambartolomei, G. H., Dennis, V. A., Lasater, B. L., Philipp, M. T. "Induction of pro- and anti-inflammatory cytokines by *Borrelia burgdorferi* lipoproteins in monocytes is mediated by CD14." *Infection and Immunity*. January 1999; 67 (1): 140–47; Giambartolomei, G. H., Dennis, V. A., Philipp, M. T. "*Borrelia burgdorferi* stimulates the production of interleukin-10 in peripheral blood mononuclear cells from uninfected humans and rhesus monkeys." *Infection and Immunity*. 1998; 66: 2691–97; Ma, Y., Seiler, K. P., Tai, K. F., Yang, L., Woods, M., Weis, J. J. "Outer surface lipoproteins of *Borrelia burgdorferi* stimulate nitric oxide production by the cytokine-inducible pathway." *Infection and Immunity*. 1994; 62: 3663–71; Morrison, T. B., Weis, J. H., Weis, J. J. "*Borrelia burgdorferi* outer surface protein A (OspA) activates and primes human neutrophils." *Journal of Immunology*. 1997; 158: 4838–45; Norgard, M., Riley, B., Richardson, J., Radolf, J. "Dermal inflammation elicited by synthetic analogs of *Treponema pallidum* and *Borrelia burgdorferi* lipoproteins." *Infection and Immunity*. 1995; 63: 1507–15; Norgard, M. V., Arndt, L. L., Akins, D. R., Curetty, L. L., Harrich, D. A., Radolf, J. D. "Activation of human monocytic cells by *Treponema pallidum* and *Borrelia burgdorferi* lipoproteins and synthetic lipopeptides via a pathway distinct from that of lipopolysaccharide by involves the transcriptional activator of NF-kB." *Infection and Immunity*. 1996; 64: 3845–52; Radolf, J. D., Arndt, L. L., Alkins, D. R., Curetty, L. L., Levi, M. E., Shen, Y. N., Davis, L. S., Norgard, M. V. "*Treponema pallidum* and *Borrelia burgdorferi* lipoproteins and synthetic lipopeptides activate monocytes/macrophages." *Journal of Immunology*. 1995; 154: 2866–77; Sobek, V., Birkner, N., Falk, I., Wurch, A., Kirschning, C. J., Wagner, H., Wallich, R., Lamers, M. C., Simon, M. M. "Direct Toll-like receptor 2 mediated co-stimulation of T cells in the mouse system as a basis for chronic inflammatory joint disease." *Arthritis Research & Therapy*. 2004; 6: R433–R446; Tai, K. F., Ma, Y., Weis, J. J. "Normal human B lymphocytes and mononuclear cells respond to the mitogenic and cytokine-stimulatory activities of *Borrelia burgdorferi* and its lipoprotein OspA." *Infection and Immunity*. 1994; 520–28; Weis, J. J., Ma, Y., Erdile, L. F. "Biological activities of native and recombinant

Borrelia burgdorferi outer surface protein A: dependence on lipid modification." *Infection and Immunity.* 1994; 62: 4632–36; Wooten, R. M., Modur, V. R., McIntyre, T. M., Weis, J. J. "*Borrelia burgdorferi* outer membrane protein A induces nuclear translocation of nuclear factor-kB and inflammatory activation in human endothelial cells." *Journal of Bacteriology.* 1996; 178: 4584–90; Yang, L. M., Ma, Y., Schoenfeld, R., Griffiths, M., Eichwald, E., Aranco, B., Weis, J. J. "Evidence for lymphocyte-B mitogen activity in *Borrelia burgdorferi*—infected mice." *Infection and Immunity.* 1992; 60: 3033–41.

252   *in skin:* Georgilis, K., Peacocke, M., Klempner, M. S. "Fibroblasts protect the Lyme disease spirochete, *Borrelia burgdorferi,* from ceftriaxone in vitro." *Journal of Infectious Diseases.* August 1992; 166 (2): 440–44. Also: Klempner, M. S., Noring, R., Rogers, R. A. "Invasion of human skin fibroblasts by the Lyme disease spirochete, *Borrelia burgdorferi.*" *Journal of Infectious Diseases.* May 1993; 167 (5): 1074–81; Ma, Y., Sturrock, A., Weis, J. J. "Intracellular localization of *Borrelia burgdorferi* within human endothelial cells." *Infection and Immunity.* 1991; 59: 671–78.

252   *and white blood cells:* Montgomery, R. R, Nathanson, M. H., Malawista, S. E. "The fate of *Borrelia burgdorferi,* the agent for Lyme disease, in mouse macrophages. Destruction, survival, recovery." *Journal of Immunology.* 1993; 150: 909–15. Also: Sambri V., et al. "Uptake and killing of Lyme disease and relapsing fever *Borreliae* in the perfused rat liver and by isolated Kupffer cells." *Infection and Immunity.* 1996; 64 (5): 1858–61.

252   *synovial cells:* Girschick, H. J., et al. "Intracellular persistence of *Borrelia burgdorferi* in human synovial cells." *Rheumatology International.* 1996; 16 (3) 125–32.

252   *At the NIH:* Dorward, D. W., Hulinska, D. LDF Conference Vancouver, BC, 1994. Also: Dorward, D. W., Fischer, E. R., Brooks, D. M. "Invasion and cytopathic killing of human lymphocytes by spirochetes causing Lyme disease." *Clinical Infectious Diseases.* July 1997; 25 Suppl. 1: S2–8.

253   *dizzying array of forms:* Warthin, A. S., Olson, R. E. "The granular transformation of *Spirochaeta pallida* in aortic focal lesions." *American Journal of Syphilis.* 1930; 14: 433–37; Balfour, Andrew, M.D. "The infective granule in certain protozoal infections, as illustrated by the spirochaetosis of Sudanese fowl." *British Medical Journal.* 1911; 1: 870; Leishman, Major General Sir William B. "The Horace Dobell Lecture on an experimental investigation of *Spirochaeta duttoni,* the parasite of tick fever." Delivered before the Royal College of Physicians of London on November 2, 1920. *Lancet.* December 18, 1920; Ovcinnikov, N. M., Delektorskij, V. V. "Current concepts of the morphology and biology of *Treponema pallidum* based on electron microscopy." *British Journal of Venereal Diseases.* October 1971; 47 (5): 315–28; Al-Qudah, A. A., Mostratos, A., Quesnel, L. B. "A proposed life cycle for the Reiter treponeme." *Journal of Applied Bacteriology.* December 1983; 55 (3): 417–28.

253   *One of the first:* Hulinska, D., Bartak, P., Hercogova, J., Hancil, J., Basta, J., Schramlova, J. "Electron microscopy of Langerhans cells and *Borrelia burgdorferi* in Lyme disease patients." *Zentralblatt für Bakteriologie.* January 1994; 280 (3): 348–59.

253   *reported by Alan:* MacDonald, A. "Concurrent Neocortical Borreliosis and Alzheimer's Disease Demonstration of a Spirochetal Cyst Form." *Annals of the New York Academy of Sciences.* 1988; 468–70.

253   *husband-and-wife team:* Brorson, Ø., Brorson, S. H. "Transformation of cystic forms of *Borrelia burgdorferi* to normal, mobile spirochetes." *Infection.* 1997; 25 (4): 240–46.

254   *from the University of Rhode Island:* Alban, P. S., Johnson, P. W., Nelson, D. R. "Serum-starvation-induced changes in protein synthesis and morphology of *Borrelia burgdorferi.*" *Microbiology.* 2000; 146: Pt. 1; 119–27.

254   *scientists from Italy:* Murgia, R., Cinco, M. "Induction of cystic forms by different stress conditions in *Borrelia burgdorferi.*" *Acta Pathologica, Microbiologica et Immunologica Scandinavica.* January 2004; 112 (1): 57–62.

254   *inoculated healthy mice:* Gruntar, I., Malovrh, T., Murgia, R., Cinco, M. "Conversion of *Borrelia garinii* cystic forms to motile spirochetes in vivo." *Acta Pathologica, Microbiologica et Immunologica Scandinavica.* May 2001; 109 (5): 383–88.

254   *scientist Judith Miklossy.* Miklossy, J., Kasas, S., Zurn, A. D., McCall, S., Yu, S., McGreer, P. L., "Persisting atypical and cystic forms of *Borrelia burgdorgeri* and local inflammation in Lyme neuroborreliosis." *Journal of Neuroinflammation.* September 2008; 5: 40.

255   *metronidazole:* Brorson, Ø., Brorson, S. H. "An in vitro study of the susceptibility of mobile and cystic forms of *Borrelia burgdorferi* to metronidazole." *Acta Pathologica, Microbiologica et Immunologica Scandinavica.* June 1999; 107 (6): 566–76.

255   *tinidazole:* Brorson, Ø., Brorson, S. H. "An in vitro study of the susceptibility of mobile and cystic forms of *Borrelia burgdorferi* to tinidazole." *International Microbiology.* June 2004; 7 (2): 139–42.

255   *grapefruit seed extract:* Brorson, Ø., Brorson, S. H. "Grapefruit seed extract is a powerful in vitro agent against motile and cystic forms of *Borrelia burgdorferi* sensu lato." *Infection.* June 2007; 35 (3): 206–8.

255   *As for Steve:* In-person interview with Stephen Barthold at UC, Davis, 2002, and by telephone, 2007.

37. MOTHER MAKES FOUR
Interviews with Sheila Statlender, 2004 and 2007.

38. THE BIG SLEEP: OUR YOUNGER SON FALLS ILL
Personal memoir.

261   Clostridium difficile. http://www.mayoclinic.com/health/c-difficile/ds00736.

39. HOUSTON CALLING
Interview with David Martz, 2007.

40. PUTTING TREATMENT TO THE TEST
267   *"What does it mean to persist?":* In-person interview with Alan Barbour, UC, Irvine, 2001.

267 *on October 18:* Consultation on Chronic Lyme Disease, National Institute of Allergy and Infectious Diseases, Solar Building, Room 3A3-4, Bethesda, MD, October 18, 1994. Meeting notes provided by Suzanne Stutman, who attended. Further descriptions through in-person interviews with Carl Brenner and Barbara Goldklang, 2002–2004.

268 *A call for proposals went out:* Interviews with Raymond Dattwyler, Ben Luft, and Carl Brenner.

268 *a sweltering day in July:* Interviews with Carl Brenner and Ken Fordyce. Also: Brenner, Carl. "Update on NIAID Intramural and Extramural Studies of Chronic Lyme Disease." *LymeLight.* VI, 1996; "NIH, NIAID, Special Emphasis Panel, RFP-NIH-NIAID-DMID-96-09." *Clinical Studies of Chronic Lyme Disease.* February 28, 1996; Comptroller General of the United States, Washington, DC. "Decision: Matter of: The Research Foundation of the State University of New York." File: B-274269. December 2, 1996.

269 *beyond the decades of bad blood:* Interviews with advisory panel members Carl Brenner and Phyllis Mervine, 2002–2007.

270 *Mervine was worried:* Mervine, Phyllis. E-mail, September 29, 2004.

270 *a daunting task:* In-person interview with Carl Brenner, Nyack, NY, 2003.

270 *entry requirements were steep:* Klempner, Mark. Eleventh Annual Diseases of Summer Conference, South County Hospital, Wakefield, RI, 2001.

270 *arranged a presentation:* Brenner, Carl. "Update on NIAID Intramural and Extramural Studies of Chronic Lyme Disease Carl Brenner (Member, Advisory Committee)." Katonah, NY, April 19, 1997.

270 *Klempner eventually rustled up:* Diseases of Summer Conference, Wakefield, RI, 2001. Clinical guidelines; Wormser, G. P., Nadelman, R. B., Dattwyler, R. J., Dennis, D. T., Shapiro, E. D., Steere, A. C., Rush, T. J., Rahn, D. W., Coyle, P. K., Persing, D. H., Fish, D., Luft, B. J. "Practice guidelines for the treatment of Lyme disease. The Infectious Diseases Society of America." *Clinical Infectious Diseases.* July 2000; 31 Suppl 1: 1–14.

270 *Donta:* From *LymeLight.* 2000. www.lyme.org/lymelight/trtcontrov.html.

271 *halted at once:* Office of Communications and Public Liaison, National Institute of Allergy and Infectious Diseases, National Institutes of Health, Bethesda, MD. "Interim Analysis of NIAID's Chronic Lyme Disease Treatment Studies Statement." November 29, 2000.

271 *published to fanfare:* Klempner, M. S., Hu, I. T., Evans, J., Schmid, C. H., Johnson, G. M., Trevino, R. P., Norton, D., Levy, L., Wall, D., McCall, J., Kosinski, M., Weinstein, A. "Two controlled trials of antibiotic treatment in patients with persistent symptoms and a history of Lyme disease." *New England Journal of Medicine.* July 12, 2001; 345 (2): 85–92.

271 *accompanied by a press release:* National Institute of Allergy and Infectious Disease. "Clinical Alert: Chronic Lyme Disease Symptoms Not Helped by Intensive Antibiotic Treatment." June 12, 2001. www.nlm.nih.gov/databases/alerts/lyme.html.

271 *announced* Time *magazine:* Gorman, Christine. "Antibiotics don't cure chronic Lyme disease, new studies show, but one dose may prevent infection." *Time.* June 25, 2001.

271 *quote of the day:* Sigal, Leonard. "Quote of the Day." *New York Times.* June 13, 2001.

272 *"How do you think it looks":* Brenner, Carl. E-mail "The Study," to John Edwards, M.D., June 14, 2001.

272 *Donta expressed concerns:* Donta, S. T. "Treatment of patients with persistent symptoms and a history of Lyme disease." *New England Journal of Medicine.* November 8, 2001; 345 (19): 1424; author reply, 1425.

273 *previously failed antibiotic therapy:* Interview with Daniel Cameron, M.D., 2007.

273 *some 75 percent of the patients:* Telephone interview with Phillip Baker, Lyme Disease Programs officer, 2003, plus e-mail clarification July 2009.

273 *As far as NIH.* E-mail interview with Philip Baker, July 2009.

273 *final disappointment:* Mervine, Phyllis. E-mail, September 27, 2004.

273 *been disbanded for good:* Heilman, Carole, Ph.D., director, Division of Microbiology and Infectious Diseases, National Institute of Allergy and Infectious Diseases, NIH. Letter to Phyllis Mervine, president, Lyme Disease Resource Center, April 16, 2002.

273 *may not have provided.* E-mail interview with Philip Baker, July 2009.

274 *next to roll:* Krupp, L. B., Hyman, L. G., Grimson, R., Coyle, P. K., Melville, P., Ahnn, S., Dattwyler, R., Chandler, B. "Study and treatment of post Lyme disease (STOP-LD): A randomized double masked clinical trial." *Neurology.* June 24, 2003; 60 (12): 1923–30.

274 *Why did Krupp's results differ:* In-person interview with Brian Fallon, 2004.

274 *A third NIH treatment study:* In-person interview with Brian Fallon, 2007. Also: Fallon, B. A., Keilp, J. G., Corbera, K. M., Petkova, E., Britton, C. B., Dwyer, E., Slavov, I., Cheng, J., Dobkin, J., Nelson, D.R., Sackeim, H. A. "A randomized, placebo-controlled trial of repeated IV antibiotic therapy for Lyme encephalopathy." *Neurology.* October 10, 2007.

276 *relapse after just ten weeks:* E-mail correspondence with Joseph Burrascano, M.D., October 2007.

276 *come out of hiding:* E-mail correspondence from Harold Smith, M.D., October 2007.

276 *Writing an editorial:* Halperin, J. J. "Prolonged Lyme disease treatment." *Neurology.* October 10, 2007.

277 *ILADS president Daniel Cameron:* Telephone discussions with Daniel Cameron on various days in October and November 2007.

277 *Writing in the journal:* Cameron, D. J. "Generalizability in two clinical trials of Lyme disease." *Epidemiological Perspectives & Innovations.* October 17, 2006; 3: 12.

277 *treatment delays:* Cameron, D. J. "Consequences of treatment delay in Lyme disease." *Journal of Evaluation in Clinical Practice.* June 2007; 13 (3): 470–72.

277 *alternative treatments:* Rosner, Bryan. *The Top 10 Lyme Disease Treatments: Defeat Lyme Disease with the Best of Conventional and Alternative Medicine.* South Lake Tahoe, CA: BioMed Publishing Group, 2007.

277 *vitamin C and salt:* See www.lymephotos.com.

277 Sputnik: See www.parasiteremedies.com/cleansing.html.

277 *A doctor from Atlanta:* Jefcoats, Kathy. "Stockbridge physician accused of health fraud. Insecticides used to treat patients, charges say." *Atlanta Journal-Constitution.* December 21, 2005.

277 *a doctor from Topeka:* Carter, Marla. "New Details in Patient's Death." *Kansas News Leader.* August 30, 2006; and Fry, Steve. "No contest plea entered in patient's death; probation recommended." *Topeka Capital Journal.* November 22, 2007.

278 *"I felt uncomfortable":* Interviews with Carl Brenner and Barbara Goldklang, 2006–2008.

279 *argues for caution:* Telephone interview with Stephen Barthold, January 2008.

279 *says Eugene Davidson:* Telephone interview with Eugene Davidson, February 2008.

41. BUSTED FLAT IN CHAPPAQUA
Personal memoir.

42. RESURRECTION
Interview with David Martz, August 2007.

285 *merit a write-up:* Harvey, W. T., Martz, D. "Motor neuron disease recovery associated with IV ceftriaxone and anti-*Babesia* therapy." *Acta Neurologica Scandinavica.* February 2007; 115 (2): 129–31.

43. LYME DISEASE AND IMMUNITY: THE SEARCH FOR THE GOLDEN FLEECE

286 *thee or me?:* Klempner, M. S., Huber, B. T. "Is it thee or me?—autoimmunity in Lyme disease." *Nature Medicine.* December 1999; 5 (12): 1346–47.

287 *The gene:* Klempner, Mark. 11th Annual Diseases of Summer Conference, South County Hospital, Wakefield, RI, 2001. (Klempner refused to grant a personal interview with me.)

287 *"molecular mimicry":* Gross, D. M., Forsthuber, T., Tary-Lehmann, M., Etling, C., Ito, K., Nagy, Z. A., Field, J. A., Steere, A. C., Huber, B. T. "Identification of LFA-1 as a candidate autoantigen in treatment-resistant Lyme arthritis." *Science.* July 31, 1998; 281 (5377): 703–6.

287 *In experiment after experiment:* Drouin, E. E., Glickstein, L., Kwok, W. W., Nepom, G. T., Steere, A. C. "Searching for borrelial T cell epitopes associated with antibiotic-refractory Lyme arthritis." *Molecular Immunology.* January 10, 2008.

288 *IVIG:* Telephone interview with neurologist Amiram Katz, November 2007. Also: Alaedini, A., Latov, N. "Antibodies against OspA epitopes of *Borrelia burgdorferi* cross-react with neural tissue." *Journal of Neuroimmunology.* February 2005; 159 (1–2): 192–95; Latoy, N., Wu, A. T., Chin, R. L., Sander, H. W., Alaedini, A., Brannagan, T. H., III. "Neuropathy and cognitive impairment following vaccination with the OspA protein of *Borrelia burgdorferi.*" *Journal of the Peripheral Nervous System.* September 2004; 9 (3): 165–67.

288 *validated in 1997:* Norris, Steven J. University of Texas Medical School at Houston, phone interview, 2002. Also: Zhang, J. R., Hardham, J. M., Barbour, A. G.,

Norris, S. J. "Antigenic variation in Lyme disease *Borreliae* by promiscuous recombination of VMP-like sequence cassettes." *Cell.* April 18, 1997; 89 (2): 275–85; Zhang, J. R., Norris, S. J. "Kinetics and in vivo induction of genetic variation of vlsE in *Borrelia burgdorferi.*" *Infection and Immunity.* August 1998; 66 (8): 3689–97; Zhang, J. R., Norris, S. J. "Genetic variation of the *Borrelia burgdorferi* gene vlsE involves cassette-specific, segmental gene conversion." *Infection and Immunity.* August 1998; 66 (8): 3698–704; Lawrenz, M. B., Hardham, J. M., Owens, R. T., Nowakowski, J., Steere, A. C., Wormser, G. P., Norris S. J. "Human antibody responses to VlsE antigenic variation protein of *Borrelia burgdorferi.*" *Journal of Clinical Microbiology.* December 1999; 37 (12): 3997–4004.

289   *In 2006, Norris:* Bykowski, T., Babb, K., von Lackum, K., Riley, S. P., Norris, S. J., Stevenson, B. "Transcriptional regulation of the *Borrelia burgdorferi* antigenically variable VlsE surface protein." *Journal of Bacteriology.* July 2006; 188 (13): 4879–89.

289   *Hoping to explore:* In-person interview with Stephen Barthold, University of California, Davis, 2002. Also: Feng, S., Hodzic, E., Barthold, S. W. "Lyme arthritis resolution with antiserum to a 37-kilodalton *Borrelia burgdorferi* protein." *Infection and Immunity.* July 2000; 68 (7): 4169–73; Feng, S., Hodzic, E., Freet, K., Barthold, S. W. "Immunogenicity of *Borrelia burgdorferi* arthritis-related protein." *Infection and Immunity.* December 2003; 71 (12): 7211–14; Barthold, S. W., Hodzic, E., Tunev, S., Feng, S. "Antibody-mediated disease remission in the mouse model of Lyme borreliosis." *Infection and Immunity.* August 2006; 74 (8): 4817–25.

291   *immunologist at the University of Utah:* In-person interview with Janis Weis, University of Utah, Salt Lake City, 2002. Also: Hirschfeld, M., Kirschning, C. J., Schwandner, R., Wesche, H., Weis, J. H., Wooten, R. M., Weis, J. J. "Cutting edge: inflammatory signaling by *Borrelia burgdorferi* lipoproteins is mediated by Toll-like receptor 2." *Journal of Immunology.* September 1, 1999; 163 (5): 2382–86; Wooten, R. M., Ma, Y., Yoder, R. A., Brown, J. P., Weis, J. H., Zachary, J. F., Kirschning, C. J., Weis, J. J. "Toll-like receptor 2 is required for innate, but not acquired, host defense to *Borrelia burgdorferi.*" *Journal of Immunology.* January 1, 2002; 168 (1): 348–55; Wooten, R. M., Ma, Y., Yoder, R. A., Brown, J. P., Weis, J. H., Zachary, J. F., Kirschning, C. J., Weis, J. J. "Toll-like receptor 2 plays a pivotal role in host defense and inflammatory response to *Borrelia burgdorferi.*" *Vector Borne Zoonotic Diseases.* Winter 2002; 2 (4): 275–78; Crandall, H., Dunn, D. M., Ma, Y., Wooten, R. M., Zachary, J. F., Weis, J. H., Weiss, R. B., Weis, J. J. "Gene expression profiling reveals unique pathways associated with differential severity of Lyme arthritis." *Journal of Immunology.* December 1, 2006; 177 (11): 7930–42.

293   *rhesus monkeys:* Telephone interview with Mario Philipp, 2004.

44. HOW I CURED MY OWN LYME DISEASE
Personal memoir.

45. PAY IT FORWARD
Interview with David Martz, August 2007.

46. A FAMILY AFFAIR

Interview with Sheila Statlender, August 2007.

47. RED-FLAGGED AT BLUE CROSS: THE ROLE OF MANAGED CARE

303   *By August 1992:* Schwartz, Matthew. "Insurers Balk at Rising Costs of Lyme Disease." *National Underwriter.* August 24, 1992; 6.

304   *The policy was:* Steere, A. C. "Lyme disease." *Transactions of the American Academy of Insurance Medicine.* 1993; 76: 73–81.

304   *By 1995, the landscape:* Public archives, Attorney General's Office, Connecticut State House, Hartford, CT.

304   *Much of what we know:* Transcript of the videotaped deposition of Dr. Richard Sanchez, M.D., New York, NY, February 23, 1999. Case heard by the Supreme Court of the State of New York, County of Westchester. *Vicki Logan, Virginia A. Philo, Deborah A. Scheid, George Nijboer, James Marino and Danny Licul, Plantiffs, vs. Empire Blue Cross Blue Shield, Defendant.* Reported by Erica L. Ruggieri, RPR, Job No. 86606. Index No. 96/20517.

307   *By 1999:* Public archives, Attorney General's Office, Connecticut State House, Hartford, CT.

307   *Testifying before:* Pat Smith, president, Lyme Disease Association. Testimony to the New York State Assembly, November 27, 2001.

307   *Throughout Lyme country:* Alan Muney, chief medical officer, Oxford Health Plans. Testimony to the New York State Assembly, November 27, 2001.

307   *"How do you explain":* New York State Assemblyman Joel Miller, questioning Muney during the New York State Assembly, November 27, 2001.

307   *"We could pay":* Alan Muney to New York State Assembly, November 27, 2001.

307   *opened his mailbox:* In-person interview with Kenneth Liegner, 2004.

308   *"I believe Vicki requires":* Liegner, Kenneth B. Letter to Mary Berlin, case manager, Empire Blue Cross Blue Shield of Greater New York, July 19, 1993.

309   *Sherwood P. Miller:* Miller, Sherwood P., M.D., F.A.C.P., assistant medical director, Medical Policy and Research, Empire Blue Cross Blue Shield of Greater New York. Letter to Kenneth B. Liegner, May 27, 1994.

309   *"deteriorated markedly":* Liegner, Kenneth B. Letter to Sherwood P. Miller, M.D., assistant medical director, Medical Policy and Research, Empire Blue Cross Blue Shield, July 9, 1994.

309   *Miller, who was:* Miller, Sherwood P., M.D., F.A.C.P., assistant medical director, Medical Policy and Research, Empire Blue Cross Blue Shield of Greater New York. Letter to Kenneth B. Liegner, August 9, 1994.

309   *And so it went:* Vicki Logan signed a release for me to see the entire file of correspondence surrounding these events.

309   *But by the summer of 1995:* In-person interview with Kenneth Liegner, 2004.

309   *did not meet:* Empire Blue Cross Blue Shield of Greater New York. Letter to Kenneth B. Liegner, July 11, 1996.

309   *$175,000 debt:* Liegner, Kenneth B., Cynthia Miller, coordinator, Utilization Review, Empire Blue Cross Blue Shield, September 11, 1997.

309   *It was in the fall of 1997:* Liegner, Kenneth B. Letter to Dr. Golonka, Blue Cross Blue Shield, October 15, 1997.

309   *Would Empire consider:* Liegner, Kenneth B. Letter to Dr. Golonka, Blue Cross Blue Shield, October 30, 1997.

310   *The treatment was "experimental":* Cavanaugh, Lori, R.N, B.S.N, C.R.N.I., team leader, Empire Blue Cross Blue Shield of Greater New York. Letter to Vicki Logan, February 12, 1998.

310   *with a specific disease:* Cavanaugh, Lori, R.N, B.S.N, C.R.N.I., team leader, Empire Blue Cross Blue Shield of Greater New York. Letter to Vicki Logan, April 7, 1998.

310   *She'd experienced the same problem before:* Liegner, Kenneth B. Letter to Geeta Chowdhary, M.D., medical director, Empire Blue Cross Blue Shield, October 29, 1998.

310   *Logan tested positive:* Liegner, Kenneth B. Letter to Franklin L. Brosgol, M.D., senior medical director, Empire Blue Cross Blue Shield, October 29, 1998.

310   *"At your request":* Brosgol, Franklin L., M.D., senior medical director, Empire Blue Cross Blue Shield of Greater New York. Letter to Kenneth Liegner, M.D., July 25, 2000.

310   *early in 2002:* Telephone interview with Kenneth Liegner, 2002.

311   *Liegner arranged to meet:* I was present at this meeting, and the description flows from my personal notes of the day. The meeting took place at the Department of Health in Albany, NY, in May 2002.

312   *In the weeks after the meeting:* Telephone interviews with Kenneth Liegner through 2002 and 2003.

312   *Hudson Valley Hospital pathologist:* Liegner, Kenneth. E-mail, December 2, 2007.

312   *"To the pathologist":* Libien, Jenny. Case presentation, Lyme Disease Association Conference. "Tick-Borne Diseases: Technology Leading the Way." Rye, NY, November 2004.

312   *Duray had a look:* In-person interview with Paul Duray, Philadelphia, November 2005.

48. THE VACCINE CONNECTION: LYME GETS A BUSINESS MODEL

In 2000, before I wrote the proposal for this book, I wrote a report, "Conflicts of Interest in Lyme Disease," for the Lyme Disease Association for which I received $4,000. Some of the material here is drawn from that report.

315   *talent for altering its outer coat:* Stephen Barthold, 2002.

315   *protect mice:* Fikrig, E., Barthold, S. W., Kantor, F. S., Flavell, R. A. "Protection of mice against the Lyme disease agent by immunizing with recombinant OspA." *Science.* 1990; 250: 553–56.

316   *killing most:* Fikrig, E., Telford, S. R., III, Barthold, S. W., Kantor, F. S., Spielman, A., Flavell, R. A. "Elimination of *Borrelia burgdorferi* from vector ticks feeding on OspA-immunized mice." *Proceedings of the National Academy of Sciences USA.* June 15, 1992; 89 (12): 5418–21.

316   *The Connaught effort:* Interview with attorney Ira Maurer at his office in White Plains, 2001. Also see: Sigal, L. H., Zahradnik, J. M., Lavin, P., Patella, S. J., Bryant, G., Haselby, R., Hilton, E., Kunkel, M., Adler-Klein, D., Doherty, T., Evans, J., Molloy, P. J., Seidner, A. L., Sabetta, J. R., Simon, H. J., Klempner, M.

S., Mays, J., Marks, D., Malawista, S. E. "A vaccine consisting of recombinant *Borrelia burgdorferi* outer surface protein A to prevent Lyme disease. Recombinant Outer-Surface Protein A Lyme Disease Vaccine Study Consortium." *New England Journal of Medicine.* July 23, 1998; 339 (4): 216–22.

316 *Steere announced the success:* Steere, A. C., Sikand, V. K., Meurice, F., Parenti, D. L., Fikrig, E., Schoen, R. T., Nowakowski, J., Schmid, C. H., Laukamp, S., Buscarino, C., Krause, D. S. "Vaccination against Lyme disease with recombinant *Borrelia burgdorferi* outer surface lipoprotein A with adjuvant. Lyme Disease Vaccine Study Group." *New England Journal of Medicine.* July 23, 1998; 339 (4): 209–15.

316 *fly in the ointment:* Gross, D. M., Forsthuber, T., Tary-Lehmann, M., Etling, C., Ito, K., Nagy, Z. A., Field, J. A., Steere, A. C., Huber, B. T. "Identification of LFA-1 as a candidate autoantigen in treatment-resistant Lyme arthritis." *Science.* July 31, 1998; 281 (5377): 703–6. Also: Trollmo, C., Meyer, A. L., Steere, A. C., Hafler, D. A., Huber, B. T. "Molecular mimicry in Lyme arthritis demonstrated at the single cell level: LFA-1 alpha L is a partial agonist for outer surface protein A-reactive T cells." *Journal of Immunology.* April 15, 2001; 166(8): 5286–91.

316 *theory provoked skepticism:* I interviewed many university-based researchers who did not think this was a big factor in Lyme, including Mario Philipp, David Persing, Stephen Barthold, and Janis Weis, among others.

317 *FDA approved LYMErix anyway:* Donlon, Jerome A., M.D., Ph.D., acting director, Office of Compliance and Biologics Quality, Center for Biologics Evaluation and Research, and Hardegree, M. Carolyn, M.D., director, Office of Vaccines Research and Review, Center for Biologics Evaluation and Research, Department of Health and Human Services, Public Health Service, Food and Drug Administration. Letter to Johan van Hoof, Ph.D., SmithKline Beecham Biologicals, December 21, 1998; www.fda.gov/cber/approvltr/lymesmi122198L .htm.

317 *"Those who did the trial":* Karzon, David. Department of Health and Human Services, Food and Drug Administration, Center for Biologics Evaluation and Research, Vaccines and Related Biological Products Advisory Committee Meeting, Tuesday, May 26, 1998; www.fda.gov/ohrms/dockets/ac/98/transcpt/ 3422t1.rtf.

317 *reconvened on LYMErix:* I attended this full-day review session in Bethesda, MD, January 31, 2001. Also: Department of Health and Human Services, Food and Drug Administration, Center for Biologics Evaluation and Research, Vaccines and Related Biological Products Advisory Committee Meeting, Wednesday, January 31, 2001; www.fda.gov/ohrms/dockets/ac/01/transcripts/ 3680t2.rtf.

317 *Huber, entered the fray:* Huber, Brigitte, and Tufts University. "Novel *Borrelia burgdorferi* Polypeptides and Uses Thereof," WO/2001/070252. Also see: Forschner, Karen. "Extended from remarks given by Karen Vanderhoof-Forschner, B.S., M.B.A., C.P.C.U., C.L.U., to the Food and Drug Administration's Vaccine Advisory Committee Meeting, November 28, 2001." www.lyme.org/ vaccine/3yrreslong.pdf.

318   *"data-gathering mode":* Telephone interview with Robert Ball, director of the FDA's Vaccine Adverse Event Reporting System (VAERS), 2001.

318   *to awaken old:* Telephone interview with Sam Donta, 2001.

318   *Western blots on fire:* This was a main topic at a Lyme Disease Foundation conference that I attended in April 2001.

318   *wide range of Borrelia-specific bands:* Telephone interview with Paul Fawcett, 2001. Also: Fawcett, P. T., Rose, C. D., Maduskuie, V. "Long-term effects of immunization with recombinant lipoprotein outer surface protein A on serologic test for Lyme disease." *Clinical and Diagnostic Laboratory Immunology.* July 2004; 11 (4): 808–10; and Fawcett, P. T., Rose, C. D., Gibney, K. M. "In vitro assessment of antiborrelial activity of OspA vaccine sera." *Clinical and Diagnostic Laboratory Immunology.* July 2002; 9 (4): 919–20.

319   *Their investigation:* Telephone interviews with Philip J. Molloy and David Persing, 2001. Also: Molloy, P. J., Berardi, V. P., Persing, D. H., Sigal, L. H. "Detection of multiple reactive protein species by immunoblotting after recombinant outer surface protein A Lyme disease vaccination." *Clinical Infectious Diseases.* July, 2000; 31 (1): 42–47.

319   *As for GlaxoSmithKline:* Telephone interview with Carmel Hogan, spokesperson for GlaxoSmithKline, 2001.

320   *potential for bias:* The Lyme Disease Association and Weintraub, P. "Conflicts of Interest in Lyme Disease: Laboratory Testing, Vaccination, and Treatment Guidelines." I researched and wrote this report for LDA in 2001, prior to writing a proposal for *Cure Unknown.* I was paid $4,000 for the work. It was minutely fact-checked and reviewed by attorneys. It is exhaustively referenced and relates to the time period under discussion here. Especially refer to the cross-referenced flow chart of conflicts. At 180 pages, this extensively documented research would require a book unto itself and is too large for extensive citation in *Cure Unknown,* but the full text online can be accessed at www.lymediseaseassociation.org/Conflicts.doc.

320   *months before the vote in Michigan:* Food and Drug Administration Center for Biologics Evaluation and Research, Open Meeting of the Vaccines and Related Biologics Products Advisory Committee, June 7, 1994.

320   *participated in clinical trials:* Steere, A. C., Sikand, V. K., Meurice, F., Parenti, D. L., Fikrig, E., Schoen, R. T., Nowakowski, J., Schmid, C. H., Laukamp, S., Buscarino, C., and Krause, D. S. "Vaccination against Lyme disease with recombinant *Borrelia burgdorferi* outer-surface lipoprotein A with adjuvant. Lyme Disease Vaccine Study Group." *New England Journal of Medicine.* July 1998; 339 (4): 209–15. Also: Sigal, L. H., Zahradnik, J. M., Lavin, P., Patella, S. J., Bryant, G., Haselby, R., Hilton, E., Kunkel, M., Adler-Klein, D., Doherty, T., Evans, J., Malawista, S. E., Molloy, P. J., Seidner, A. L., Sabetta, J. R., Simon, H. J., Klempner, M. S., Mays, J., and Marks, D. "A vaccine consisting of recombinant *Borrelia burgdorferi* outer-surface protein A to prevent Lyme disease." *New England Journal of Medicine.* 1998; 339 (4): 216–22; Sikand, V. K., Halsey, N. Krause, P. J., Sood, S. K., Geller, R., Van Hoecke, C., Buscarino, C., and Parenti, D. "Safety and immunogenicity of a recombinant *Borrelia burgdorferi* outer surface protein A vaccine against lyme disease in healthy children and adolescents: a randomized controlled trial." *Pediatrics.* 2001; 108 (1): 123–28.

321 *"there was the feeling"*: Phillip J. Baker, e-mail, April 24, 2009.

316 *Food & Drug Administration*: Open meeting of the vaccines and related biologics products advisory committee, Silver Spring, MD, June 7, 1994.

321 *resides on the same plasmid*: Persing, D., "Method for detecting *B. burgdorferi* infection." *Mayo Foundation for Medical Educational Research*. April 4, 2000; 18.

321 *made clearly by Raymond Dattwyler*: Food & Drug Administration, open meeting of the Vaccines and Related Biologics advisory committee, June 7, 1994, Silver Spring, MD Transcript, pages 37–38.

322 *Stanley M. Lemon*: Food & Drug Administration, open meeting of the Vaccines and Related Biologics advisory committee, June 7, 1994, Silver Spring, MD Transcript, pages 37–38.

322 *special meeting with the FDA*: See www.lymediseaseassociation.org/Lymerix_Meeting.html.

322 *ultimate vaccine whistle-blower*: Marks, Donald H., M.D., Ph.D. Presentation at the Food and Drug Administration, January 22, 2002, in Bethesda, MD.

323 *written answers*: Meyer, Mary T., director, Office of Communications, Training and Manufacturers Assistance, Center for Biologics Evaluation and Research, Food and Drug Administration. Letter to Patricia V. Smith, president, Lyme Disease Association, February 2002. Also see: http://lymediseaseassociation.org/Vaccine_LYMERIXMeeting.html. Click on the bottom link for the response.

323 *"poor sales"*: LYMErix Lyme Disease Vaccine, Center for Biologics Evaluation and Research, FDA, May 21, 2002. www.fda.gov/ ohrms/dockets/AC/02/slides/3854S1_06.ppt.

323 *suit was settled*: Interview with Stephen A. Sheller, 2003.

324 *At Baxter*: In-person interview with John Dunn, Brookhaven National Laboratory, 2003. Also: Combination Lyme Disease Vaccine Proteins Patented, Brookhaven National Laboratory, April 9, 2007.

324 *Another possibility*: Telephone interview with Eugene Davidson, 2008.

324 *Stephen K. Wikel*: In-person interview, University of Connecticut, 2008. Pennington, Carolyn. "Ticks' tactics for spreading disease are focus of Health Center study." *The UConn Advance*. July 24, 2006.

49. OVER AND OUT, COLORADO
Interview with David Martz, August 2007.

50. THE FALMOUTH REUNION
Interview with Sheila Statlender, Falmouth, MA, August 2007.

51. GETTING DR. JONES
This chapter is based on Dr. Charles Ray Jones's hearings in Hartford, CT, from 2006 to 2007. I was either in attendance or am quoting the transcript for everything cited. In addition, I interviewed Dr. Jones on these issues in December 2007. Additional interviews with Lorraine Johnson, 2007 and 2008.

335 *There to bear witness*: Lyon, Kay, and Lyon, Meredith J. E-mail to author, January 13, 2008.

52. THE NEVER-ENDING STORY: WHAT HAPPENED TO MY FAMILY

Personal memoir.

53. STARTING OVER: DON'T GET SLYMED AGAIN

347 *Jonas Salk:* I interviewed Jonas Salk over the course of a year in La Jolla and New York City, from 1983 to 1984.

347 *"Quite to the contrary":* Telephone interview with Ben Beard, 2007.

   a study documenting this: Bacon, R. M., Biggerstaff, B. J., Schriefer, M. E., Gilmore, R. D., Jr., Philipp, M. T., Steere, A. C., Wormser, G. P., Marques, A. R., Johnson, B. J. "Serodiagnosis of Lyme disease by kinetic enzyme-linked immunosorbent assay using recombinant VlsE1 or peptide antigens of *Borrelia burgdorferi* compared with 2-tiered testing using whole-cell lysates." *Journal of Infectious Diseases.* April 15, 2003; 187 (8): 1187–99.

347 *"the study is circular":* Telephone interview with Kenneth Liegner, 2007.

   input on the recommendation: Wormser, G. P., Dattwyler, R. J., Shapiro, E. D., Halperin, J. J., Steere, A. C., Klempner, M. S., Krause, P. J., Bakken, J. S., Strle, F., Stanek, G., Bockenstedt, L., Fish, D., Dumler, J. S., Nadelman, R. B. "The clinical assessment, treatment, and prevention of Lyme disease, human granulocytic anaplasmosis, and babesiosis: clinical practice guidelines by the Infectious Diseases Society of America." *Clinical Infectious Diseases.* November 2006; 43 (9): 1089–134.

347 *treat a tick bite:* Nadelman, R. B., Nowakowski, J., Fish, D., Falco, R. C., Freeman, K., McKenna D., Welch, P., Marcus, R., Agüero-Rosenfeld, M. E., Dennis, D. T., Wormser, G. P. "Tick Bite Study Group. Prophylaxis with single-dose doxycycline for the prevention of Lyme disease after an Ixodes scapularis tick bite." *New England Journal of Medicine.* July 2001; 345 (2): 79–84.

347 *Nordin Zeidne:* Interview by phone, April 2008. Also: Zeidner, N. S., Massung, R. F., Dolan, M. C., Dadey, E., Gabitzsch, E., Dietrich, G., Levin, M. L. "A sustained-release formulation of doxycycline hyclate (Atridox) prevents simultaneous infection of *Anaplasma* phagocytophilum and *Borrelia burgdorferi* transmitted by tick bite." *Journal of Medical Microbiology.* April 2008; 57 (Pt 4): 463–68; Zeidner, N. S., Brandt, K. S., Dadey, E., Dolan, M. C., Happ, C., Piesman, J. "Sustained-release formulation of doxycycline hyclate for prophylaxis of tick bite infection in a murine model of Lyme borreliosis." *Antimicrobial Agents and Chemotherapy.* July 2004; 48 (7): 2697–99.

348 *got a call from:* Phone conversations and e-mails from Gary Wormser, April 2008.

348 *how can Dr. Wormser know:* Discussion by phone and e-mail with David Volkman, professor emeritus at Stony Brook, April and May 2009.

348 *from Stony Brook:* Interviews with Daniel Dykhuizen, Raymond Dattwyler, and Ben Luft, 2003, and Ben Luft, 2004, all at SUNY Stony Brook, and with Ben Luft in 2007 in Newton, MA. Also: Qui, W. G., Bosler, E. M., Campbell, J. R., Ugine, G. D., Wang, I. N., Luft, B. J., Dykhuizen, D. E. "A population genetic study of *Borrelia burgdorferi* sensu stricto from eastern Long Island, New York, suggested frequency-dependent selection, gene flow and host adaptation." *Hereditas.* 1997; 127 (3): 203–16; Wang, I. N., Dykhuizen, D. E., Qui, W., Dunn, J. J., Bosler, E. M., Luft, B. J. "Genetic diversity of OspC in a local population of *Borrelia burgdorferi* sensu stricto." *Genetics.* January 1999; 151 (1): 15–30; Seinost, G.,

Dykhuizen, D. E., Dattwyler, R. J., Golde, W. T., Dunn, J. J., Wang, I. N., Wormser, G. P., Schriefer, M. E., Luft, B. J. "Four clones of *Borrelia burgdorferi* sensu stricto cause invasive infection in humans." *Infection and Immunity.* July 1999; 67 (7): 3518–24; Seinost, G., Golde, W. T., Berger, B. W., Dunn, J. J., Qiu, D., Dunkin, D. S., Dykhuizen, D. E., Luft, B. J., Dattwyler, R. J. "Infection with multiple strains of *Borrelia burgdorferi* sensu stricto in patients with Lyme disease." *Archives of Dermatology.* November 1999; 135 (11): 1329–33; Gomes-Solecki, M. J., Dunn, J. J., Luft, B. J., Castillo, J., Dykhuizen, D. E., Yang, X., Glass, J. D., Dattwyler, R. J. "Recombinant chimeric *Borrelia* proteins for diagnosis of Lyme disease." *Journal of Clinical Microbiology.* July 2000; 38 (7): 2530–35; Qiu, W. G., Dykhuizen, D. E., Acosta, M. S., Luft, B. J. "Geographic uniformity of the Lyme disease spirochete (*Borrelia burgdorferi*) and its shared history with tick vector (*Ixodes scapularis*) in the Northeastern United States." *Genetics.* March 2002; 160 (3): 833–49; Qiu, W. G., Schutzer, S. E., Bruno, J. F., Attie, O., Xu, Y., Dunn, J. J., Fraser, C. M., Casjens, S. R., Luft, B. J. "Genetic exchange and plasmid transfers in *Borrelia burgdorferi* sensu stricto revealed by three-way genome comparisons and multilocus sequence typing." *Proceedings of the National Academy of Sciences USA.* September 28, 2004; 101 (39): 14150–55.

54. AND THE BANDS PLAY ON

354   *appeared like a vision:* International Lyme and Associated Diseases Society, Lyme Scientific Session, October 21–22, 2006, Crowne Plaza, Philadelphia. Also: MacDonald, A. B. "Plaques of Alzheimer's disease originate from cysts of *Borrelia burgdorferi,* the Lyme disease spirochete." *Medical Hypotheses.* 2006; 67 (3): 592–600; and telephone interviews, 2006 and 2007.

355   *updated* Clinical Practice Guidelines: Wormser, G. P., Dattwyler, R. J., Shapiro, E. D., Halperin, J. J., Steere, A. C., Klempner, M. S., Krause, P. J., Bakken, J. S., Strle, F., Stanek, G., Bockenstedt, L., Fish, D., Dumler, J. S., Nadelman, R. B. "The clinical assessment, treatment, and prevention of Lyme disease, human granulocytic anaplasmosis, and babesiosis: clinical practice guidelines by the Infectious Diseases Society of America." *Clinical Infectious Diseases.* November 1, 2006; 43 (9): 1089–134.

356   *heretic ILADS guidelines:* Cameron, D., Gaito, A., Harris, N., Bach, G., Bellovin, S., Bock, K., Bock, S., Burrascano, J., Dickey, C., Horowitz, R., Phillips, S., Meer-Scherrer, L., Raxlen, B., Sherr, V., Smith, H., Smith, P., Stricker, R.; ILADS Working Group. "Evidence-based guidelines for the management of Lyme disease." *Expert Review of Anti-Infective Therapy.* 2004; 2(1 Suppl): S1–13.

357   *antitrust investigation:* Miller, Robert. "Lyme disease activists to protest." *Times-News.* Danbury, CT. November 28, 2007. Also: Hathaway, William, and Waldman, Hillary. "Lyme disease experts: butt out, Blumenthal." *Hartford Courant.* March 21, 2007.

357   *another set of guidelines:* Halperin, J. J., Shapiro, E. D., Logigian, E., Belman, A. L., Dotevall, L., Wormser, G. P., Krupp, L., Gronseth, G., Bever, C. T., Jr.; Quality Standards Subcommittee of the American Academy of Neurology. "Practice parameter: Treatment of nervous system Lyme disease (an evidence-

based review): Report of the Quality Standards Subcommittee of the American Academy of Neurology." *Neurology.* July 3, 2007; 69 (1): 91–102.

357   *duly subpoenaed:* Phillips, Lisa. "Guidelines on trial: AAN subpoenaed as part of investigation into treatment parameters for Lyme disease." *Neurology Today.* October 16, 2007; 7 (20): 1, 12–13.

358   *blistering response:* Feder, H. M., Jr., Johnson, B. J., O'Connell, S., Shapiro, E. D., Steere, A. C., Wormser, G. P.; Ad Hoc International Lyme Disease Group. "A critical appraisal of 'chronic Lyme disease.'" *New England Journal of Medicine.* October 4, 2007; 357 (14): 1422–30.

358   *the paper's flaws:* Telephone interview with Daniel Cameron, November 2007.

359   *Florence Griswold:* Florence Griswold Museum, Old Lyme, CT. See www.flogris.org.

359   *Driving into Lyme myself:* Coming back from Brown University, where Jason was in school, I took Exit 70 off Interstate 95 one fall day in 2004, and explored the area, including the streets Polly Murray mentioned in her classic, *The Widening Circle.* This recounts my experience.

54. EPILOGUE

362   *I write this note:* Personal memoir.

363   *By Burrascano's reckoning:* Talk with Joe Burrascano, 2007.

363   *A meeting with Richard Horowitz:* Personal memoir.

363   *Richard Horowitz grew up in Queens:* In-person interview with Richard Horowitz, Hyde Park, NY, May 30, 2009.

367   *flows freely from the journals:* Feder, Jr., H. M., Johnson, B. J., O'Connell, S., Shapiro, E. D., Steere, A. C., Wormser, G. P.; Ad Hoc International Lyme Disease Group, Agger, W. A., Artsob, H., Auwaerter, P., Dumler, J. S., Bakken, J. S., Bockenstedt, L. K., Green, J., Dattwyler, R. J., Munoz, J., Nadelman, R. B., Schwartz, I., Draper, T., McSweegan, E., Halperin, J. J., Klempner, M. S., Krause, P. J., Mead, P., Morshed, M., Porwancher, R., Radolf, J. D., Smith Jr., R. P., Sood, S., Weinstein, A., Wong, S. J., Zemel, L. "A critical appraisal of 'chronic Lyme disease,'" *New England Journal of Medicine.* October 2007; 357 (14): 1422–30.

367   *Psychiatric comorbidity:* Hassett, A. L., Radvanski, D. C., Buyske, S., Savage, S. V., Gara, M., Escobar, J. I., Sigal, L. H. "Role of psychiatric comorbidity in chronic Lyme disease." *Arthritis and Rheumatism.* December 15, 2008; 59 (12): 1742–49.

367   *similar train:* Wormser, G. P., Shapiro, E. D. "Implications of gender in chronic Lyme disease." Journal of Women's Health (Larchmont, NY). June 2009; 18 (6): 831–4.

368   *work on strains:* Phone interview with Ben Luft, May 2009.

368   *could alter how:* E-mail interview with Alan Barbour, February 2009.

369   *At New York University:* E-mail interview with David Younger, June 2009

370   *At Columbia:* E-mail interview with Brian Fallon, June 2009.

370   *At UC Davis:* Steven Barthold talk, LDA, San Francisco, plus phone interview with Ben Luft and e-mail with Joseph Nayfach, 2008.

370   *Lyme disease in the South:* Regional Conference to Assess Research and Outreach Needs in Integrated Pest Management to Reduce the Incidence of Tick-Borne

Diseases in the Southern U.S., January 2009, sponsored by the Southern Region Integrated Pest Management Center, Centers for Disease Control and Prevention, Bayer Environmental Science, Focus Diagnostics, and Novozymes Biologicals, Inc.

370 *Karen Newell:* Phone interview with Karen Newell, June 2009.

371 *Charles Ray Jones:* In-person interview with Charles Ray Jones, New Haven, CT, May 2009.

372 *Connecticut doctors:* "Governor Rell Signs Bill That Shields Doctors in Treatment of Lyme Disease," State of Connecticut Executive Chambers, Hartford, CT, June 22, 2009.

Index